SPORTSFITNESS FOR WOMEN

SPORTSFITNESS FOR WOMEN

Sandra Rosenzweig

Illustrated by Melissa Mathis

HARPER & ROW, PUBLISHERS, New York
Cambridge, Philadelphia, San Francisco,
London, Mexico City, São Paulo, Sydney

1817

Grateful acknowledgment is made for permission to reprint:

Excerpt from *The Aerobics Way* by Kenneth H. Cooper, M.D., M.P. Copyright ©
1977 by Kenneth H. Cooper. Reprinted by permission of the publisher, M. Evans
& Co., Inc.

Table from *The Wonderful World Within You* by Dr. Roger J. Williams. Copyright
© 1977 by Dr. Roger J. Williams. Reprinted by permission of Bantam Books, Inc.
All rights reserved.

Table for use with "Kasch Pulse Recovery Test: Women Ages 18–26 Years and
Women Ages 27–60 Years" from article "The Kasch Pulse Recovery Step Test,"
1976. Reprinted by permission of the author, Fred W. Kasch.

Table on page 24, originally titled "Percent Fat Estimates for Women, Sum of
Triceps, Suprailium and Thigh Skin Folds" from "Measurement of Cardiorespiratory Fitness and Body Composition in the Clinical Setting" by Michael L. Pollock,
Ph.D., Donald H. Schmidt, M.D., and Andrew S. Jackson, P.E.D. from *Comprehensive Therapy*, vol. 6, no. 9, September 1980: 20, courtesy of The Laux Company, Inc. and Michael L. Pollock, Ph.D.

FIRST EDITION

Designer: C. Linda Dingler

Library of Congress Cataloging in Publication Data

Rosenzweig, Sandra.
    Sportsfitness for women.
    Bibliography: p.
    Includes indexes.
    1. Physical education for women.
2. Physical fitness for women.   I. Title.
GV439.R77   1982   613.7′045   81-48048
                        AACR2
ISBN 0-06-014966-3   82 83 84 85 86 10 9 8 7 6 5 4 3 2 1
ISBN 0-06-090937-4 (pbk.)   82 83 84 85 86 10 9 8 7 6 5 4 3 2 1

To Michael Taylor, Rachel Carroll, Shana Carroll, David Rosenzweig, and Isabelle Rosenzweig. This book is yours. You earned it.

Contents

III: THE INNER WOMAN

8. Menstruation and Menopause   277

9. Birth Control and Pregnancy   296

Acknowledgments

I am deeply indebted to the hundreds of people—the most respected and innovative experts in the fields of women's sports, fitness, and sports medicine as well as countless athletes of all ages and experience—who sacrificed hours from their busy schedules to supplement and bring to life my almost three years of research for this book.

Special thanks go to Dorothy V. Harris (the perfect interview), Paula Cabot (a graciously accommodating and knowledgeable resource), and Forrest Smith, M.D. (a patient teacher of the principles of exercise physiology and the limitless possibilities of the human body).

In addition, the following people were incalculably helpful and will always have my gratitude: Lynn Adams; Ransom Arthur, M.D.; Major Jeremy J. Beale; Albert R. Behnke, M.D.; Rosemary Bellini; Harmon Brown, M.D.; Susan Borger Budge; Mildred Burke; Royer Collins, M.D.; David Costill, Ph.D.; Kathleen O'Brien Di Felice; Sue Dooley; Dan Dorman; Barbara L. Drinkwater, Ph.D.; Mary Phyl Dwight; Carol Elsner; June Everett; Maggie Faulkner; Kenneth E. Foreman, Ph.D.; Rose Frisch, Ph.D.; Deborah Gellerman; Evalyn Gendel, M.D.; Sadja Greenwood, M.D.; Marcia Hall; William L. Haskell, Ph.D.; Christine Haycock, M.D.; Bobby Hinds; Paul Hutinger, P.E.D.; Ellen Jacob; Rusty Kanokogi; Fred W. Kasch, Ph.D.; Victor L. Katch, Ph.D.; Marty Kennedy; Keith Kingbay; Kenneth W. Kizer, M.D.; June Krauser; Darlene Lanka, M.D.; Peggy L. Lau; Patricia Lo; Lori Maynard; Patricia McCormick; Heather McKay; Don Meucci; Dick Mulvihill; Margo Oberg; Michael Pollock, Ph.D.; Mabel Rader; Jack Rockwell, R.P.T.; Richard Ruoti, R.P.T.; Allan J. Ryan, M.D.; Maren Seidler; Harold Sexton, M.D.; Mona Shangold, M.D.; Liz Allen Shetter; Pete Snyder; LaVada Staff, R.N.; Laura Stamm; Pat Sweeney; Glenn Swengros; Barbara Swenson; Clayton L. Thomas, M.D.; Sue Torok; Ann Valentine; Jackie Walker; Michelle Warren, M.D.; Eunice E. Way, Ph.D.; Christine L. Wells, Ph.D.; Roger J. Williams, Ph.D.; Jack H. Wilmore, Ph.D.; and the people at the Women's Sports Foundation. Roger M. Katz, M.D., and Ernest M. Vandeweghe, M.D., supplied the latest information on exercise-induced asthma.

Richard Huttner and Peg Cameron originated this project and then nudged, cajoled, and encouraged me until the book took shape. I'm going to miss them both.

My editor, Carol Cohen, massaged and coached this book into shape, all the while becoming a friend by long distance. She is the writer's dream: supportive, enthusiastic, sensitive, perceptive, and savvy. Michael Taylor, critic and crutch, accepted no excuses for hackneyed phrases or blown deadlines. My mother was right. . . .

Melissa Mathis created clean, precise, vigorous drawings under less than optimal conditions. Marcy McGaugh somehow managed to turn my acervate manuscript into flawless typescript. Chris Hayden's patience and understanding during the writing of this book were capped by a vintage act of generosity rivaling the long and multi-layered finish of a 1961 Château Petrus.

And, saving the best for last, Ellen Weber, friend, writer, doctor, set me on innumerable right tracks and slipped me countless leads. Words are but empty thanks.

Introduction

When I was playing badminton on the women's team in college, my boyfriend was on the men's team. One day he was bragging about his power shot, and I challenged him to a match. I realized very soon that he had more power, but I was faster and in better shape. I ran him all over the court, and when I made that last kill shot for the final point of the last game, I felt like an atomic bomb was exploding inside of me. There he stood—or, rather, stooped— bent over, red as a lobster, and gasping for breath.

—A forty-year-old housewife

You can play any sport a man can, although you may not always be able to beat him. If he is bigger and stronger, he probably runs faster, throws farther, and jumps higher. (Both speed and power require strength.) However, you have greater endurance and extra fuel resources for energy, you cool your body more efficiently in hot weather, and you insulate it better against the cold.

Women are participating in some form of exercise or athletics in ever-increasing numbers. Twenty years ago, most women exercised just to improve their figures. Now, women play soccer or ride bicycles or swim for the sense of challenge, accomplishment, and sensuality it gives them. And, of course, for their health.

The women coming into every popular sport today far outnumber the trickle of male newcomers. Three out of every five new runners or bicyclists are women, and so are four out of every five baseball and basketball players. Women comprise 49 percent of all tennis players, 44 percent of all downhill skiers, 39 percent of all backpackers, 36 percent of all squash players, 33 percent of all high school athletes, and 30 percent of all college athletes. In 1980, 135 women from twenty-seven countries competed in the first Women's World Judo Championships in New York City. There are some 150 women's rugby clubs in the United States—playing not last-minute pick-up scrimmages but regular league games—and more than 300 noncollegiate competing women's ice hockey teams under the aegis of the American Hockey Association. In 1978 an all-women climbing team conquered Annapurna I, the tenth-highest mountain in the world.

The number of adults exercising regularly in the United States rose from 28 million (or 24 percent) in 1961 to 93 million (60 percent) in 1979, and manufacturers reported $15.4 million in sales of running shoes, graphite tennis rackets, reflectorized bicycling suits, digital read-out gadgets for clocking laps, pulse beats, or calories expended, and even "sports fragrances"—a six-fold increase over 1960 sales. And yet magazines, newspapers, and television programs still crank out a jumble of information and misinformation about what women can and cannot do and how they should or should not do it. Here are the facts.

Pound for pound, inch for inch, you are likely to have narrower shoulders, shorter arms, and smaller bones than a man has. This means that there is less room for muscles on your skeleton and less length to apply leverage against a force. (The longer the lever, the less work you have to do to lift something, even if it's just your own weight.) About 23 percent of your body mass is muscle tissue, versus 40 percent of his. Your smaller frame and muscle mass are both due to your high levels of estrogen, the primary female hormone. Around the time your menstrual period first begins, the amount of estrogen in your system rises. Because estrogen closes the growth plates, or epiphyses, at the ends of the long bones, women stop growing at about fourteen or fifteen years of age, whereas men may continue to grow until they are close to twenty. Estrogen also encourages the laying down of body fat for fuel storage, whereas the male hormones, such as testosterone, encourage the growth of muscle fiber. Therefore, you naturally have more fat than a man, and less muscle.

Every woman does produce some testosterone, just as every man has some estrogen; the amounts vary with one's genetic makeup. So some women will show muscle definition approaching that of men, but most women cannot develop bulky muscles no matter how hard they train.

Tradition—as well as hormones—has kept women weak in their upper bodies. In the past, women simply didn't do the push-ups, chin-ups, pull-ups, and other exercises with which men strengthen the muscles in their arms, shoulders, and chests. But Jack H. Wilmore, Ph.D., of the University of Arizona has shown that women in a weight-training program can increase their strength by the same percentages as men, and his studies indicate that you have the same strength—sometimes more—in your abdomen, hips, and legs as a man of the same size. Women, you see, use their legs as much as men do, and their wider pelvises allow extra room to attach more muscle fibers.

As a woman you have 10 to 12 percent more fat than a man has, tucked away in your breasts, buttocks, inner thighs, and genitalia to support your reproductive functions and protect the fetus during pregnancy. Although this sex-specific fat, as Albert R. Behnke, M.D., calls it, is a burden when you are trying to run fast or jump high, it is a real advantage when you are running 100 miles or swimming the English Channel or doing any other kind of long-distance sport; you are still drawing on it for fuel when a man is starting to run out of energy.

Moreover, this extra fat layer insulates you against cold and helps make you buoyant in water, so that you float and swim more efficiently. For these reasons, most open-water long-distance swimmers have been women, from Gertrude Ederle, the first woman to swim the English Channel (August 1926) to Penny Dean, who holds the record for crossing it the fastest (7⅔ hours in July 1978).

What women yield to men in strength, they make up in flexibility. Women are naturally more limber and loose-jointed than men, an advantage in ballet dancing and sports such as gymnastics and figure skating. (Many women also use their ability to reach lower and twist farther to defeat otherwise superior male opponents in enclosed court games such as racquetball and squash.)

Trained women are no more subject to injury than trained men. It was once thought that a woman's wider hips and looser joints made her more likely to wrench her knee or twist her ankle, but that doesn't seem to be true. "Women are better structured for contact sports than men for two reasons," says Dorothy V. Harris, Ph.D., director of the Center for Women and Sport at the Pennsylvania State University. "First, they have their own built-in protective layer of fat stored between their skin and their muscles, so their bony projections are protected. Second, women's sex organs are internal, and almost invulnerable to any injury short of a puncture." Your ovaries and uterus float entirely inside your body in sacs of fluid, much better protected than a man's testicles. And there is no proof that blows to the breasts, although painful, cause cancer or other diseases. "Breast protectors," Harris notes, "are the first thing male coaches worry about, but they are usually unnecessary. Women's breasts are handled more roughly during sexual contact than during any contact sport."

But women athletes, we are told, lack the competitive drive; they crumble in adversity. Or they are competitive, all right, but just until they have children (Evonne Goolagong and Madeline Manning, take note). Or they are competitive, but only against other women; they are afraid to beat men. (Right, Billie Jean?) Or they can't endure the pain necessary for top-level competition (only for having babies). "Anyone who believes that women are frail and noncompetitive has never watched the Roller Derby," says Dorothy Harris.

Unfortunately, very few studies have been made of female athletes, and most existing research is badly out of date. Women are only now beginning to train with the concentration and technical guidance that men have always received. No one can predict their potential. Each year, women's performances improve by quantum leaps. In 1970, who would have thought that in ten years a woman would lift 540 pounds (Jan Todd), or drive a golf ball 308 yards (Alice Ritzman), or run a marathon in two hours, twenty-four minutes, and forty-one seconds (Grete Waitz)? Within a few years, women may be able to develop upper-body strength comparable to men's. Certainly, women will catch up to men, and surpass them, in distance events.

For now, the myths live on: that women are innately weaker, especially during their periods; that they need stress tests before they start exercising; that they can't throw or run like men because their shoulders and pelvises are proportioned differently.

Sportsfitness for Women refutes this follydiddle. You can do anything you want to do, whether it's starting to dance again, improving your soccer game, or exercising in your bedroom to trim your figure and regain the sleek, bouncy feeling of being strong, limber, and full of energy. However, you must train as a woman. You may not have as much strength as a man, but you have greater potential endurance, more flexibility in your joints, and more stretch in your muscles. Using this book, you can:

- Choose an exercise program tailored to your age, physical condition, and life-style
- Improve your skills in the sports you already play
- Combine sports for year-round conditioning
- Balance the strength and flexibility of your muscle groups for overall fitness and fewer injuries
- Learn the basic principles of training and conditioning for peak physical fitness and top performance
- Design a diet specifically suited to your own needs
- Control your weight for the rest of your life by using exercise to reset your metabolism and your appetite
- Find answers to all those questions men never have to ponder (about bras, menstruation, birth control, pregnancy, menopause, special equipment, local clubs)
- Diagnose your own injuries and learn how to treat, rehabilitate, and prevent them

Now you no longer have to model yourself after male jocks. Instead, you can play and exercise in the most effective and comfortable ways for you—as a woman.

I / THE BASICS

The first time I went cross-country skiing, we were out on this huge meadow covered with snow. It was so isolated and white—a huge marshmallow. I was freezing cold, and I felt clumsy on those skinny skis. After a few minutes, though, I started gliding along following a deer trail, almost floating between evergreens and leafless maples. I've never felt so peaceful and so excited at the same time. All I knew was the rhythm of my kick, the bite of the cold on my nose, and the sound of snow falling off the pine boughs. I was hooked. Still am.

—A thirty-eight-year-old secretary

1 / Choosing Your Own Fitness Program

If you've ever raced the wind across a lake in a kayak or done a perfect cartwheel on the lawn, you know how good it feels to exercise. Your body was *made* to move. It feels cramped and sluggish when forced to be still. Your blood pressure rises, your appetite goes askew, your bones become brittle, your muscles ache, you feel tired and become moody, depressed, or ill-tempered. If you had lived in prehistoric times—or even in pioneer days—you would have exercised as you found food, built your home, made your clothes, and gathered your fuel. In between, just for fun, you might have run races, square-danced, staged throwing contests, slid down hills, and otherwise entertained yourself with games of physical prowess. In the modern world, you no longer have to do physical labor to feed and clothe yourself, but you still need exercise to be fully alive.

WHY EXERCISE?

When you move your body vigorously, you bring oxygen to every cell. Exercise makes your skin glow and sometimes even makes pimples disappear as your circulation improves. Your reflexes become quicker. Exercise tones up your muscles, so that your body looks trimmer and more attractive. You become more graceful, because your joints learn to move through their whole range of motion. Exercise helps you achieve and maintain your ideal weight in a way that diet alone never can. And exercise helps control your appetite by increasing the amount of endorphins your brain secretes. (These recently discovered chemicals are often called "the brain's opium" because they tone down pain sensations, but they also prevent you from feeling hungry unless your body actually needs refueling.)

Exercise actually combats chronic fatigue by increasing your energy and your capacity for handling work. It brings extra oxygen to your brain, making you more alert during the day. But it also enables you to sleep more soundly at night because it produces sleep-inducing endorphins and releases the day's nervous tensions while making you physically tired (rather than washed out, the way inactive people feel). Exercise prevents depression not only by releasing nervous tension but by breaking down excess adrenaline and other stress-produced chemicals stored in your brain and heart. It also boosts your self-confidence and self-image by showing that you can improve yourself, no matter what your age or physical condition.

Exercise stimulates your digestion and helps with bowel function. It may encourage you to stop smoking, since nicotine cuts your wind. (Athletes also report that giving up cigarettes is easier when they exercise strenuously, because the extra oxygen they draw decreases their craving for tobacco. Many smokers, it seems, take drags on a cigarette as a way of inhaling extra oxygen.) Exercise helps prevent or eliminate varicose veins. It also speeds your recovery after surgery, because strong muscles have a greater capacity to use oxygen than flabby ones, and the more oxygen they get, the faster they heal. (Many hospitals now put prospective chest and abdominal surgery patients on an exercise program several weeks *before* a scheduled operation.)

You may decide to exercise because it relaxes you or raises your spirits. Tests by M. A. Carmack and R. Martens show that people who run for these reasons tend to be more highly committed and to feel they are getting more benefits than people who exercise only because someone said it was good for them. Or you may play sports because it is an excuse to get out of the house or office, to see old friends and make new ones.

Everyone should find her own compelling reason for exercising. One New York woman whose close friend was mugged spent a year lifting weights and studying karate for self-defense. Another woman decided to conquer her tension backaches by swimming a mile and a half five days a week and doing special calisthenics to strengthen her abdominal and back muscles. Yet another woman read an article about women body builders in a sports magazine and decided to train in order to enter a local body-building contest. (After only nine weeks of full-time training and dieting, she won second prize for the overall competition as well as first place in four trophy events.)

You are never too old or infirm to exercise, or even to compete. Most Ys and national sports associations have masters' programs for people middle-aged or older. Where necessary, these competitions are age graded so that sixty-year-old swimmers or gymnasts, for example, are not competing against thirty-year-olds. Many of these programs contribute teams to the Senior Olympics, held each year in various locations around the country.

Several organizations promote athletics for people with chronic illnesses or handicaps. For more information, contact the organizations listed in Appendix A or your local chapter of the association devoted to research and education specializing in your problem.

Exercise and Your Heart

The most important reason to exercise is to strengthen your heart. Along with other muscles, your heart can be trained to do a larger amount of work. Whenever you exert yourself, if only to carry a sack of groceries upstairs, your heart pumps extra oxygen-rich blood to your moving parts, for your muscles need oxygen in order to contract. At first, your heart beats faster and faster to carry more blood (more oxygen) to the arm muscles lifting that shopping bag. However, if you carry groceries every day, after a few weeks your heart and muscles become trained. The heart pumps more blood with each beat, and the muscles use their oxygen more effectively. Eventually, your heart doesn't need to beat as fast to do the same amount of work.

If, in addition to carrying groceries, you run, bicycle, or do some other sport which provides a high level of training, the exercise stretches the size of the chambers in your heart. The larger chambers pump out more blood with each stroke so, again, your heart is trained to beat slower and your pulse slows down, during exercise and at rest.

EXERCISE AND HEART SIZE

It has been known for at least fifty years that the hearts of well-trained athletes are bigger than those of sedentary people. At first, doctors confused these larger hearts with the enlargements associated with congestive heart failure, but now any physician familiar with sports medicine knows that vigorous exercise increases the size of the heart in one of two ways. In weight lifters and other athletes who emphasize isometric and sudden-burst types of exercise, the muscular walls of the heart become *thicker*. In distance runners and others who exercise steadily, the chambers of the heart are *stretched* to hold a greater volume of blood. Either way, the heart responds to exertion by fortifying and strengthening itself to withstand any pressure.

Strenuous exercise helps you control high blood pressure. Instead of causing a sharp rise in both your resting (diastolic) and pumping (systolic) pressures, as it does in untrained bodies, exercise in a trained body raises only the systolic rate. Because the aorta and larger arteries stretch to hold a larger volume of blood, the diastolic pressure in trained athletes during exercise may even become lower than it is at rest. Thus blood vessels remain elastic and the heart doesn't have to overwork.

A study from Tufts University School of Medicine revealed that endurance athletes have thinner blood plasma than sedentary people. (Plasma is the liquid component of blood.) This, again, makes it easier for your heart to pump blood through the small blood vessels in your muscles and near your skin. (Thicker than normal plasma has been found in people with acute and chronic inflammations, rheumatoid arthritis, and tuberculosis. One Australian study even linked it to the spread of some cancers.)

Exercise also trains your body to send extra blood quickly and efficiently only to the muscles you're moving and not willy-nilly to every part of your body.

Even relatively mild exercise such as walking or climbing a flight of stairs helps dissolve potentially dangerous blood clots. In a study directed by R. Sanders Williams, M.D., at Duke University Medical Center, regular mild physical exercise in men and women stimulated the lining of the blood vessels to release greater amounts of plasminogen activators than when these people were sedentary. (Plasminogen activators stimulate the production of plasminogen, which dissolves fibrin, the stringy clotting blood protein. Clots in important blood vessels cause heart attacks and strokes.) Exercise also lowers the level of "bad" cholesterol (LDLs) in your blood, raises the level of "good" cholesterol (HDLs), and reduces the amount of cholesterol plaque already in your arteries. (See chapter 2.)

JOGGERS WHO DROP DEAD

The sudden deaths of people—mostly men—during jogging or other strenuous exercise have been used as proof that exercise is dangerous for the heart. However, as Dr. Jeffrey Koplan of the Center for Disease Control in Atlanta pointed out in a 1980 article in the *Journal of the American Medical Association,* "Given the millions of persons now running in the United States, some number of them could be expected by chance to die while running—just as some die while eating, reading, and sleeping."

Pre-menopausal women already have a head start in their defense against coronary artery disease. A 1980 article in the *Journal of the American Medical Association* estimated that there are probably less than 3,000 heart attacks a year in the United States in women under the age of forty-six, while the Royal College of General Practitioners in Great Britain reported only nine heart attacks in a study review of 200,000 women (and seven of the nine women were taking birth-control pills). After menopause, a woman's risk of heart disease increases, but it never quite matches a man's.

Exercise may slow down the aging process. A study by Dr. John O. Holloszy and colleagues at Washington University School of Medicine in St. Louis showed that middle-aged runners had greater cardiovascular performance than their sedentary age mates and achieved a cardiovascular fitness level only 14 percent lower than that of trackmen in their early twenties—a 4 percent decline per decade of age instead of the 8 percent decline researchers expected. Dr. Ralph S. Paffenbarger, Jr., of Stanford University says his study of 17,000 Harvard University alumni shows that you keep this advantage only if you stay in shape. People who were in good cardiovascular condition in college but became sedentary in later life aged like other sedentary people.

You are an individual biochemically. No one else has the same enzymatic balances, the same digestive, nervous, or circulatory reactions. Exercise can't change the hereditary blueprint you were born with. If your parents lived to a vigorous old age, chances are you will too. If your parents were cursed with high blood pressure, atherosclerosis, or other forms of heart disease, you probably will be too. However, if you do have a heart attack, your good physical condition will make it milder and may even save your life. If you are lucky, exercise may even prevent heart disease altogether. It certainly will make your life more fun and more satisfying.

WHICH SPORTS ARE BEST?

Know Your Goals

Before choosing a new activity, decide what you want to accomplish. Most women want to improve their appearance, to firm up flabby bodies or fill out scrawny figures. If that is your goal, choose sports and exercises that work on the areas you worry about most. If you want to lose weight, choose aerobic exercises, the kind that get your heart beating quickly and your lungs huffing and puffing. Only when you elevate your heart rate do you speed up your metabolism enough to burn up calories. Michael Pollock, Ph.D., director of the Cardiac Rehabilitation and Human Performance Laboratory at Mount Sinai Medical Center in Milwaukee, has found that to lose weight you must exercise at least three times a week for thirty minutes at a time at 60 to 80 percent of your maximum heart rate, and burn about 300 calories per session. Depending on your condition, vigorous walking, jumping rope, running, bicycling, swimming, cross-country skiing, or rowing will fit the bill. (For more on weight loss, see chapter 4.)

MAXIMUM HEART RATE

Your maximum heart rate equals the number 220 minus your age in years (220 is a statistical abstraction based partially on the known heart rates of small children). No matter how hard you work, your heart can't beat at this maximum rate for very long. After a minute or two of full-bore effort, you simply collapse from exhaustion.

A significant number of women take exercise like a bitter tonic—because it's good for them. These are generally the ones who don't keep it up; they aren't really motivated. It takes hard work to strengthen your heart and improve your circulation, metabolism, and digestion. You don't strengthen your heart unless you exercise it, and you don't actually start exercising it right away. Pollock's formula applies here too. In order to get a cardiovascular training effect, you must exercise at least three times a week for thirty minutes a session at 60 to 80 percent of your maximum heart rate. This is also, not coincidentally, the formula for turning exercise into a habit.

THE THIRTY-MINUTE BONUS

No matter what your sport or condition, if you are exercising strenuously, you will be out of breath for the first ten minutes or so. This is the most uncomfortable time of the whole workout. After that, your body pays back the oxygen debt it has incurred, replenishes the oxygen and fuel it burned in each muscle cell, and becomes more efficient. Your breathing becomes more regular, your heart settles into a comfortable elevated rate, and the pleasure begins. You get your second wind. If you exercise only for ten or twelve minutes a day, you never enter the enjoyable phase. The whole workout is an exercise in pain and exhaustion—and that's enough to discourage anybody.

If you have exercised this way for a month or more, your body comes to depend on it. Your digestive processes become more regular, you sleep more soundly, your hands and feet don't get as cold at night, and your joints don't ache nearly as much at the end of each working day. You wake up one morning and realize that you can't live without your exercise fix; it has become a permanent part of your life. On cold mornings, you may still have to force yourself out onto the track or into the pool, but you know you'll feel much better with your workout than without it. From then on, you'll resent missing a day.

Play Several Sports

Some women exercise throughout their lives but still think of themselves as novices. A woman may say, "I'm just not athletic. I tried tennis for a year, but my tennis partner moved away, so I switched to running. But when winter came along, I couldn't get myself out onto the icy streets. I did calisthenics for a few weeks, but I got bored. Everyone laughs at me because I've tried so many things, so now I just stay home. I wish I could find an exercise I liked."

This woman is really very active. She just doesn't understand that it's better to have several different sports than to concentrate on one. The more games she plays, the more muscles she will move, the more joints she will flex, and the more she will strengthen her heart, lungs, and bones. She should feel free to move back and forth between sports as the seasons—and her whims—dictate, as long as she understands how to prepare her muscles and joints for each one.

Prepare for Each Sport

In order to avoid injury and play at your best, you should either practice special training exercises to condition the key muscles used in each sport or choose complementary sports, activities which use the same muscles in the same ways. If you are a skier, running during the summer strengthens the backs of your thighs but not the fronts. In the winter before you go downhill, you should do specific exercises aimed at strengthening the fronts of your thighs or you won't have the stamina to enjoy your days on the slope. If, on the other hand, you ride a bicycle in the summer, you develop the fronts of your thighs in a manner similar to skiing, so you don't need pre-ski conditioning. Special conditioning or complementary sports—the effect is the same; the choice is up to you.

Even seasoned athletes may overlook the importance of preparing for each sport. Most injuries happen to novices, many of whom are already adept at another sport and assume that their training will carry over to the new one. Unfortunately, it doesn't work that way. Every sport makes its own unique demands on your body. (Part II describes the training needed for over fifty sports and lists complementary activities; should injuries occur anyway, Part IV explains how they are caused and how you and your doctor should treat them.)

If you are looking for new sports to complement present ones, therefore, it is not enough to figure that one sport uses your arms so any other arm sport will do. You must know *what part* of your arms each sport uses. Does it use the muscles in the back (the triceps) to straighten your elbow, or the muscles in the front (the biceps) to bend it? Does the sport use slow powerful muscular contractions for maximum lift or quick bursts of power for speed? (The way you use your muscles is as specific as which muscles you move.) Does the sport require short periods of intense effort (sprinting, or throwing a heavy object such as the shot put) or long periods of sustained effort (swimming laps, running, or bicycling)? A sprint uses one kind of energy, and a distance event uses another. Unless trained otherwise, your body prefers one kind of energy over another.

Find Ways to Keep Going

No matter what sports you choose, you won't stick with them if they aren't fun. The sports I've settled down with as an adult are the ones I loved as a child—bicycling, dancing, gymnastics, kayaking, and jumping rope. Some women have told me that the sports they love now are the ones their mothers or doctors forbade them to play as kids—scuba diving, tackle football, skiing, or weight lifting. No one has ever told me that they are devoted to a sport they once hated. If you are looking for sociability or fresh air, calisthenics aren't for you, nor is swimming laps in an indoor pool. If you are the kind of person who never misses your office's Saturday morning volleyball game, joining a tennis or racquetball club or a weight training gym might be a sensible investment.

Choose your partners carefully. When you play any sport intensely, you may sweat and smell and make rude bodily noises. In cold weather, your nose will run or drip. You may suddenly have to run behind a bush if the exercise speeds up your digestion or jostles your bladder. People who are exercise buffs themselves will understand; boyfriends, husbands, or business associates may not. That's why many women prefer to exercise with other women.

If you want to exercise alone as an escape, without an audience to evaluate your every move, you will be uncomfortable with competitive sports. Choose an activity you can do at home. If you have to take lessons before you can begin to play, or if you have to travel to a court or gym, or rely on partners to play with, or keep equipment in proper working order, the game may become too much trouble. The weather, your car, your friend's son's chicken pox, even a broken racket string becomes an excuse to sit out a day . . . or five. On the other hand, you can jump rope in any space larger than a closet, you can run around your basement until you are confident enough to go outdoors; you can lift weights in front of the television set, and you can do calisthenics and gymnastics floor exercises just about anywhere.

Set short-range goals so that you can feel you've accomplished something each day. As you grow, your goals become higher and more sophisticated. In rope jumping, for example, your first goal could be to do 100 jumps without stopping, which might take you two weeks or a month to reach. After two months, aim for fifteen minutes of jumping, and three months later, work up to thirty minutes. When you start getting bored, teach yourself trick steps and fancy routines. If you write down your goals and workout schedules and file them away, you can reread them every few months. You'll be surprised at how much progress you've made.

Be creative in finding time to exercise. Use your lunch hour to run or swim instead of eating a fattening lunch. Trade baby-sitting with another mother who needs time off. Exercise very early, before you go to work, and benefit from the added energy you'll feel all morning. Or exercise right after you get home from work or school, or while dinner is in the oven, and come away feeling relaxed, with renewed vigor. Form an exercise club with a few friends and obligate yourself to show up. Or exercise alone so that you can do it at a moment's notice. Just don't accept the excuses of your lazy self. Believe in your soul that you *must* exercise at least three days a week.

EXERCISE TESTS

Before you begin an exercise program or change from one sport to another, rate yourself with the following tests. With them, you will learn exactly what your muscles and joints can do, what condition your heart is in, and where your weaknesses lie. Then select the most suitable sports for your present fitness level (chapters 5 and 7) or develop a conditioning program to bring your body up to the requirements of any sport you choose (chapter 6). Many people have overblown ideas of their physical condition. Running for the bus every morning or playing two rounds of golf on Saturday has not kept you in shape.

If you fail in one or more categories, don't give up. Strong muscles are not just for men. In only a few weeks, you can make dramatic changes in your physical condition and even learn the joy and satisfaction of doing a push-up with ease. If you do well, the urge to beat your old record may be irresistible. Either way, retest yourself every few months to chart your progress.

Caution: **If you feel pain or tightness in your chest during the course of any of these tests, or severe breathlessness, light-headedness, or dizziness, nausea, or loss of the control of your muscles, stop immediately and consult your doctor. These tests are for healthy women only.**

Heart-Lung Tests

PULSE

To take your wrist, or radial, pulse, press the first and second fingers of your right hand—left hand, for southpaws—into the depression about an inch above your other wrist, below the thumb. (This hollow lies between the outside bone and the hard tendon down the middle of the wrist.) Press hard enough to feel the thumping of the blood coursing through your artery, but not hard enough to block it off. Watch the second hand of a clock as you count the beats, starting with the first beat as *zero*. Unless you must be very precise, count your pulse for ten seconds, and multiply by six for the total heartbeats per minute. If you must be extremely accurate, count for a full minute.

Some people find the carotid pulse, in the neck, easier to count. Hold the first three fingers of your hand flat against your neck just below the angle of the jaw. Lengthen your neck and move your fingers slowly down toward your collarbone until you feel the beat. Do not actually press on this pulse because it is very easy to block it off.

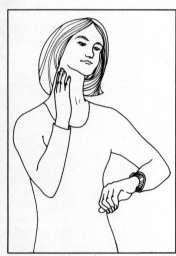

WRIST PULSE

CAROTID PULSE

Kasch Step Test

If you are in poor athletic condition and haven't been training for a while, the Kasch Step Test, developed by Fred W. Kasch, Ph.D., professor of exercise physiology at San Diego State University, is the easiest way to take stock of your cardiovascular fitness. Find yourself a bench or large sturdy stool that rises 12 inches off the floor. (Most stairs won't work because they are only 7 or 8 inches high.) Step up onto the bench in a four-count sequence: up with one foot, up with the other, down with the first foot, down with the second. Step at the rate of two complete sets of ups and downs every five seconds, twenty-four sets every minute, for three minutes. Immediately sit down on the bench and take your pulse for a full minute.

TABLE I: KASCH STEP TEST*

	Pulse Beats per Minute	
Classification	Women Ages 18 to 26	Women Ages 27 to 60
Superior	73	74
Excellent	74–82	75–83
Good	83–90	84–92
Average	91–100	93–103
Fair	101–107	104–112
Poor	108–114	113–121
Very poor	115	122

* Fred W. Kasch, Ph.D., San Diego State University

You must count your pulse *for the full minute* because you are not only measuring how fast your pulse races but also the rate at which your heart recovers from its exertion and slows down. Compare your pulse with Table I below to see how fit you are. Then record the result on the fitness profile at the end of the chapter. (If you are taller than five feet six inches, you will probably find this test too easy and so will score better than your true fitness level. Although Kasch may disapprove, you can compensate for this by adding two inches to the height of the stool for every three inches of height you have over five feet.)

One-and-a-Half-Mile Run/Walk Test

Anyone can take the Kasch Step Test. However, according to Kasch, the test isn't very accurate if you are in fairly good shape. If you have been working out for at least three months and are comfortable running, the One-and-a-Half-Mile Run/Walk Test devised by Kenneth H. Cooper, M.D., of aerobics fame will give you a much better indication of your cardiovascular fitness level.

Find a track whose distance you know and then run until you are winded. Slow down and walk until you catch your breath, then go back to your fastest pace again, slowing and speeding until you have covered 1½ miles. Since this is a test of your stamina and your maximum capacity, you should push yourself as much as you can, short of hurting

TABLE II: ONE-AND-A-HALF-MILE RUN/WALK TEST°

Age

Rating	13–19 Years	20–29 Years	30–39 Years	40–49 Years	50–59 Years	Over 60 Years
Superior	Less than 11 min. 50 sec.	Less than 12 min. 30 sec.	Less than 13 min.	Less than 13 min. 45 sec.	Less than 14 min. 30 sec.	Less than 16 min. 30 sec.
Excellent	12:29 to 11:50	13:30 to 12:30	14:30 to 13:00	15:55 to 13:45	16:30 to 14:30	17:30 to 16:30
Good	14:30 to 12:30	15:54 to 13:31	16:30 to 14:31	17:30 to 15:56	19:00 to 16:31	19:30 to 17:31
Fair	16:54 to 14:31	18:30 to 15:55	19:00 to 16:31	19:30 to 17:31	20:00 to 19:01	20:30 to 19:31
Poor	18:30 to 16:55	19:00 to 18:31	19:30 to 19:01	20:00 to 19:31	20:30 to 20:01	21:00 to 20:30
Very Poor	More than 18:31	More than 19:01	More than 19:31	More than 20:01	More than 20:31	More than 21:01

°Adapted from Kenneth H. Cooper, *The Aerobics Way* (New York: M. Evans & Co., 1977).

yourself. Compare your performance with Table II below to find your fitness category and record the result on the fitness profile at the end of the chapter.

Strength Tests

Before beginning the following strength and flexibility tests, warm up your heart and muscles by doing a few minutes of the universal warm-ups in chapter 2. In addition to protecting your heart and muscles, the warm-ups will enable you to perform better on the tests themselves.

The following six exercises measure the power in various parts of your body. If you can do only one or two repetitions of each, consider yourself in poor shape; three indicates fair shape; four, good shape; and five earns you excellent marks.

Bent-Knee Curl-up (Abdomen)

Lie on your back with your knees bent and your feet flat on the floor. Put your hands behind your head, and your chin on your chest. Leading with your head, curl up into a sitting position. If it is necessary, and only if it is necessary, someone may hold your feet down.

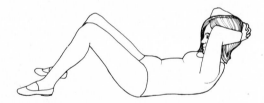

BENT-KNEE CURL-UP

Push-up (Arms and shoulders)

Lie on the floor, face down, with your hands under your shoulders and your elbows bent and pointing toward the ceiling. Keeping your body

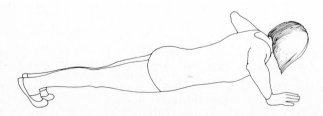

STANDARD PUSH-UP

stiff as a board, straighten your arms and push your body up until the entire weight of your body is resting on your extended arms and your flexed toes. Return to starting position without collapsing in a heap. If you can do even one push-up, you have more arm and shoulder strength than most American women.

Chin-up (Biceps)

Grasp a chinning bar with your hands, palms facing toward you. Pull yourself up with your arms so that your chin comes above the bar, then lower yourself slowly. Most women can't do two chin-ups, and of the few who can, many cheat by swinging their bodies or kicking their legs. (If you don't have a chinning bar, child's jungle gym, loft-bed beam, or other sturdy structure to hang from, skip this test.)

Pull-up (Triceps)

This is a chin-up with the palms facing away from you, and it is even harder to do.

Back Arch (Back)

Lie on the floor, face down, with your hands behind your head. Keeping your legs straight and on the floor, arch your back so that you can

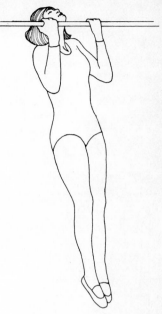

CHIN-UP

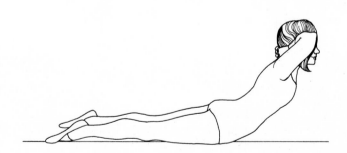

BACK ARCH

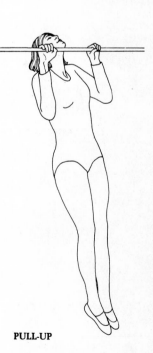

PULL-UP

lift your head and upper body off the floor. If this is difficult, ask someone to hold your buttocks and legs down. Do not attempt this exercise if you have lower back problems.

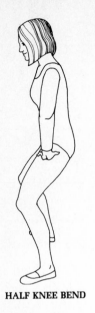

HALF KNEE BEND

Half Knee Bend (Legs)

Stand with your back straight and your hands on your hips or upper thighs. Bend your knees as far or farther than in the figure. Return to a standing position. Don't squat all the way into a deep knee bend, for that makes the test much harder, brings other muscles into play, and can damage your knees.

Record the results of these tests on the fitness profile at the end of the chapter by noting whether or not you could do the exercise and how many repetitions you achieved.

Flexibility Tests

These seven exercises measure how far you can bend and stretch the muscles around your joints. Do each one only once. Either you will be able to do it or you won't.

Toe Touch (Lower back and hamstrings of leg)

Stand with your feet together and your knees locked. Without bending your knees, try to put your palms flat on the floor. If you can, you are acceptably flexible. If you can barely touch your toes with your fingertips, you pass by the skin of your teeth. (If you have exceptionally long legs, you may not be able to put your palms flat on the floor, but be honest. Are your legs really too long, or are you just so stiff that they feel that way?)

Knee-Nose Touch (Neck and upper back)

Lie on your back, knees bent, and try to pull one knee up to touch your nose as you bend your head and upper body forward to meet your knee. (Grasp your leg *behind* the knee to avoid stressing your knee joint.) Repeat with the other leg.

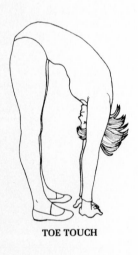

TOE TOUCH

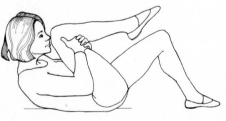

KNEE-NOSE TOUCH

Posture Clasp (Shoulders)

Sit or stand and place one arm over your shoulder and down behind your back. Try to grasp that hand from below and behind with your other hand. Repeat, reversing arms.

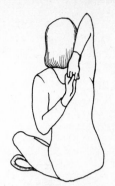

POSTURE CLASP

Heel and Toes (Ankles and calves)

Stand with your toes on a thick telephone book (about two inches) and try to touch your heels to the floor.

Stork (Front of the thighs)

Stand up and place one hand against a wall (or on a table) for support. From behind grasp your left leg with your left hand, holding it where the ankle and foot meet. Bending at the hip, pull your heel up, as close to your buttocks as you can, and try to point your bent left knee directly behind you. Do not arch your back or let your knee move out to the side. Repeat with the opposite leg and arm.

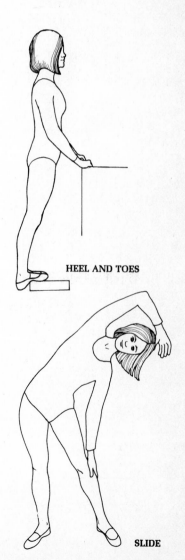

HEEL AND TOES

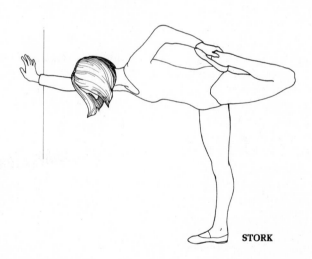

STORK

Slide (Sides of the trunk)

Stand with your feet about shoulder width apart, or whatever is comfortable, and bend to the left as you slide your left arm down the outside of your left leg. Try to get your hand below your knee. You may bring your right arm over your head to help. Repeat, bending to the other side.

SLIDE

Rocker (Abdomen and back)

Lie down on your stomach and reach back to grasp one foot in each hand. (Your head will have to come up in order to do this.) Arch your back enough to rock back and forth on your belly.

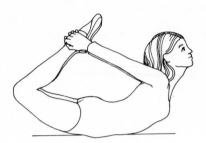

ROCKER

Record the results of these tests by writing "yes" or "no" under each flexibility exercise profile at the end of the chapter.

PERCENTAGE OF FAT TESTS

The height-weight charts published in insurance brochures and fashion magazines vary enormously from one to the next and have little to do with determining how *fat* you are. Traditionally, these charts reported what the *average* American woman already weighed, not what she should weigh.

Exercise physiologists today are less interested in what you weigh compared to your height than in what percentage of your weight is fat. Twenty-three to 24 percent fat is healthy for women, although trained athletes often carry only 10 to 15 percent fat on their frames. (Men put on less fat than women. A healthy inactive man should have between 15 and 19 percent body fat, and athletes often get down to 6 or 8 percent.)

Weight and ratios of body fat do not always run parallel. Women suffering from anorexia nervosa, having starved themselves down to living skeletons by feeding off their own muscles, frequently still have a very high proportion of fat to lean on their bones. Conversely, a formerly flabby woman can start exercising, firm up, and slim down from a size twelve, say, to a size eight, lose 5 percentage points of body fat, and still not lose a pound. She has added muscle, and muscle, although smaller and more tightly packed, weighs more than fat—as any football player knows.

Laboratory Fat Tests

Body fat percentages have been a controversial issue for over twenty years. One researcher develops a new, more precise way of calculating these ratios, and another comes along and pokes holes in the method. The problem is that no one can see inside you to pinpoint where you've hidden all your fat, nor can they weigh your bones, muscles, and organs individually. Their formulas are mere generalities, based on assumptions of how sex, age, and ethnic origin determine what your lean body mass really is.

While some labs rely on skin-fold measurements, others use hydrostatic, or underwater, weighing—seating you in a sling attached to a scale and then completely immersing you in a tub of water. (Because fat floats, the thinner you are, the denser you are under water.) A few labs even try fat biopsies, drawing fat from your thigh into a syringe and then counting the number of fat cells. All three techniques seem equally accurate.

Three Quick Fat Tests

1. Stand undressed with your arms down at your sides, feet comfortably apart, in front of your mirror. Take a good look. Lift your arms to expose bat wings hanging from your upper arms. Turn and note any ripples of fat on your back, butt, and thighs. If you look fat, you *are* fat.

2. Stand up, arms hanging loosely at your sides. Ask a friend to grab a vertical pinch of skin and fat from the back of your dominant arm, midway between your shoulder and your elbow, and measure the thickness of the skin fold. (Be sure she doesn't also measure her fingers.) Next, measure a horizontal pinch of skin from your right or left side, halfway between your lower rib and your hip—about an inch below your waist and parallel to your belt line. Finally, measure a vertical skin fold from the front of your upper thigh. If two out of three are greater than an inch, you have too much fat on your body.

This test works because you store much of your nonessential fat immediately under your skin. The more fat under your skin, the thicker the skin folds.

3. Stand up. Have a friend carefully measure, in millimeters, pinches of skin from your triceps area (the back of your arm, halfway between shoulder and elbow), from the bottom tip of your scapula (shoulder blade), and from a spot on the front of your thigh (about halfway between hip and knee and just slightly toward the inside of your thigh). Pinch all skin folds vertically.

Mark down each measurement and add them together. Find your

percentage of body fat under your age group in Table III (below). If you want to be much more accurate, use a skin-fold calipers to pinch and measure the skin at the same time (see Appendix B for sources).

Record the results of your fat tests. List all obvious areas of fat and flab. Your completed profile tells you at a glance what you need to work on. But start gradually. Pretending you're an elite athlete not only strains your heart but also stresses your bones, muscles, tendons, and joints.

TABLE III: PERCENTAGE OF FAT ESTIMATES*

Sum of Skinfolds (mm)	Age								
	22 and under	23–27	28–32	33–37	38–42	43–47	48–52	53–57	58 and over
23–25	9.7	9.9	10.2	10.4	10.7	10.9	11.2	11.4	11.7
26–28	11.0	11.2	11.5	11.7	12.0	12.3	12.5	12.7	13.0
29–31	12.3	12.5	12.8	13.0	13.3	13.5	13.8	14.0	14.3
32–34	13.6	13.8	14.0	14.3	14.5	14.8	15.0	15.3	15.5
35–37	14.8	15.0	15.3	15.5	15.8	16.0	16.3	16.5	16.8
38–40	16.0	16.3	16.5	16.7	17.0	17.2	17.5	17.7	18.0
41–43	17.2	17.4	17.7	17.9	18.2	18.4	18.7	18.9	19.2
44–46	18.3	18.6	18.8	19.1	19.3	19.6	19.8	20.1	20.3
47–49	19.5	19.7	20.0	20.2	20.5	20.7	21.0	21.2	21.5
50–52	20.6	20.8	21.1	21.3	21.6	21.8	22.1	22.3	22.6
53–55	21.7	21.9	22.1	22.4	22.6	22.9	23.1	23.4	23.6
56–58	22.7	23.0	23.2	23.4	23.7	23.9	24.2	24.4	24.7
59–61	23.7	24.0	24.2	24.5	24.7	25.0	25.2	25.5	25.7
62–64	24.7	25.0	25.2	25.5	25.7	26.0	26.7	26.4	26.7
65–67	25.7	25.9	26.2	26.4	26.7	26.9	27.2	27.4	27.7
68–70	26.6	26.9	27.1	27.4	27.6	27.9	28.1	28.4	28.6
71–73	27.5	27.8	28.0	28.3	28.5	28.8	28.0	29.3	29.5
74–76	28.4	28.7	28.9	29.2	29.4	29.7	29.9	30.2	30.4
77–79	29.3	29.5	29.8	30.0	30.3	30.5	30.8	31.0	31.3
80–82	30.1	30.4	30.6	30.9	31.1	31.4	31.6	31.9	32.1
83–85	30.9	31.2	31.4	31.7	31.9	32.2	32.4	32.7	32.9
86–88	31.7	32.0	32.2	32.5	32.7	32.9	33.2	33.4	33.7
89–91	32.5	32.7	33.0	33.2	33.5	33.7	33.9	34.2	34.4
92–94	33.2	33.4	33.7	33.9	34.2	34.4	34.7	34.9	35.2
95–97	33.9	34.1	34.4	34.6	34.9	35.1	35.4	35.6	35.9
98–100	34.6	34.8	35.1	35.3	35.5	35.8	36.0	36.3	36.5
101–103	35.3	35.4	35.7	35.9	36.2	36.4	36.7	36.9	37.2
104–106	35.8	36.1	36.3	36.6	36.8	37.1	37.3	37.5	37.8
107–109	36.4	36.7	36.9	37.1	37.4	37.6	37.9	38.1	38.4
110–112	37.0	37.2	37.5	37.7	38.0	38.2	38.5	38.7	38.9
113–115	37.5	37.8	38.0	38.2	38.5	38.7	39.0	39.2	39.5
116–118	38.0	38.3	38.5	38.8	39.0	39.3	39.5	39.7	40.0
119–121	38.5	38.7	39.0	39.2	39.5	39.7	40.0	40.2	40.5
122–124	39.0	39.2	39.4	39.7	39.9	40.2	40.4	40.7	40.9
125–127	39.4	39.6	39.9	40.1	40.4	40.6	40.9	41.1	41.4
128–130	39.8	40.0	40.3	40.5	40.8	41.0	41.3	41.5	41.8

*From Michael L. Pollock, Ph.D., Donald T. Schmidt, M.D., and Andrew S. Jackson, P.E.D., "Measurement of Cardiorespiratory Fitness and Body Composition," *Comprehensive Therapy*, vol. 6, no. 9, September 1980, p. 20.

Test yourself every few months and keep a dated record of the results. The scores will indicate whether you have overlooked some aspect of your training and will also serve as a history of your progress.

MEDICAL STRESS TESTS

If you are healthy and test at fair level or above, you can probably start exercising without medical supervision. If you have any doubts, call your doctor. According to the AMA, if you have any of the following conditions or symptoms, you should definitely talk to your doctor *before* you begin *any* exercise program.

- Chest pain from the slightest activity
- Angina pectoris or moderate to severe coronary heart disease
- Congenital heart diseases
- Severe anemia
- High blood pressure not controlled by medication, or readings of 180/110 even with medication
- Significant disease of the heart valves or larger blood vessels
- Blood clots in veins—in medical terminology, phlebothrombosis or thrombophlebitis
- Lung disease
- Kidney disease
- Liver disease
- Central nervous system diseases
- Diabetes or other metabolic diseases which are not well controlled
- Obesity (more than 35 pounds overweight)
- Acute or chronic infectious diseases
- Psychosis or severe neurosis
- Severe heartbeat irregularities which require medication or medical attention
- Enlarged heart from high blood pressure or other progressive heart disease
- Convulsive disease not completely controlled by medication
- Arthritis severe enough to require frequent pain-killing medication
- Current use of any of these drugs: reserpine, propranolol hydrochloride, guanethidine sulfate, quinidine sulfate, nitroglycerin or other vascular dilators, procainamide hydrochloride, digitalis, catecholamines, ganglionic blocking agents, insulin, psychotropic drugs

It will help if your doctor is a fitness buff too, preferably interested in the same sports you are. Although sports medicine has become a recognized subspecialty—see Appendix A for how to find such a spe-

---

SELF-TESTING WITH A FIT-KIT

The Canadian National Ministry of Health has created an ingenious self-testing packet called a Fit-Kit. You choose a cut on a record and perform specified exercises in rhythm to the recorded cadences. You then take your pulse for ten seconds afterward. Accompanying posters, charts, and booklets help you design a tailor-made fitness program. To order a Fit-Kit; send check or money order for $9.55 (United States residents) or $7.95 (Canadian residents), payable to S.S.C. Publishing Centre, to: The Canadian Home Fitness Test, Operation Lifestyle, Supply and Services (Printing Operations), Ottawa, Canada K1A 0S7.

---

cialist near you—many doctors are still timid about the effects of sports on their patients. Someone who isn't up on the latest in sports medicine, for example, may not understand why a basketball player insists on exercising while her mild sprain heals, or why a diver with multiple sclerosis still insists on scuba diving. (The woman with multiple sclerosis was told by one doctor that scuba diving was out of the question. However, when she sought a second opinion, this doctor, also a diver, designed a program that permitted her to dive under strict supervision.) Or an unathletic physician might not know how to analyze an athlete client's playing form to find the cause of a recurrent injury.

Asked whether you are healthy enough to start exercising or to increase your exercise load, your doctor may suggest that you come in for a routine exercise stress test to detect hidden coronary artery disease. However, a study published in *The New England Journal of Medicine* in 1979 recommended a stress test only if you have symptoms of heart disease or high blood pressure or have a family or medical history which indicates some danger. Another study published the same year in the same journal pointed out that exercise stress tests of people *without symptoms* may produce false-positive or false-negative results. In other words the tests may say you have coronary artery disease when you don't, or may say you don't have coronary artery disease when you do. It is difficult to *predict* "underlying" heart disease in some patients even with extensive testing. Since such a small number of pre-menopausal women suffer heart attacks, the exercise stress test for coronary artery disease in women without symptoms is probably unnecessary under the age of forty-five. If you are over forty-five, consult a doctor whose judgment you trust.

If your age or heart condition indicates that a stress test is in order, expect to spend a couple of hours in the doctor's office working very hard. You will probably wear running clothes and rubber-soled shoes. You will answer detailed questions about your family's medical history

FITNESS PROFILE

Date	Step or 1½ Mile Test	Strength				Flexibility									Percent Body Fat	Problem Areas
		Sit-up	Push-up	Chin-up	Pull-up	Back Arch	Half Knee Bend	Toe Touch	Knee-Nose Touch	Posture Clasp	Heel and Toe	Stork	Slide	Rocker		

and your own. You will probably have a chest x-ray, a urinanalysis, and a Pap smear as part of a complete physical work-up. You will be weighed and measured to determine what percentage of your body weight is actually fat. You will take a resting electrocardiogram, and then you will perform a few sit-ups or other exercises to test the strength of various parts of your body. Finally, you'll be hooked back up to the electrocardiogram, as well as to the blood-pressure cuff and, in some laboratories, a mouthpiece which measures how much oxygen you exhale. For eight or ten minutes, you will either jog on a treadmill, ride a stationary bicycle, or climb up and down stairs.

This part is exhausting. (Dr. George Sheehan thought it was about as close as he would ever come to the pain of childbirth.) Unless you are already a cyclist, request the treadmill test, because your untrained thigh muscles may give out on a stationary bicycle long before your wind and you won't get an accurate measurement of your heart and lung capacity.

The completed stress test, coupled with your medical history and general physical, provides you with a fitness profile: maximum heart rate, target heart rate, ideal body weight, aerobic capacity (how efficiently you use oxygen), contraindications to playing one or more sports. With these figures, you and your doctor can design a safe exercise program tailor-made to your needs.

2 / Fourteen Principles of Conditioning

No matter who you are and what your goals, the ways you get into condition are the same. The fourteen principles that follow apply as much to a woman firming up a flabby tummy as to a Chris Evert Lloyd or a Nancy Lieberman training for the biggest contest of her career. Learn to apply them to every aspect of your daily life. They not only help you derive the maximum effect from the minimum effort but also help you keep free of injury.

I. DEVELOP ENDURANCE, STRENGTH, AND FLEXIBILITY

Endurance gives you stamina, strength gives you power, and flexibility gives you resiliency. Some sports develop all three, while others build only one or two. You should make up for what your sport lacks by playing a complementary game or by doing specific training exercises.

Endurance

Also called cardiovascular endurance, cardiorespiratory endurance, heart/lung capacity, or aerobic capacity, endurance refers to your ability to use oxygen to burn fuel for vigorous activity over long periods. Endurance sports are those lasting longer than three minutes—such as many track events, lacrosse, field hockey, swimming, cross-country skiing, rowing, and cycling. (Sports using quick bursts of speed or power and lasting less than ninety seconds rely on anaerobic energy reactions.) Although it may appear that you don't need aerobic capacity to put the shot, steal a base, swing a golf club, or spike a volleyball, in fact you will be a better player if your lungs have been trained to take in deep draughts of oxygen, and your heart has been trained to pump efficiently no matter how big the workload and to send blood quickly and directly to the muscles that need it. Activities such as the 880-yard dash, gymnastics events, and wrestling matches that typically last between one and a half and three minutes use a combination of aerobic and anaerobic energy systems.

AEROBIC AND ANAEROBIC METABOLISM

When you burn wood in a fireplace, you get heat. When you "burn" fuel in your muscle cells, you get heat and work. Although the reactions inside your cells may seem different from those in your fireplace, they share one crucial similarity—they both need oxygen in order to occur.

Making energy in your cells in the presence of oxygen is called aerobic metabolism, a very efficient process in which a sugar (glucose), stored in your muscles and liver, and fatty acids, stored in your hips, buttocks, and other fat depots, are continually recycled to produce energy and more fuel. Almost every bit of energy in your body comes from aerobic reactions.

However, during your first couple of minutes of exercise (or during that final kick at the end of a race or if you have exhausted all your fuel), your system can't pump enough oxygen to your muscle cells. So you have a backup mechanism to create oxygen-less energy for a minute or two: Your body breaks down a small amount of muscle glycogen (a starchy chain of glucose molecules) in what is called anaerobic (without oxygen) metabolism. Unfortunately, this is not a recycling system the way aerobic metabolism is, and anaerobic energy reactions produce lactic acid as a waste product. Lactic acid accumulates in your muscles and makes them weak and achy.

Because of lactic acid, your body can tolerate anaerobic metabolism for only a minute or two. If your body doesn't adjust to the exercise, or if you work at a flat-out pace (a heart rate over 80 percent of your maximum), your muscles fill with lactic acid, you run out of muscle glycogen, and you cramp up and become so uncoordinated you can barely move.

If, on the other hand, you work at a moderate steady pace (between 60 and 80 percent of your maximum heart rate), aerobic metabolism kicks into gear to run side by side with the anaerobic for a few minutes and then takes over. For the first few minutes of aerobic metabolism, however, you still hurt and can't get your breath because you are still paying off the oxygen debt you incurred during your anaerobic phase. During this time, your body needs oxygen not only to burn energy but also to flush out the unwelcome load of lactic acid and recycle it into more fuel. Only after about ten minutes of aerobic work is most of the lactate recycled, and then you become comfortable and hit your second wind.

Strength

Strength refers to how much force a muscle can exert or how much work it can do against some kind of resistance. Speed is a function of strength because it requires power. You need strength for any sport using short explosive bursts of effort (as in weight lifting or sprinting 100 yards), for jumping (as in basketball or skipping rope), and for any sport where your arms must support your weight (as in gymnastics) or pull your body against gravity (as in pole vaulting) or against water (as in rowing or swimming). You build up your strength by forcing selected muscle groups to work against weights or by lifting parts of your body against gravity, as in chin-ups, sit-ups, and push-ups.

Flexibility

In athletics, flexibility refers to how far you can move your arms, trunk, and legs around each joint. You must be flexible to perform well in gymnastics, dancing, swimming, hurdles, and in any sport that requires reaching and bending. Flexibility is the opposite of strength; strength shortens muscles, while flexibility lengthens them. When you stretch your muscles, you are actually making them longer, and as they elongate they become looser, less taut. Long, loose muscles move through their full range of motion without pulling or tearing. Your genes have already determined the basic stretchiness of your muscles and their enveloping connective tissue, the looseness of the ligaments (fibrous bands) connecting the bones, and the shape of these bones as they meet at your joints. However, with training you use your full potential for flexibility. Age is no reason to become stiffer. "You can be just as flexible at age sixty as you are at age six," says Fred Kasch, developer of the Step Test, who is himself sixty-eight years old. (I did the first splits of my life—all the way down to the floor—when I was thirty-nine, so it's not impossible for an adult woman to reclaim the flexibility of her youth.) The way to become more flexible is to do gradual, progressive stretching exercises over several months. The exercises must be done slowly, without bouncing or rocking, because sharp, quick movements cause your muscles to contract, not relax. Some vigorous sports, such as lifting weights, running, and playing football, actually make your muscles tighter and less flexible the more you do them. Stretching counteracts this tendency and prevents soreness and injury after each game.

II. BUILD YOUR CAPACITY FOR ENDURANCE

No matter what your sport, you need endurance, not only for stamina but for all-around physical fitness. Even in sports such as bowling and golf, which require great skill but very little strength, flexibility, or aerobic capacity, the athlete with the better endurance has an advantage. More important, without good circulatory and respiratory endurance, you will never be truly healthy, no matter how active you are.

Improve your aerobic capacity by practicing one of the endurance sports (distance swimming, cycling, running, jumping rope, or walking) at least three times a week. If you are under fifty years old and in good health, work for at least fifteen minutes at a target pulse of 80 percent of your maximum heart rate. If you are over the age of fifty or have health problems, develop your cardiovascular condition by working for at least thirty minutes at a target pulse of 60 percent of your maximum heart rate. (See chapter 1 for fitness self-testing.)

TARGET PULSE RATE

To find your target pulse, first calculate your maximum heart rate—220 minus your age in years—and then multiply your maximum rate by 60 to 80 percent, depending on age and physical condition. For example, a thirty-five-year-old woman has a maximum heart rate of 185 (220 − 35 = 185). If she is in poor condition, her target pulse rate should be 185 × .60 = 111. If she is in very good condition, her target rate is 185 × .80 = 148.

In endurance training, your muscles use oxygen to burn glycogen. Working out at target pulse rates forces your body to use oxygen more efficiently, and that's the ultimate goal of endurance training. Over the weeks, as you huff and puff for air, the lack of oxygen stimulates your bone marrow to manufacture more red blood cells to carry oxygen to the muscles. At the same time, your body synthesizes more enzymes to separate the oxygen from your blood and give it to your muscles. Your heart muscles become stronger, so that with each newly powerful heartbeat they pump more oxygen-rich blood to your muscles. Your arteries widen to carry this greater blood flow, and you actually grow new capillaries, the tiniest of blood vessels, to carry all this extra blood to every part of each muscle. Exercise physiologists express these cumulative changes as "max VO_2": the maximum volume of oxygen you consume during heavy work. Marathoner Grete Waitz, for example, uses 73.5 milliliters of oxygen per kilogram of body weight each minute. In contrast, an average 110-pound woman endurance athlete has a max VO^2 of 44.0 ml/kg/min.

Smoking cigarettes, however, makes your heart pound 5 to 25

beats faster each minute, narrows your blood vessels and raises your blood pressure 10 to 20 points, reduces the amount of blood sent to your heart and other muscles, and lowers the amount of oxygen in your blood by binding 10 percent of it to carbon dioxide, a waste product of breathing. Thus, if you smoke, you tire more easily and can't develop your maximum training effect. If you quit smoking, you will regain some or all of your lung function within eight months—unless you have permanent lung damage.

When you first begin to exercise, it's a good idea to check your heart rate by taking your pulse every few minutes. For this, the six- or ten-second count you learned in chapter 1 is certainly sufficient. Your pulse tells you whether you are working hard enough to get any training effect or whether, in fact, you are overdoing the exertion. (If you feel very uncomfortable, no matter what your target pulse rate is, *stop.*) After a few weeks, you won't need to take your pulse anymore. You'll know when you have reached your target rate just by feel.

THE TALK/SING TEST

The talk/sing test keeps you hovering around your target heart rate without the nuisance of constant pulse counting. If you can talk to a partner or sing out loud to yourself—but just barely—you are probably working at your target rate. If you are going at a pace which makes conversation or singing impossible, and you feel muscle tightness, rapid pulse, rapid breathing, or the overall sensation of *too much,* you are working beyond your target rate. Slow down. (Obviously, this test is nonsense for swimmers. They must rely on pulse counting.)

As you get into better and better condition, your body will recover more and more quickly from each workout. In fact, your recovery time is a measure of your fitness. Even a beginner should be able to catch her breath within ten minutes. (If you find yourself badly winded, get down on all fours, with your head hanging down between your arms, and pant like a dog.) Your pulse should come down to around 120 within five minutes after you stop exercising, and should be down to 100 or below within ten minutes. If you are in good shape, your pulse should sink to below 100 within five minutes. However, even if you are in good shape, your recovery time will decline if you drastically overexert. One woman who cycles 45 miles a week had a pulse of 100 for three days after riding in her first century (hundred-mile race).

If you hang out with other athletes at the local pub, you are likely to hear a lot of banter about resting pulses. As people get into better and better cardiorespiratory condition, their resting or basal pulse (the number of times their heart beats when they are completely relaxed) often drops by half from the American norm of 80 or 90. If your pulse has come down to the low 50s or 40s when you first wake up in the morning, you can brag with the best of them. However, if it is still up in the 70s, just remind your friends that, according to George Sheehan, Jim Ryun's resting pulse was 72 when he ran his world-record mile.

III. FIND THE RIGHT TIME TO EXERCISE

Try to wait at least two hours after a meal before exercising. If you exercise right after eating, you may feel weak because some of the blood your muscles need has been shunted to your busy intestinal tract. In addition, some people become nauseated or get stitches from intestinal gas if they exercise immediately after a meal. Finally, you may discover what a male friend of mine delicately calls the Army Evacuation. (Recruits in his outfit sent on ten-mile marches right after breakfast discovered that exercise speeds up intestinal contractions, making the call of nature almost as insistent as the shouts of the drill sergeant.) Drinking water immediately before—or during—exercise, on the other hand, is highly recommended.

Exercise at the time that feels "right." Like all plants and animals, human beings are divided into those who are more active in the morning and those who are more active in the afternoon or evening. You run on an approximately twenty-four-hour cycle that Franz Halberg at the University of Minnesota called circadian (from the Latin *circa dies*, about a day). These daily biochemical patterns control when you sleep and wake, when you're hungry, when your body temperature is high or low (it varies 1½ or 2 degrees in a day), when your blood pressure and heart rate are high or low, when your memory is keen, your energy high . . . even how fast your cells divide. You even urinate more frequently during some parts of the day than others. Night people, or owls, run about two hours behind morning people, particularly in body temperature and food intake, and their sluggish hormones in the morning make major physical exertion almost impossible. Morning people, or larks, will spring out of bed and into vigorous exercise, but they should remember that people are stiffer in the morning and so require a longer warm-up to prevent injuries.

IV. LEARN HOW TO OVERLOAD

Any gain in endurance, strength, or flexibility comes from overloading the muscles involved. The idea is to make each muscle group work against a resistance *a little* greater than the amount it is used to. De-

YOUR BODY CLOCK AND JET LAG

When your body clock goes out of synch, you may suffer from insomnia or indigestion, bad temper or moodiness, experience menstrual cramps, lose interest in sexual relations, become forgetful, sluggish, and unable to judge the passage of time, be more or less sensitive to medications, and be unable to perform in your sport with your usual quickness, speed, strength, and endurance.

Any number of factors can throw your circadian cycle out of whack, but the most common are a change of work shifts from day to night or vice versa, sleeping pills (because they interfere with the cyclical hormonal secretions of the adrenal cortex), illness, and traveling across several time zones within a day or two.

Jet lag can be irritating. In a city whose time zone is three hours ahead of (or behind) yours, you may have to ride in a bicycle race or play an important tennis match three hours earlier (or later) than your body's peak of oxygen uptake, heart rate, body temperature, or metabolism. People who are up and active early in the day have more trouble adjusting to jet lag than night people. The older you get, the more sensitive you become to the rigors of time changes.

If you schedule an important game or workout while traveling and want to be at your best, you have only a few options. Fly to your destination a few days before the contest to have time to adjust. (Allow one day for each hour of time change.) Or try to make the time shift while you are still at home. Beginning five days or a week before your trip, go to bed and wake up one half hour earlier each day (to simulate moving to a more easterly time zone) or one half hour later (for a western time zone). Before you actually leave, you will be falling asleep (not just lying in bed) according to the new time zone. Or minimize the effects of jet lag by eating your meals and scheduling your games according to your home clock. Otherwise, if you travel eastward, your performance is likely to be under par in the morning hours because you would be asleep at home, and if you travel westward, your performance may be less than satisfactory in the late afternoon or evening hours because your internal clock is telling you it's bedtime.

pending on your sport, that resistance can be the weight of your own body against weights, gravity, or distance. Swing overweight bats. Throw an overweight shot put, discus, or javelin. Hold a one-pound dumbbell while simulating tennis strokes. When you actually play the game, your regular equipment will seem blissfully light.

But note: The extra stress should be small. Use weights just large enough to feel slightly heavy, and increase their weight only when they begin to feel light. If you add too much weight at once, you will damage your muscles and they will take longer to repair themselves and build. If your muscles start to quiver during exercise, they are trying to tell you they are exhausted. Back off for a few minutes and let them rest.

V. FOLLOW THE LAW OF SPECIFICITY

The best way to get better at your sport is to play it. If you want to do additional exercises to become stronger or move faster, choose exercises that duplicate the movements you use when you actually play your sport. It's taken years for trainers to realize that bench presses will not help their quarterbacks pass farther, nor will walking in ankle weights help their guards jump higher in basketball. (In fact, ankle weights alone, without a structured, progressive weight training program, can hurt you by creating traction at your knees and hips.) In simplest terms, the best exercise for a sucked-in gut is sucking in your gut, the best exercise for running longer is running longer, and the best exercise for a strong backhand is hitting a lot of backhand shots.

There is a physiological basis for this. Much like a Thanksgiving turkey, your muscles are composed of light meat and dark meat. Your light or fast-twitch muscle fibers contract very quickly, with immense force for very short bursts of effort, but light muscles lack myoglobin, the red-colored oxygen-carrying muscle pigment similar to the hemoglobin in your blood. Without myoglobin, these muscles have no oxygen and must burn their small supply of muscle sugar in anaerobic nonrecyclable chemical reactions. The fuel is depleted within ninety seconds, and the muscles simply stop working. Slow-twitch muscle fibers contract more slowly and with less power than fast-twitch fibers, but their myoglobin provides them with a constant supply of oxygen which they use to continually recycle fuel for long-term aerobic energy. Just as the turkey uses its slow-to-tire dark leg and back muscles for basic standing and strutting and the light muscles in wings and breast for short desperate flights to escape predators, you use the dark fibers in your muscles for long walks along the beach and your light fibers for lifting heavy objects and sprinting for the bus.

The proportions of dark and light fibers in each muscle are preordained by your genes. (Muscle biopsies will tell you whether you have a higher percentage of fast-twitch explosive fibers or slow-twitch endurance fibers.) However, when you combine the principles of overload and specificity, you stress your body enough to actually enlarge the fibers you already have and even, some scientists speculate, to provoke the growth of new fibers. In addition, highly concentrated training converts fibers from one sort to the other. These fibers don't completely ignore your genetic blueprint, because they change back to their original type when you stop stressing them. Nonetheless, no matter what nature ordained, you can increase your endurance and strength by intelligent practice.

VI. HONOR THY ANTAGONISTS

Groups of muscles come in pairs, and each has its own job. The biceps muscles in your arms, for example, bend your elbows, but can't straighten them out again. For that, you use your triceps. These pairs are called antagonists, and you should exercise all members of each set of muscles as well as the muscles that oppose them. If you strengthen a muscle, it becomes thicker, tighter, and shorter. If you don't strengthen its antagonist at the same time, the antagonist remains longer and weaker and can't keep the joint it operates in alignment. Misalignment is a common cause of injury in athletes. (Although it is a second-best solution, instead of strengthening the antagonist, you can try to stretch out the agonist—or contracting muscle—with concentrated flexibility exercises. This is the rationale behind many pre- and post-exercise stretching programs and is quite effective. The ideal, however, is still to strengthen all members of a muscle group and then stretch them out equally.)

VII. OBEY THE ORDER OF EXERCISE

The sequence of your exercise depends on your emphasis. If you just want to stay in shape, do your strength or resistance work first, your endurance work next, and your flexibility work last. If you are concentrating on weight training, for body building or power lifting, you can also follow this schedule. However, if you are a dancer or a gymnast, interested in flexibility above all else, put your flexibility routines first, then do your weight training, and save the endurance workouts for last. On days when you have a hot squash game or swim meet scheduled, just stretch. Don't do your full workout, or you will be too tired to play at top form.

    You are strongest at the beginning of your workout, before your aerobic work cranks out high quantities of lactic acid. Since stretching exercises do not produce much lactic acid or require "clean" muscles, you can do them last and enjoy the bonus of warm, already supple muscles willing to stretch much farther. Vary the order if you discover that long hard workouts leave you too weak to touch your toes.

VIII. USE IT OR LOSE IT

According to Forrest Smith, M.D., medical director of the Total Health Medical Center in Oakland, California, it takes only three or four weeks for your body to lose its conditioning, whether you are a world-class athlete who has been training all her life or a woman who just started cross-country skiing three months ago.

If muscles aren't stressed constantly, they quickly lose their ability to use oxygen efficiently. This happens faster in endurance sports than in anaerobic events; for a while after they stop training, sprinters and weight lifters can run as fast or lift as powerfully, although their stamina is impaired. But after an extra week or two, laziness takes its toll on them too.

The unmistakable symptoms of detraining are:

• You can't do the things you once could
• You're breathless at a pace you used to find comfortable
• Your muscles are sore

It takes much more work to get into shape than to stay in shape. If you work out four or five times a week, you will *improve* your skill and fitness. If you do the same workout three times a week—preferably every other day—you will *maintain* your present level of fitness and skill, assuming you have achieved a moderate level of conditioning in the first place.

IX. WARM UP PROPERLY

Before any kind of workout, you must warm up your muscles with stretches and light exercises. Never, never neglect your warm-ups. A gradual stretching program raises your body temperature slightly by increasing your breathing and circulation and, in the process, gently lengthens your ligaments and limbers your muscles. Warm-ups also prepare your joints for action by thickening the tissue and by lubricating the articular surfaces and tendons with additional viscous synovial fluid.

Don't forget to give your heart some gradual warm-up time. Your heart is a muscle too, and the harder it works the more oxygen it needs; however, it takes the arteries a few minutes to dilate enough to bring in an increased supply of oxygen-rich blood from the lungs. Sudden strenuous exercise may leave the heart deprived of oxygen, causing irregular blood flow and abnormally high blood pressure. This is particularly dangerous for people with coronary artery disease (and that group includes most middle-aged men and women and some younger men).

Three or four serves or ten jumping jacks won't suffice. To warm up your heart, do two to five minutes of very light jogging or the equivalent *after* your stretching exercises. On very cold days, warm up your heart *before* you try to stretch your muscles. (A very cold body can't stretch out effectively.) Run slowly in place or do a few jumping jacks first and then begin your stretching regimen.

JUMPING JACKS

Stand with your feet together and your arms at your sides. On the count of one, jump up and as you land with your feet comfortably apart, simultaneously swing your arms up and clap your hands above your head. On the count of two, jump back to your starting position and swing your arms back down to your sides for one full jumping jack.

Throughout most of your stretching warm-up, don't bounce. The so-called ballistic movements of old-fashioned toe touches and knee bends actually tighten rather than loosen unprepared muscles. Smooth sustained static stretches, similar to those used in ballet and yoga, prevent as well as relieve muscle soreness while they improve your flexibility. They really act as a kind of massage, as professional football, basketball, and baseball players have recently discovered. However, if you play an aggressive reaching sport such as hockey or racquetball, perform a second, brisker round of warm-ups to prepare your muscles for sudden twists and turns but stop well short of pain.

STATIC STRETCH

In a static stretch, you get your body into a position in which your joints are locked while your muscles are stretched to their greatest possible length. You hold this position for one to three minutes, letting gravity pull or push you farther. In other words, if you are bending over to touch your toes, go as far as you can with your knees locked. Stop when you feel a slight pull and it becomes a little uncomfortable, and rest there until your muscles relax and the strain is gone. Then move a little farther down until you feel that *slightly* uncomfortable tension again.

Universal Warm-ups

The following universal warm-ups come from Jack Rockwell, registered physical therapist and associate director of the Center for Sports Medicine at St. Francis Memorial Hospital. He recommends them for every healthy person, man or woman, no matter what their age or sport. "We have used these same exercises," he says, "for girls in gymnastics and swimming, for runners, and for women in their sixties, seventies, and eighties who have had myocardial infarctions or open-heart surgery and are now enrolled in our program for cardiac rehabilitation."

Keep the following instructions in mind:

- Don't bounce; work slowly
- Work from the feet up, doing all the exercises on one part of your body before moving on to the next and stretching out any muscles still sore from your previous workout
- Stretch until you feel a solid pull, but stop short of pain
- Do each warm-up once at first (unless otherwise noted) and progress to three to five times per session
- Hold each exercise for a count of ten to twenty, depending on your condition, unless otherwise noted
- Warm up your heart by doing a slow version of your sport—a slow jog or an easy rally or just running in place—for five to ten minutes

Remember: If you have health problems, see your doctor before embarking on *any* exercise program.

1. Toe Flexer

Loosens and stretches the muscles around your ankles. Sit on the floor (or the ground), legs extended. Keep your heels on the floor. Flex your

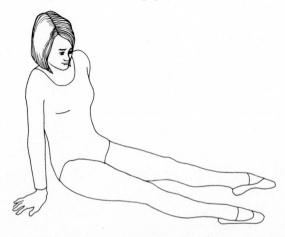

TOE FLEXER

toes toward your body and then point them away, back and forth, twenty times for each foot.

2. Ankle Roll

Stretches the muscles around your ankles. Sitting with legs straight out in front, lift one foot slightly and move that ankle in large circles, first clockwise and then counterclockwise, twenty circles in each direction. Repeat with other foot.

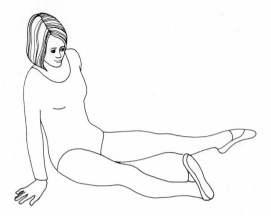

ANKLE ROLL

3. Foot Twister

Stretches the muscles on the outside of the lower leg. Still sitting, cross the lower leg of your left foot over your right thigh. Grasp your left foot with both hands, holding the outside and sole of your foot with your left hand and the top of your foot with your right hand. Without moving your leg or knee, and bending only the ankle, try to turn your foot so that the sole points upward and you feel a pull along the outside of your skin. Exert force—"as if you are twisting your foot off," Rockwell says. Repeat with the other foot.

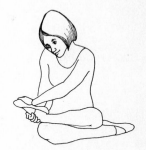

FOOT TWISTER

4. Calf Stretch

Stretches the Achilles tendon, the lower hamstrings, and the shin muscles. Stand about 18 inches from a wall, facing it. Place both hands on the wall, about shoulder height and shoulder width apart. Stretch one leg out behind you, keeping the knee straight and the heel firmly on the floor. Keep the forward leg beneath you, knee bent slightly, heel

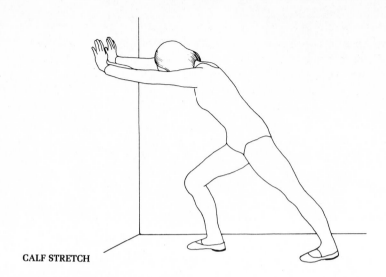

CALF STRETCH

flat on the floor. Slowly lean into the wall, sliding your hips forward and bending your arms as if you were doing a push-up against the wall, until you feel a real pull. Hold for a slow count of fifteen. Repeat with the other leg.

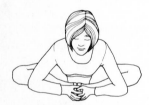

GROIN STRETCH

5. Groin Stretch

Stretches the muscles of the groin area. Sit on the floor or the ground. Bend your knees and bring the soles of your feet together. Grasp your feet with your hands and pull up on them while you try to bring your head down to touch your toes. As you get more flexible, bring your forehead down to the floor ahead of your feet, reaching farther in front of your feet each day.

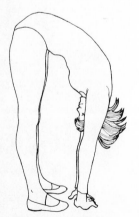

GRAVITY TOE TOUCH

6. Gravity Toe Touch

Stretches the hamstrings. Stand up with your feet comfortably close together and your knees locked. Bend over at the hips and try to touch your toes or the floor. Go down just as far as you can until you feel a stretch; then hang there, letting gravity pull you farther down, for a count of fifteen. Don't bounce. When you release to stand up, bend your knees a bit to prevent a strain on your lower back.

7. Stork

Stretches the quadriceps, the large muscle running down the front of your thigh. Standing, place your right hand against a wall or table for support. From behind, grasp your left leg with your left hand, holding it where the ankle and foot meet. Bending at the hip, pull your heel

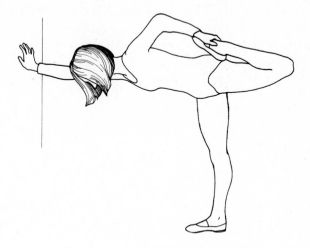

STORK

up, as close to your buttocks as you can, and try to point your left knee directly behind you. Don't let your leg swing out to the side. Keep your body straight; do not bend your back or arch your neck. When you are truly limber, your body will form a T on your supporting leg. Reverse position for the other leg.

8. Knee-Nose Touch

Stretches the lower back. Lie on your back on the floor or ground. Bend your knees. Reach forward with both hands and grasp one leg

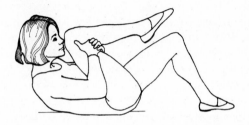

KNEE-NOSE TOUCH

behind the knee. (If you hold the top of the knee, you may put too much stress on it.) Bring the knee toward your head as you bend your neck and back to meet it. Repeat with the other leg.

9. Killer Sit-up

Strengthens the abdominal muscles. Lie on your back, knees bent, feet flat on the floor. Flatten the small of your back into the floor. (This is called a pelvic tilt.) Put your hands behind your head, tuck your chin into your chest, and slowly roll yourself up to a 30- or 40-degree angle from the floor. The angle is critical—too little or too much, and the exercise isn't effective. For some people, the perfect position comes right after their shoulder blades leave the floor. For others, it feels as if it is halfway down the spine. For still others, the sweet spot is an open hand span—a friend's hand—from the base of the neck to the floor.

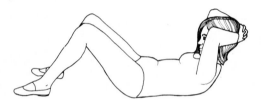

KILLER SIT-UP

The way you know you've hit the spot is that it should be misery incarnate. In fact, if your abdominal muscles aren't in top condition, they will start to quiver about halfway through the exercise. That's all right. Hold the position for a slow ten count, then relax back to the floor very slowly. Keep your knees bent to prevent injury to your lower back. Move at an even pace without jerky movements. One killer sit-up is enough unless you want to firm up your middle; then do as many as you can tolerate. Tests at Southern Illinois University at Carbondale showed that one killer sit-up is the physiological equivalent of twenty regular sit-ups. Ordinary ballistic sit-ups strengthen the abdominals during only a fraction of your up-and-down movement. The rest of the time, they develop your back, upper legs and the hip flexors that move your thigh. Killer sit-ups, on the other hand, concentrate 93 percent of your effort on the upper and lower abdominal muscles.

10. Standard Push-up

Strengthens the muscles of your chest, shoulders, and triceps. Lie on the floor, prone, with the weight of your body supported on your flexed toes and your hands. Keep your hands under the outer edges of

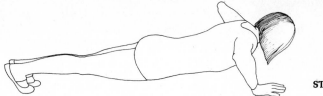

STANDARD PUSH-UP

your shoulders and your whole body stiff as a board. Slowly straighten your arms to raise your body; then slowly return to a prone position. Take a count of ten to get up and a count of ten to get down again. Don't let your fanny flap up and down, don't bend at the waist, and don't droop your head toward the floor. Work up to twenty.

If this is too hard for you at first, remember that the higher your hands are in relation to your trunk, the shorter the distance you have to lift your weight. Thus, if you are very weak, start by pushing off a sturdy table or even the side of a wall. On the other hand, if you are looking for a real challenge, keep your hands on the floor and rest your feet on a stool or table. Good luck!

Killer Push-up (Alternate)

Lie on the floor in the usual push-up position, but place your hands flat on the floor under your chest instead of at shoulder level, forefinger tips touching and pointing toward your head, thumb tips touching and pointing toward your feet. Keeping your body rigid, push yourself

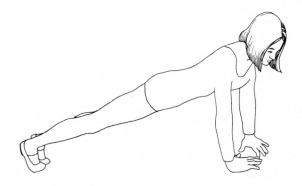

KILLER PUSH-UP

slowly up and down, taking a ten count on each stroke. One killer push-up is the equivalent of several standard push-ups. Work up to twenty.

11. Airplane

Loosens the muscles of the trunk. Stand up, feet comfortably apart. Extend your arms to the sides, shoulder height. Turn slowly to the right and then to the left, taking a five count in each direction. Do three to five times.

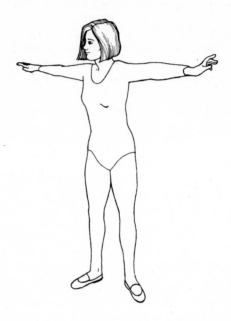

AIRPLANE

12. Windmill

Loosens the muscles of the trunk and adds a little upper body rotation. Stand with feet about shoulder width apart. Extend your arms out to the sides. Keeping your legs straight, slowly reach down with your right hand to touch your left toe as your left arm goes straight up in the air behind you. Work slowly, taking a four count to get down and another four count to get up again. Repeat with your left arm and right foot. Do three to five pairs.

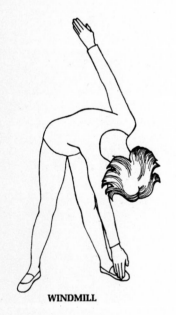

WINDMILL

13. Reach-for-the-Sky

Loosens the upper arms and shoulders and stretches the whole body. Stand with feet comfortably apart. Raise your hands over your head. With one hand, try to touch the ceiling, going up on tiptoes and stretching that whole side of your body. Repeat with your other arm. Do this slowly four or five times. Rockwell suggests you repeat this four or five times a day to relieve tension in your shoulders.

14. Chicken Flap

Loosens the arms. Stand with feet comfortably apart. With elbows bent, swing and flap your arms around, hug yourself, reach your arms back behind you as far as you can go without strain, and then flap your arms again. Many people do this as they run their warm-up jog or take their practice swings with racket or bat. Since most of us stretch, reach, and grasp things in our daily lives, we don't have to be as specific in our arm and shoulder warm-ups as we do in our other exercises.

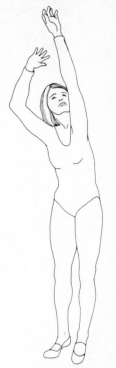

REACH-FOR-THE-SKY

X. ALWAYS COOL DOWN

To prevent muscle soreness, cooling down after exercise is just as important as warming up before it. As you exercise, your muscles tighten up. A cool-down after every workout stretches the muscles out again and massages the lactic acid wastes back to the liver for recycling. Ballet dancers have known this for years and stretch for about twenty minutes after every class, rehearsal, or performance.

Cool-downs may be the same as warm-ups, but the key is always slow and easy. To cool down, just repeat each warm-up exercise once—three times if you have taken an unusual pounding or lifted weights (these activities shorten your muscles).

Your heart also needs this cool-down period. While you exercise, your heart valiantly pumps all that extra blood into your leg and arm muscles. The muscles, in their turn, push the blood back to the heart. (The heart only pumps blood out; muscles massage the blood back.) When you suddenly stop moving, your heart continues to pump blood at an accelerated rate for a few minutes. The blood pools in your arms and legs and not enough gets back up to the heart—and thence to the brain. Whenever your brain runs low on oxygen, you faint. That's your body's way of forcing fresh blood to the brain. If you slow down your activity gradually, walking after you run or playing a lazy, friendly game of volleyball, your muscles continue to force your blood back to your heart at a rate compatible with your gradually declining heartbeat. After a few minutes, your pulse is back to within 20 beats of normal, and so is your circulation.

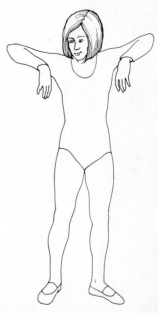

CHICKEN FLAP

XI. ALTERNATE HARD AND EASY DAYS

Each time you push your muscles beyond their ordinary limits, you tear down muscle tissue. Your body needs a day of rest to rebuild these fibers and make them bigger and better than before. Furthermore, during a hard workout you exhaust the supply of fuel in your muscles. It takes ten hours or more to replenish it. Finally, if you sweat, your body loses potassium, a mineral essential for body heat control, proper muscle functioning, and the transfer of nerve impulses. It takes your body up to a day (or two, in extreme cases) to restore your potassium balance. When you work out strenuously one day and ease off the next, you give your body time to recuperate and, in fact, come back stronger than before.

On a hard day, you go all out—an hour of jumping rope, perhaps, or swimming a mile and a half or pressing 55 pounds. An easy day may mean just a relaxed workout or even the day off. Twenty-four hours usually is enough time to recover, but if your workout was particularly strenuous, you may need an extra day. You'll know if you do, you'll still be exhausted and achy the second morning after. Marathoners and ultra-long-distance swimmers sometimes take as long as two weeks to recover from a race.

If you are lifting weights, three days, spaced evenly throughout the week, is ideal; your strength and muscle mass will grow on your off days. Play other sports on the intervening days if you like, or divide your weight or resistance workouts so that you work on your chest and legs, say, on Monday, Wednesday, and Friday, and your arms and shoulders and abdomen on Tuesday, Thursday, and Saturday. This system allows you to have shorter and more intense training sessions.

XII. DON'T OVERTRAIN

It *is* possible to overdo. Since exercise is a stress, your body needs time to rebuild. If it hurts to exercise, or if it makes you feel sick or exhausted afterward, you are overtraining. Pain is nature's way of telling you to stop. Shorten your workouts or reduce your workload, and make sure you give yourself one or two days a week off.

These are signs of overtraining:

- Your early morning resting pulse is more than ten beats higher than usual
- You are exhausted, rather than exhilarated, after a workout, or still tired from a workout twenty-four hours later
- Your legs or arms feel heavy or your muscles and joints ache and feel stiff while you exercise or for several days afterward

- Your glands are swollen, you lose your appetite, you are always tired, your allergies flare up, you feel headachy, jittery, or weepy, have diarrhea or constipation, can't relax, and have trouble concentrating
- Your performance takes a nose dive even though you are working out as much or more than before
- You develop insomnia or have trouble staying asleep (do not consider inability to sleep as a sign that your newly fit body now needs less sleep; athletes in heavy training need more sleep)
- You get colds frequently
- You vomit or feel nauseated after a workout
- You lose interest in exercise or feel unaccountably depressed

XIII. USE SAFETY EQUIPMENT

Fortunately, the reckless, death-defying athletic machismo of the first half of this century has given way to the chic, sensible, protective styles of today, and kids seem to have led the way. When roller skating became a fad, cushioned gloves, knee pads, and elbow pads were as essential as cool wheels. Skateboarders now wear helmets, as do cyclists and white-water kayakers. Sailors wear flotation jackets, joggers wear reflective vests at night, home gymnasts roll and tumble on mats, racquetball and squash players wear eye guards or goggles. It's the fashion. And it's the only intelligent thing to do.

XIV. OBEY WARNING SIGNALS

Stop exercising and consult your doctor if you feel:

- Pain or tightness in your chest
- Severe breathlessness
- Light-headedness or dizziness
- Nausea
- Loss of control of your muscles
- Severe pain from any injury
- Persistent pain in a bone or joint or muscle due to a fall, a blow, or a wrenching, tearing, or twisting
- Any bone or joint pain that persists for longer than two weeks
- Any injury that doesn't heal in three weeks
- Any skin infection that shows pus, red streaks, swollen lymph nodes, or fever

Follow these general rules:

1. If any part of your body hurts when at rest, don't exercise without a physician's okay.
2. If that part of your body doesn't hurt at rest, try exercising it. If it doesn't hurt when you exercise it, keep going.
3. If that body part hurts when you exercise again, stop.
4. If you have any questions at all, call your physician. (See chapter 10.)

3 / Sound Nutrition

Vigorous exercise is one of the two keys to good health. The other is an intelligent diet. Everyone is looking for the magic combination of foods that will ensure glowing skin, boundless energy, and eternal youth. As an active woman, you want a diet that gives you all this and also helps you to run faster, have greater endurance, muscle up quicker, and lose (or gain) body fat.

WHAT MAKES A WINNING DIET?

Nutritional deficiencies show up more quickly and more sharply when you are active, because you make more demands on your body. But when it comes right down to it, everyone needs the same nutrients in the same basic proportions. Although an active woman may be able to eat more calories overall than a sedentary one, nothing short of the basic well-balanced diet—tailored to your body's individual demands, of course, and supplemented, if necessary, with vitamins and minerals—will keep you in peak condition.

In the fifties and sixties, nutritionists taught us that a balanced daily diet consisted of a prescribed number of servings from each of four basic food groups: meats, dairy products, fruits and vegetables, and cereals. However, in 1977 the Senate Committee on Nutrition and Human Needs, chaired by George McGovern of South Dakota, cited evidence that the high-protein, high-fat, low-complex-carbohydrate diet of affluent twentieth-century America had actually increased the incidence in the United States of heart disease, digestive cancers, diabetes, and other degenerative diseases. Americans, the committee said, typically make protein 40 percent of their diet (some go as high as 60 percent) and fat another 40 percent. This has two effects. First, if you eat so few complex carbohydrates, you get very little plant fiber, or roughage. (Fiber speeds the passage of food through your intestines and, as a result, prevents bowel cancer. Fiber also traps some of the cholesterol particles from the meat you eat and prevents them from entering the bloodstream.) Second, any excess protein you consume beyond your basic need is converted into fat and stored in layers in your body (along with the extra fat you eat).

The McGovern committee redefined the concept of a balanced diet in the light of modern nutritional and biochemical research. It suggested eating 15 to 20 percent in the form of protein, another 20 to 30 percent in the form of fats—only one third of which should be saturated (solid or animal) fats—and the remaining 50 to 65 percent as complex carbohydrates—that is, fruits, vegetables, seeds, nuts, and whole grains. You use the carbohydrates and fats as fuel, the protein to replace and build body tissue, and the vitamins and minerals contained in your food as catalysts or prompters to power the chemical reactions occurring in every cell of your body.

You have unique nutritional needs, affected by your genetic and emotional makeup, your environment, your health and level of activity, and the drugs you are taking. There isn't a scientist on earth who can dictate a diet to suit both you and your next-door neighbor equally well. The McGovern formula is merely a set of guidelines. To use it, first calculate the total number of calories you need each day (see "Your Plus Diet" in chapter 4). Then figure out the minimum and maximum number of calories of protein, fat, and carbohydrates you can allow yourself. For example, let's say you need 1,625 calories each day. Your protein allowance is 15 to 20 percent of 1,625 calories, or 244 to 325 calories per day (1625 × .15 = 243.75; 1625 × .20 = 325). Your fat allowance is 20 to 30 percent of 1,625 calories, or 325 to 488 calories per day (1625 × .20 = 325; 1625 × .30 = 487.5). Your carbohydrate allowance is 50 to 65 percent of 1,625 calories, or 813 to 1,056 calories per day (1625 × .50 = 812.5; 1625 × .65 = 1056.25).

That's what the McGovern guidelines say, but unfortunately that's not what you put into your mouth. No food is pure protein or pure carbohydrate or pure fat. If you consult a chart of nutrients in one of the books listed in the back under Selected Readings, you'll see that most animal and vegetable protein foods have a significant amount of fat, and most carbohydrates contain at least small amounts of protein. If you eat 300 calories of chicken breast, for example, you don't get 300 calories of protein; you get 238.1 calories of protein and 61.8 calories of fat. In fact, half a pound of chicken breast contains 149.2 calories (37.3 grams) of protein and 38.7 calories (4.3 grams) of fat. The rest of the weight is water, carbohydrates, and trace nutrients. Other examples:

- Half a pound of choice T-bone steak contains 118.4 calories (29.6 grams) of protein and 671.4 calories (74.6 grams) of fat

- Half a pound of roasted shelled peanuts contains 237.6 calories (59.4 grams) of protein and 994.5 calories (110.5 grams) of fat
- Half a pound of brook trout contains 85.6 calories (21.4 grams) of protein and 21.6 calories (2.4 grams) of fat

The easiest way to use the McGovern guidelines is to add up the total calories in each protein and carbohydrate food you eat, cut down on extra fat (in the form of the butter, cream, and oil you cook with or spread on top of your food), and let the hidden fat make up your 20-odd percent daily fat allowance. Thus, if you need 1,625 calories each day and you eat 500 calories' worth of protein foods and 1,100 calories' worth of carbohydrate foods, you will probably wind up eating 20 to 30 percent fat calories.

If you are on a low-fat diet to lose weight or reduce your serum cholesterol, or if you are worried that you are not eating enough protein to rebuild your muscles, you can, in fact, calculate the actual amount of protein, fat, and carbohydrate in each food you eat. Most nutrient charts list the amounts of each nutrient by weight in grams. One gram of protein or carbohydrate contains 4 calories; 1 gram of fat contains 9 calories. Thus, if you multiply the number of grams of protein or carbohydrate by 4, or the number of grams of fat by 9, you come out with the number of actual calories of each constituent in your food. An extra-large egg, for example, contains almost equal weights of protein and fat (7.4 grams and 7.2 grams respectively). However, it contains 29.6 calories of protein (4 × 7.4) and 64.8 calories of fat (9 × 7.2).

There's a lot of juggling you can do within these guidelines. Want butter on your baked potato? Fine. Just have chicken for dinner, with its 38.7 calories of fat per half pound, instead of steak, with its 671.4 calories of fat. Can't resist that steak after all? Compensate over the next few days by eating chicken and fish and avoiding butter and oil. Whatever you do, however, don't try to compensate by eliminating one or more of the essential nutrients. You need them all.

Fat

Although too much fat makes you obese, you must eat some fat every day in order to stay alive. Fat is your heart's favorite fuel. Of the two types of building blocks in fat, saturated and unsaturated fatty acids, the unsaturated fatty acids, especially linoleic, arachidonic, and linolenic acid—the three the body can't manufacture for itself—build nerves, carry oxygen to vital organs and every other tissue in the body, and combine with protein and cholesterol, a lipid or fatlike substance, to make up the walls of every cell in your body. (Unsaturated fatty acids are liquid at room temperature and come from vegetable sources.

Saturated fatty acids, the second type of building block, are usually solid at room temperature and come from animal sources. Among the few exceptions, palm and coconut oil contain saturated fatty acids and yet come from vegetable sources.) Fat also keeps your skin from drying out and carries the fat-soluble vitamins A, D, E, and K throughout your system. Cutting your fat intake to less than 20 percent of your total daily calories can lead to serious health hazards and possibly even to dangerously irregular heartbeats.

Protein

Your body needs protein to build and replace the muscle cells you break down with constant use. Protein maintains and repairs every cell in your body—muscle, nerve, blood, skin, heart, brain. It also forms hormones to control the chemistry of growth, metabolism, and development; enzymes for digestion and other body functions; and antibodies to fight disease. Protein is used as an energy source only if the body is starving and has no fat or carbohydrate to draw on. Your body doesn't store excess protein. If you eat more protein than your body needs to replace blood or other body tissues, your liver either breaks down the excess into storage fat or converts it into ammonia and excretes it in your urine. Therefore, if you eat more protein than the 15 to 20 percent your body needs to rebuild itself, the surplus becomes ugly fat.

An athlete's need for protein is no greater than a sedentary person's, male or female. Unless you are a serious weight lifter, you need only the standard allowance of 15 to 20 percent. If you are a power lifter, add 5 percent more (about 28 additional calories, or 7 grams, per day), to support muscle growth.

Carbohydrates

Complex carbohydrates—fruits, vegetables, seeds, nuts, and whole grains—are your body's most important source of energy. They are, in fact, the only fuel your brain and nerve cells will accept. Your body also needs carbohydrates to break down and burn its other fuel source, fat, and to construct those amino acids (or protein building blocks) the body knows how to make for itself.

In the human body, the fundamental carbohydrate is glucose. Only glucose can be used directly for energy. In order to use any other carbohydrate, the intestine must first break it down into simple sugars, and then the liver converts those sugars into glucose. With the exception of lactose (milk sugar) and glycogen (stored glucose molecules strung together), all carbohydrates come from plants and arrive in three basic forms: sugar, starch, and cellulose.

CHOLESTEROL

There is some good news, after all! Exercise reduces the amount of "bad" cholesterol you have in your bloodstream and increases the amount of "good" cholesterol. The bad cholesterol is called low-density lipoprotein (LDL)—large clumpy fatlike particles that form deposits on the walls of your arteries, encourage the platelets (clotting cells) in your blood to lump together, and cause blocked and hardened arteries. The good cholesterol is called high-density lipoprotein (HDL)—particles that are smaller, heavier, and less fatty. (Lipoproteins are compounds made of blood protein, cholesterol, and fat.) HDLs prevent atherosclerosis in two ways: They chemically block a blood cell's ability to absorb LDLs, and they scavenge LDLs out of the bloodstream and carry them to the liver for excretion in the feces, reducing the amount of LDLs circulating through your system.

Cholesterol isn't your enemy. Both types are vital for building cell membranes and keeping cell walls stable. You need between 100 and 200 milligrams of cholesterol per 100 cubic centimeters of blood in order to survive, and 55 percent of your total serum cholesterol should exist in the form of HDLs. To guarantee an adequate supply of cholesterol, your liver manufactures about 75 percent of your stock. Only 25 percent comes from the meat and dairy products you eat. For this reason, reducing the amount of cholesterol in your diet doesn't always lower your levels enough to reduce your chances of stroke and heart attack. Exercise does.

Women naturally have higher HDL levels in their bloodstreams than men, and women (and men) who exercise regularly have higher HDL levels and lower LDL levels than their sedentary neighbors. When you do efficient aerobic exercise, you burn up fat (the doctors call it triglyceride) which might otherwise be combined with cholesterol to form LDL. Thus, moderate aerobic workouts are best for lowering your LDL count. Work at 60 to 80 percent of your maximum heart rate for at least one half hour (longer to encourage fat burning), at least three days a week.

There are two kinds of sugars, the simple sugars, or monosaccharides, and the double sugars, or disaccharides. Simple sugars, including fructose, galactose, and glucose, are found in fruit and honey and are processed so quickly they provide instantaneous energy. Double sugars such as sucrose (table sugar), maltose, and lactose are broken down almost as quickly. Starches, or polysaccharides, such as those found in flour and other grain products, are chains of simple sugars. They take longer to digest (it takes the digestive enzymes longer to break the chain apart), so they stay longer in your digestive system and you feel full longer. Cellulose, the fiber found in raw fruits and vegetables, is also a polysaccharide, but your digestive enzymes can't break it down.

Simply because it is indigestible, though, cellulose is essential to your diet, providing the bulk necessary to move food through your intestinal tract and out the bowel.

Some of the glucose from the carbohydrates you eat circulates in your bloodstream to supply immediate energy. Another small amount is converted into glycogen and stored in your muscles and liver for future use. Any excess is converted into fat and stored away in those ugly saddlebags and beer bellies.

The key word in the McGovern committee's carbohydrate recommendations is "complex." You should eat fewer simple and double sugars and more starch in the form of whole grains and unprocessed (that is, raw or lightly cooked) fruits and vegetables because they have cellulose and many nutrients in them. The committee objected to table sugar, white flour, white rice, and other highly processed foods (including most breakfast cereals) because they provide no nutrients of their own and rob you of B vitamins you already have. Your intestines require B vitamins in order to break down and use carbohydrates. Many whole foods come equipped with their own supply of B vitamins, but highly refined foods don't. They draw on the stock of Bs already in your system and leave you with a deficit.

After a strenuous workout, you may crave sugars, starches, and foods heavy in B vitamins because you've used up much of your stored carbohydrates. Go ahead. Indulge. Whole-grain breads, potatoes, and fresh fruit won't make you fat as long as you decrease your intake of fat and protein accordingly. It isn't the slice of whole wheat toast that's fattening. It's the butter and jam you pile on top.

Vitamins and Minerals

The old-fashioned balanced diet included at least two servings each day of meat or vegetable protein, two servings of dairy products, four servings of fruits and vegetables, including at least one serving of dark leafy green or deep yellow vegetables (when was the last time you ate kale or collard or mustard greens, or even spinach?), and four servings of bread or cereals.

To get maximum value from these foods, they should be raw or very lightly cooked. Overcooking destroys delicate vitamins. Cooking foods in water dissolves all the water-soluble vitamins and many of the minerals; in order to get the full benefit you must drink the soup or "pot likker" too. Processing foods also removes water-soluble vitamins. According to *Consumer Reports*, for example, frozen orange juice contains only 20 to 40 milligrams of vitamin C in a three-and-a-half-ounce glass. Fresh orange juice has 60. Canned peas lose 94 percent of their vitamin C, while reheated frozen peas lose 83 percent. Peas fresh from the garden, by contrast, have 100 percent of their vitamin C if eaten raw and 50 percent if heated quickly in a bare minimum of water.

The ideal balanced diet, furthermore, is grown in soil undepleted by chemical fertilizers, and the ideal people who eat it don't drink alcohol (it disrupts the absorption of vitamins B_1, B_6, and folic acid), smoke cigarettes (they reduce the levels of vitamin C in your blood by 30 to 40 percent), or take birth-control pills (they increase your need for vitamins B_1, B_2, B_{12}, C, and folic acid—all necessary for building blood cells to carry precious oxygen to your working muscles).

Vitamins help you use your food more efficiently. They form chemical compounds which, in their turn, stimulate your digestive enzymes to break down food particles into components your intestine can absorb. Minerals are essential for the chemical reactions that contract your muscles, transmit nerve impulses to your brain and back, control your heartbeat, regulate the amount of water your body retains and where it is stored, and give structure to your bones, teeth, hair, and fingernails. In addition, at least one nutritional researcher, Michael Colgan, M.D., a professor at the University of Auckland in New Zealand, believes that adding a vitamin and mineral supplement to your diet may markedly improve your speed and endurance and increase your strength during training. In a series of "double blind" experiments designed to eliminate the bias of the scientist and the suggestibility of the athletes, he gave marathoners and weight lifters either vitamin/mineral supplements or placebos (matching fake pills) for three months. Then he reversed the order for another three months, all the while measuring how much each athlete improved during a normal training program. Neither he nor the athletes knew who was getting what when. During each three-month supplement interval, these experienced athletes knocked 10 to 20 seconds off their mile runs, ran marathons an average of 17 minutes and 44 seconds faster, and lifted 30 to 55 percent more weight. When they took placebos, the athletes made little progress and sometimes lost ground. In addition, when they were on the supplements, their blood pressure, LDL cholesterol levels and heart rates decreased—all signs of improved fitness—and they suffered fewer injuries.

The amount of vitamins and minerals you need each day depends on your height and weight, your age and sex, the state of your health, whether you smoke or take birth-control pills or other drugs, what you eat, your genetic makeup, and how active you are.

With all these variables—and more—at work, there is no way anyone can establish a single daily allowance for everybody. No one person in the whole country fits the protocol for the "average American" used by the U.S. Food and Drug Administration as the basis of their Recommended Dietary Allowances (RDAs) for vitamins and minerals. "We all have different body chemistries," says Roger J. Williams, Ph.D., professor emeritus of chemistry at the University of Texas in Austin, "so it's hard to say what each person needs and how much. We need about forty different nutrients in our food each day. Most people don't eat a perfectly balanced ideal diet every day—I don't think even I do. If we don't get all forty of these things in the right balance, we need a vitamin supplement." (Williams discovered pantothenic acid, an essential B vitamin, and was involved in isolating and naming folic acid, another member of the B complex.)

As an active woman, you need more of most vitamins and minerals because training speeds up your metabolism to produce energy and you go through your supplies more quickly. You lose minerals and possibly some vitamins in your sweat during hot weather and heavy exercise. Both a high-carbohydrate diet and the stress of intensive exercise increase your need for B vitamins. Here is a rundown of vitamins and minerals of particular interest.

B complex vitamins

The B vitamins power the digestion and conversion of carbohydrates and fats into energy to be directly used by the muscle cells. The more energy a cell processes, the faster the B vitamins are used up. Therefore, the more active you are and the more carbohydrates (and fats, heaven forfend) you eat, the more B vitamins you will need. In addition, vitamin B_{12} and folic acid are necessary for making new red blood cells to carry oxygen to the muscles. Pregnant and nursing mothers and women on birth-control pills have an increased need for all B vitamins. Good natural sources are liver, brewer's yeast, peanuts, whole grains, wheat germ, and sunflower seeds.

Vitamin C

Vitamin C is "absolutely essential to the production of collagen, which is the most abundant connective tissue in the body," says Dr. Williams. (Collagen is the body's cement for holding cells together, particularly those of the bones and teeth.) Vitamin C also strikingly improves your body's ability to absorb iron, B complex vitamins, and vitamins A and E. It may be able to reduce the amount of cholesterol and other fats in your bloodstream. It stimulates your body's immune system so that you have greater resistance to infections and other diseases. It is involved in the production of adrenaline and other hormones in the glands lying around your kidneys. Adrenaline instructs the liver to release glycogen as glucose into the bloodstream to boost your energy level during exercise and helps remove lactic acid from your muscle cells. It also appears to help the body release fatty acids for muscle energy and to decrease muscle stiffness after exercise. Thus, vitamin C is indirectly involved in maintaining your stamina during a workout. In addition, it quickens your reaction time and provides resistance to heat and cold.

Each of us is different. Some people need only 250 milligrams of vitamin C a day for optimal health, others need 2,000 or 4,000 mg each day, and very sick people may need as much as 10,000 mg, or 10 grams, in order to recover. Dr. Williams says there is no way to estimate how much vitamin C you need, but he suggests that 2,000 mg (2 grams) a day is a good average figure. Experiment. If you take enough to prevent colds, he says, you are probably taking enough. On the other hand, if you develop diarrhea, you are taking too much. Although there is some health-food propaganda to the effect that the body can't use the so-called synthetic forms of vitamin C as thoroughly as the "natural" ones, Nobel laureate Linus Pauling says any ascorbic acid sold in this country is biologically active and works as well, dose for dose, as any other.

Unless you already have kidney trouble, you will not develop kidney stones, the only worrisome side effect of vitamin C, if you take less than 4,000 mg a day, but you probably will start urinating more frequently. That is perfectly harmless, although it can be inconvenient during competition. People who have sickle-cell anemia or glucose-6-phosphate dehydrogenase deficiency, a rare hereditary blood abnormality, should stick to doses under 1,000 mg per day. Diabetics who must monitor their blood-sugar levels with urine tests will get skewed results if they take high doses of C.

Good old-fashioned orange juice is one source of vitamin C, but there are much better ones, such as Brussels sprouts, broccoli, collard greens, and strawberries.

Vitamin E

Many athletes believe that vitamin E grabs onto extra oxygen, thereby increasing the oxygen-carrying capacity of hemoglobin. However, there is no proof that large doses of E will increase your strength or your endurance. The body's need for this vitamin is small. A healthy diet including cold-pressed oils, nuts, sunflower seeds, peanuts, whole wheat flour, and wheat germ probably will give you sufficient amounts. Very large doses of E can cause skin sores, lower thyroid output, and decrease the body's absorption of calcium and vitamin K.

Vitamin K

Vitamin K aids in converting glucose to glycogen and helps to form prothrombin, a blood-clotting chemical. About half the vitamin K you need is manufactured by friendly bacteria living in your own intestines. The other half comes from dark-green leafy vegetables such as mustard and collard greens, from members of the cabbage family, and a little from liver and egg yolks. Yogurt, kefir (cultured curdled milk), and acidophilus milk supply bacteria for your intestinal vitamin K factory. Vitamin K supplements have no effect on athletic performance.

Iron

The most important mineral of all to women between the beginning of menstruation (menarche) and menopause is iron. Dorothy Harris of Penn State estimates that 32 percent of all moderately active women are anemic, although it doesn't always show up on routine red-blood-cell counts. (Sometimes, the deficiency can be found only by taking painful bone-marrow assays.) For this reason, it's better to judge by your feelings of chronic fatigue, inexplicable staleness, pale complexion, drop in performance, or inability to progress rather than by a blood test.

As an active woman, you need an adequate supply of iron. Women have 600,000 fewer red blood cells per milliliter of blood than men do, and they store about 250 milligrams of iron while the average adult man stores about 850. The number of red blood cells you have is important because each cell contains hemoglobin, the oxygen trapper in your blood, and the more oxygen carriers you have, the higher your aerobic capacity. (Iron is also necessary to form myoglobin, the oxygen-carrying pigment in muscle fibers.) Less iron means less hemoglobin, which means fewer oxygen-carrying red blood cells, putting an active anemic woman at a distinct disadvantage.

Every woman loses about 30 milligrams of iron during a menstrual period. IUDs, pregnancy, childbirth, exercise, and sweating also cause marked iron losses. Your diet supplies only small amounts of iron. Meats, especially liver, and fish are moderate sources. Egg yolks, spinach, and kidney beans also supply iron, but packaged in a form that your body may not be able to use. The iron in iron-enriched foods is often equally unabsorbable. Ample supplies of vitamin C and minute amounts of copper in the diet help the iron travel through the intestinal membranes and into the bloodstream. What's more, a recent study by the U.S. Plant, Soil, and Nutrition Laboratory suggests that when you eat large amounts of raw fruit, the fructose (fruit sugar) makes iron more absorbable. Conversely, tea, milk products, and egg whites interfere with iron absorption.

No matter what your diet, your body absorbs only a tiny fraction of the iron you eat each day, usually much less than 10 percent. For this reason, Clayton Thomas, M.D., vice-president of medical affairs for Tampax, Inc., and a specialist in preventive medicine for athletes, says the Recommended Dietary Allowance of 18 milligrams is too low for women. You need two to four times as much daily iron as a man, he says. With the RDA, even if you do absorb the maximum—10 percent—you won't break even over a month of iron loss.

Therefore, an active woman needs an iron supplement in addition to her dietary sources of iron. If you are taking iron simply as a preventive, start out with 20 milligrams a day and increase the amount gradually. If you are already anemic or if you wear an IUD or if you have just had a baby, start with 30 mg and go as high as 100, divided into two or three doses a day. As long as you menstruate regularly, any excess you take will be eliminated in your menstrual fluid, but don't exceed 100 mg a day without consulting your doctor, and cut back your dosage to half or one quarter after menopause.

Natural forms of iron such as dessicated liver and yeast are expensive but not highly concentrated, so you can gradually increase your intake until you feel more energetic. Synthetic forms such as ferrous gluconate or the slightly less absorbable ferrous fumarate are less expensive but more potent, so you can't take small incremental doses as easily. Read the labels when you shop for supplements. Many drugstore formulas offer iron in the form of ferrous sulfate or other compounds your body can't absorb well. Time-release iron capsules are a waste of money too, for the mineral is absorbed only in the duodenum, the uppermost section of the intestine, and the part scheduled for release hours later passes untouched through the lower intestine and out.

About one quarter of all people who take moderate to heavy doses of iron develop diarrhea, constipation, or stomach cramps or feel faint. If this happens to you, take the iron with meals to minimize the side effects or switch brands or types of iron or cut back on the dosage.

Enormous megadoses of iron will do you no good and may damage your liver, kidneys, and heart. Don't take any iron without medical supervision if you have sickle-cell anemia, thalassemia, or hemochromatosis.

Calcium

Calcium is the most prevalent mineral in your body. Ninety-nine percent of all the body's calcium is found in your bones and teeth, with only one percent in your muscles and other soft tissues, but although this amount appears to be small, your muscles can't contract without it. Calcium keeps your bones strong, maintains cell membranes, and helps cement your cells together. It is vital for blood clotting. A calcium deficiency can cause your muscles to go into spasm. (So can an insufficiency of potassium or magnesium.) When soft tissues (including muscles) need calcium, they draw it out of your bones. For this reason, the amount of calcium in your bones isn't static. Adults lose and replace about 700 milligrams of calcium each day. A shortage of calcium or the inability to absorb it leads to thin, porous, fragile bones (called osteoporosis, a common condition in postmenopausal women).

MILK INTOLERANCE

If you suffer from cotton mouth, cactus throat, side stitches, or gas when you exercise, the solution may be as close to your refrigerator. Milk may be the culprit.

Many adults can't break down the double sugar called lactose in milk. The undigested sugar passes into the lower intestine, where bacteria ferment it until it produces gas and cramps. The solution for the 50 to 90 percent of adults who can't tolerate milk (some ethnic groups are more intolerant of lactose than others) is to give it up entirely and replace it with other natural sources of calcium, or avoid it within a few hours of strenuous exercise.

If you want to continue drinking milk, use cultured fermented milk products such as yogurt, sweet acidophilus milk, and buttermilk, in which the milk sugar is already broken down by bacteria, or eat cheese, in which the milk sugar has been removed. Or buy an enzyme powder called Lact-Acid in drugstores and health-food stores and let it break down the lactose for you into easily digestible glucose and galactose. Just mix the powder into milk and let it stand in the refrigerator for a day.

You can't use calcium unless you have enough vitamin D. Your diet supplies some D and your own body manufactures more whenever you head and skin are exposed to sunlight (D is actually a hormone rather than a true vitamin); women who have spent much of their lives outdoors have a lower incidence of osteoporosis. Your body absorbs calcium more efficiently in the presence of milk sugar (lactose), which is why dairy products are such a good source of calcium. It's hard to improve on the elegance of nature's designs.

On the other hand, your body has difficulty absorbing calcium if you eat large amounts of animal protein or fat. (If you eat 100 grams of protein, you need 1,000 milligrams of calcium.) In addition, your body reacts as if you have a calcium deficiency if you take proportionately too much magnesium, phosphorus, or other minerals. (Dr. Williams's formula in Table IV gives a rough proportion for each of these minerals.)

Cod- and halibut-liver oils, vitamin-D-fortified milk, and dark-fleshed fish are good sources of vitamin D. Dairy products, chicken bones (doesn't everyone gnaw on the soft, sweet ends of leg and wing bones?) soybean products (including tofu), dried beans, dark-green leafy vegetables (collard and mustard greens again, but not spinach, because its oxalic acid ties up calcium and makes it unabsorbable), soft fish bones found in canned salmon and sardines, and "hard" water are good sources of calcium. Bone meal, a popular health-food supplement made from sterilized and pulverized leg bones of cattle, is also loaded with calcium, but some batches have been found to be contaminated with dangerously high levels of lead.

Magnesium

Magnesium activates enzymes to convert carbohydrates into muscle and liver glycogen. It also helps release this stored energy when you exercise. It aids in the manufacture of proteins, keeps muscle fibers in working order, and helps conduct nerve impulses.

Magnesium is necessary for regulating body temperature, which is particularly important if you are exercising in hot or cold weather. An insufficiency of magnesium causes muscle cramping. Since large quantities of magnesium are lost in sweat during exercise, heat cramps may be caused, in part, by magnesium deficiency. Magnesium must be present in proper proportions for the body to absorb calcium, and also to use vitamin C. The best natural sources of magnesium are foods containing good supplies of calcium, vitamin C, and B vitamins: Brussels sprouts, wheat germ, brewer's yeast, peanuts, nuts, dark-green leafy vegetables, whole grains, and beans.

Potassium

Like calcium and magnesium, potassium is necessary for the smooth operation of the heart and skeletal muscles. It helps transmit nerve impulses and triggers the release of energy from carbohydrates and fats. It is the principal mineral inside the cells of soft body tissues and, along with sodium, controls the amount of water in those tissues. It offsets the effects of sodium in high blood pressure. You lose significant amounts of potassium in your sweat and during strenuous exercise, leaving you feeling weak and extremely tired, but a glass of orange juice, a banana, or even a cup of coffee will restore potassium levels quickly. You also lose potassium when you have diarrhea. Because the mineral is distributed so widely through plant and animal foods, a well-balanced diet should provide enough potassium unless you boost your calcium and magnesium intake with supplements. Good natural sources of potassium are bananas, dried fruits (particularly apricots), oranges, peanuts, dark-green leafy vegetables (again), potatoes, and chicken and liver. If possible, keep your intake of potassium equal to that of sodium.

Sodium

Table salt (sodium chloride) controls the amount of water between your cells, but American diets are so high in salt that it has become a killer mineral among the 30 percent of the population susceptible to high blood pressure. Although we need only 1 to 3 grams of sodium a day, most of us eat 4 to 5 grams (2 to 2½ teaspoons), and people with a salty tooth may consume 30 grams on some days. When sodium levels are high, extra fluids build up in the heart and blood vessels, increasing the volume of blood pushing on the sides of your arteries, increasing your blood pressure, and forcing your heart to work harder. Even if you don't have high blood pressure, eating a lot of salt, particularly around your menstrual period, makes you retain fluids and can make you feel waterlogged, logy, and clumsy.

Although it is true that you lose quantities of salt when you sweat, you don't need salt tablets to prevent heat injury. In fact, the better trained you are, the more your body learns to keep the sodium inside your body instead of releasing it in your perspiration.

Vitamin and Mineral Supplements

Since everyone has her own unique body chemistry, as Dr. Williams says, it is impossible at this stage of nutritional science to prescribe a vitamin and mineral supplement suitable for everyone. Dr. Williams's formula for twenty-nine essential vitamins and minerals (Table IV) lays the groundwork for your own experimentation. "It gives you a pretty good supply of most nutrients," he says, "even if you don't eat as well as you should."

Whenever you take any vitamin and mineral supplement—whether it is Dr. Williams's formula or separate nutrients—follow these rules:

- Take the fat-soluble vitamins (A, D, E, and K) during meals containing fat so that they will be absorbed by the gut.
- Take water-soluble vitamins (Bs, including the named vitamins, and C) with food, either during a meal or immediately afterward. If you are taking large amounts of vitamins C and B_{12} as separate pills, save the B_{12} for two hours later. Large quantities of vitamin C destroy B_{12}.
- If you take a single multivitamin pill, take it with the meal containing the largest amount of fat.
- If you take your vitamins in several individual pills, take the water-soluble ones in small doses throughout the day. Vitamins help you process your food. If you take a single large dose at one meal, your body may not be able to absorb the whole amount and will eliminate the excess in your urine.
- If you start to take vitamins, tell your doctor. Some vitamins and medications don't mix happily, and others make urine or blood tests appear abnormal unless the laboratory is informed.
- Even if you do take vitamins and minerals, try to eat a balanced diet. If your diet changes or if you know that you have eaten an abundance of some vitamin in its natural form, eliminate it from your pill popping that day.

TABLE IV: SUGGESTED DAILY AMOUNTS OF VITAMINS AND MINERALS[*]

Nutrient	Amount
Vitamin A	7,500 IU
Vitamin D	400 IU
Vitamin E	40 IU
Vitamin K (menadione)	2 mg
Vitamin C (ascorbic acid)	250 mg[1]
Vitamin B$_1$ (thiamin)	2 mg
Vitamin B$_2$ (riboflavin)	2 mg
Vitamin B$_6$ (pyridoxine)	3 mg
Vitamin B$_{12}$ (cobalamine)	9 mcg
Vitamin B$_3$ (niacin or niacinamide)	20 mg
Pantothenic acid	15 mg
Biotin	0.3 mg
Folic acid	0.4 mg[2]
Choline	250 mg
Inositol	250 mg
Para-amino benzoic acid (PABA)	30 mg
Rutin	200 mg
Calcium	250 mg
Phosphate	750 mg[3]
Magnesium	200 mg
Iron	15 mg[4]
Zinc	15 mg
Copper	2 mg
Iodine	0.15 mg
Manganese	5 mg
Molybdenum	0.1 mg
Chromium	1 mg
Selenium	0.02 mg
Cobalt	0.1 mg

[*] From Roger J. Williams, *The Wonderful World Within You.* (New York: Bantam Books, Inc., 1977). Reprinted by permission.

A few manufacturers produce multivitamins approximating this formula, but none follow it exactly. The two closest are Vitamin and Mineral Formula by Bronson Pharmaceuticals and Strong Cobb and Arner, ICN Pharmaceuticals (see Appendix B).

[1] Dr. Williams says that many people need more vitamin C than this; two grams (2,000 mg) a day is a good average figure.

[2] Dr. Williams says it is probably better to take much more folic acid, 5 mg a day, but the FDA restricts the sale of amounts that large. In Canada, folic acid is available over the counter at much higher levels than in the United States. (It is safe for most of us, but it is dangerous for people with pernicious anemia to take folic acid because it masks the symptoms of that disease. People with pernicious anemia need vitamin B$_{12}$ instead.)

[3] Equivalent to 250 mg phosphorus.

[4] See text discussion of iron requirements for women.

Some of the fat-soluble vitamins, such as A, D, and K (but not E), are toxic in large amounts over long periods of time because they are not excreted in the urine the way water-soluble vitamins are. Instead, they build up in the liver to dangerous levels.

Dosages above 25,000 to 50,000 IU per day of vitamin A over weeks or months can cause nausea, diarrhea, dry flaky skin, hair loss, headaches, bone thinning, enlargement of the liver and spleen, and blurred vision.

Dosages above 50,000 to 100,000 IU per day of vitamin D over weeks or months can cause nausea, diarrhea, dizziness, loss of calcium and phosphorus from the bones, and calcification of the soft tissues and the walls of the blood vessels and kidney tubules. Your body can't make use of vitamin D without adequate amounts of calcium. If you step up your vitamin D intake, you must also increase your calcium.

If you have high blood pressure, diabetes or rheumatic heart conditions, don't take more than 100 IU of vitamin E per day.

Unspecified megadoses of synthetic vitamin K at one time can cause flushing, sweating, chest constrictions, and a kind of anemia.

Vegetarian Diets

Many women who become seriously involved in endurance athletics wake up one day to discover that they don't like the taste of red meat as much as they did when they were sedentary.

You certainly don't need meat in order to have enough stamina and recuperative ability for exercise and athletics. Several national studies performed on athletes and sedentary people show that balanced vegetarian diets provide more than enough protein, B vitamins, iron, and other nutrients as long as dairy products are included. In a Swedish test, people increased their endurance capacities by an hour or more when they switched from a diet heavily loaded with meat to a totally vegetarian one.

Whether they are strict vegans, who eschew all animal products and eat only vegetables, fruits, nuts, grains, seeds and legumes; ovo-lacto-vegetarians, who add eggs and milk to their diet; fruitarians, who eat only fruits; or halfway vegetarians, who prefer the ovo-lacto-vegetarian regimen but occasionally eat chicken or fish, vegetarians say they feel lighter and less sluggish and have more energy, stamina, and drive. Their food digests quickly and easily, so that they can eat nearer to game time. They feel safer not eating the chemicals and antibiotics fed as growth stimulators to beef cattle, pigs, and other animals. They cut the amount of saturated or animal fat they eat, reducing the amount of cholesterol in their bloodstreams and thus reducing their chances of developing atherosclerosis. *Women's Sports* magazine reported that a study of runners conducted by the Institute of Health Research in San Francisco showed that running vegetarians consistently had the lowest cholesterol and triglyceride levels, nonrunning vegetarians had the next lowest, running meat eaters the third lowest, and nonrunning meat eaters the highest.

Because seeds, grains, and nuts are high in protein and fat, vegetarians have no problem getting enough of these vital nutrients. However, vegetable protein may not be fully balanced. Each protein is made up of several amino acids in proper propotions. One type of food—such as corn—may be deficient in one amino acid, while another—such as beans—may be strong in it but weak in something else. Combined together (as the Mexicans do when they stuff corn tortillas with beans), they make a balanced protein source as good or better than animal ones. (For the principles of protein balancing and appetizing recipes, read Frances Moore Lappé's *Diet for a Small Planet*.)

A high-carbohydrate diet requires extra thiamin, niacin, and riboflavin to help break down and use the starches and sugars. Vitamin B_{12}, necessary for making new hemoglobin in your blood cells, is found in only a few vegetable products; more frequently, it is produced by microorganisms in animals. Therefore, if you are a vegetarian, eat brewer's yeast, peanuts, whole grains, wheat germ, and sunflower seeds for most of the B-complex vitamins, and milk, eggs, seaweeds, or fermented foods such as tamari, miso, and yogurt for your B_{12}. Microorganisms in your own intestines also produce some B_{12}, but you may want to take a B_{12} vitamin supplement to make sure you have enough hemoglobin and, therefore, oxygen-carrying ability, in your blood cells. In addition, if you eat only small quantities of beans and cheese, you may develop a zinc deficiency. Zinc, found abundantly in red meat, liver, and oysters, helps you absorb vitamins, especially B-complex. It also is an ingredient of at least twenty-five digestive and metabolic enzymes and plays a particularly important role in carbohydrate digestion and phosphorus metabolism. It is essential for the proper development of sexual organs, promotes the healing of burns and wounds, and is active in the formation and activity of almost every cell in your body. Diets high in protein and B-complex-rich foods supply ample zinc. Otherwise, 15 milligrams per day is a good protective dose, although you may need 20 if you are a vegan or fruitarian.

EATING FOR COMPETING

In order to plan a feeding program for important contests, you must understand how your body stockpiles and burns its fuel—both the fats stored as fatty acids in your muscles and in layers beneath the skin and the carbohydrates stored as glycogen in your muscles and liver.

When your body needs energy, it converts these stored fuels into glucose (also called muscle sugar) and sends it to your muscle cells. There, oxygen helps break it down into adenosine triphosphate. Within a few seconds, this ATP mixes with water, then also breaks down, releasing heat. Part of this heat contracts your muscles. The rest makes you hot. (This explains how shivering—uncontrollable muscular contractions—warms you.)

In order to convert fats into glucose for fuel, your body needs both carbohydrates and oxygen. Therefore, the amount of carbohydrate (in the form of glycogen) you have stored in your liver and muscles determines how long you can go on. When you run out of liver glycogen, you run out of your brain's primary fuel—you become dizzy, weak, shaky, confused, and break out into a cold sweat—but you can recover from this "bonk" (or "knock," as the British call it) by immediately eating carbohydrates. If you run out of muscle glycogen and "hit the wall," that's it, because it takes at least ten hours to replenish your muscle stores. (One controversial theory says that drinking a dilute sugar solution during—not before—a race may replace this muscle glycogen, but no one knows for sure. It *is* known, however, that this process can cause dehydration, a real danger in hot weather.)

The metabolism of exercising muscles isn't an either/or proposition. Even during your most efficient aerobic stage, there is some anaerobic metabolism occurring and some lactic acid being produced. As your muscles continue to contract, they massage the lactic acid into your bloodstream and away from the muscles you are using most heavily. As long as you take in enough oxygen, your liver recycles the lactate into more fuel. If you exercise beyond your capacity, your liver can't keep up; lactic acid fills your muscles and you become exhausted and can't go on.

Precompetition meals

What you ate about twelve hours earlier determines how much glycogen you have stored for your workout. (Anything you eat within four hours of activity barely has enough time to circulate through your system, much less become stored energy.)

Races and other contests require careful planning. Because many are scheduled for early in the day, dinner the night before is usually your last chance to stockpile fuel. Go heavy on the potatoes, whole-grain breads, pastas, rice, and other carbohydrates—as long as you don't pig out and gain weight. Eat very little fat (it slows down your digestion) and avoid spices, if they give you dyspepsia, and gassy foods such as beans, cabbage, broccoli, and Brussels sprouts. Make this last dinner low on fiber by avoiding salads and raw fruits, because fiber eaten within twenty-four hours of any hard exertion can cause diarrhea. (If you still get diarrhea, cut out whole-grain breads, milk, and/or coffee.) Cut down on your salt intake by eliminating sausages and other salted foods. Salt your food normally as you cook it, so that you will have enough to prevent heat exhaustion, but don't add extra amounts at the table. Salt causes your cells to retain enough extra water to make you waterlogged, clumsy, and slow.

As a general rule, don't eat less than two hours before any exercise. For important events, have your last meal (breakfast or lunch) at least four hours before you compete. If you exercise strenuously before your food is completely digested, you may become nauseated, develop stitches in your side from intestinal gas, or come down with a hefty case of the runs.

Many people are too nervous to eat anything at all within five or six hours of a big race. You will have to find out by trial and error which foods make you lean and mean and which foods send you running to the toilet. If you eat, keep the meal light. Simple and refined carbohydrates such as white flour and fruit juices digest more quickly and have less fiber than complex carbohydrates such as whole-grain cereals. Avoid fats and proteins because they delay the emptying of your stomach. (Protein also produces extra urine.) The idea is to get the food out of your stomach and into your bloodstream as soon as possible. You want to exercise on a virtually empty stomach. A pregame meal will provide no energy for sprinters, because their whole contest is over by the time the carbohydrates are available for fuel, but endurance athletes may be able to use some newly deposited glycogen late in the day.

If you want to eat before competition but have trouble holding down solid food, try the liquid diets designed specifically as pregame meals. They provide an adequate amount of nutrients to the muscles and leave the stomach quicker than a solid meal does, so you can eat them closer to game time. (One study, performed at the University of Southern California, suggests that you can drink a liquid meal only thirty minutes before maximal exertion without any ill effects.) Liquid meals offer particular advantages to sprint athletes, who often exercise empty in order to feel as light as possible. They are also useful as snacks during rest periods between games in a tournament—a track meet, tennis, or wrestling match, for example. Do not use liquid meals over a long time, because even the ones made of so-called natural ingredients are an artificial compilation of nutrients, totally devoid of fiber. Check the labels to find one approximating the proportion of carbohydrates, protein, and fat you want and then test it ahead of time to make sure your body can handle it.

The one liquid meal you should avoid is the three-martini lunch. Just one beer lowers your heat tolerance and makes you tire sooner. Even moderate quantities of alcohol decrease the amount of blood your heart can pump with each stroke, while increasing the amount of oxygen your heart muscles need. Alcohol also prevents the breakdown of fat for fuel. Net result: Your heart and other muscles get less oxygen and less fuel.

Whether or not you eat before competition, be sure to drink one to three cups of water—more if you can stand it—before and after an event. For endurance athletics or long-lasting matches, drink during the event too. Although this extra water makes you urinate more frequently, it is your last line of defense against heatstroke. If you can stomach it, fruit juice will replenish some of the potassium you are losing in your sweat.

If you do anaerobic (nonendurance) sports, these are the only dietary preparations you need make before that life-or-death game. However, if you are a cyclist, marathon runner, channel swimmer, or cross-country ski racer, there are three ways you can train your body to start burning fat sooner, spare your glycogen stores, and at the same time increase the amount of glycogen your muscles can hold: depletion sessions, carbohydrate loading, and simple stockpiling.

Depletion Sessions

Once a week, deplete your muscles of all their glycogen by exercising to exhaustion and then a little beyond. Make yourself hit the wall. Your muscles will ache and feel heavy and lose their coordination. (You'll probably need someone to pick you up and take you home.) When your muscles refill—which will take anywhere from twelve hours to a week—they will fill up with more glycogen than before. At the same time, repeatedly hitting the wall will train your body to switch to fat earlier in the run.

Carbohydrate Loading

Another way is to trick your muscles into temporarily accepting more glycogen by using the controversial and dangerous carbohydrate-loading diet six days before the race. Carbohydrate loading has two phases. In the first phase, you deplete the glycogen your muscles have already stored by exercising to exhaustion, the way you would for depletion sessions. For days six, five, and four before the race, you starve your muscles of carbohydrate by eating a high-protein low-carb diet and exercising to exhaustion. Then, on days three, two, and one, you eat extremely high-carbohydrate low-protein foods and exercise only a little bit. When you finally start feeding your muscle cells carbohydrates again, they react like a starving kitten and consume much more fuel than they would normally hold, as the muscle fibers swell with glycogen and become very stiff. On the day of the race, you're loaded with glycogen and can presumably last longer.

Carbohydrate loading has become popular among athletes, but in fact it is quite dangerous and may not give you any more muscle glycogen than ordinary stockpiling. During the depletion phase, you may become nauseated, headachy, weak, bad-tempered, and unable to sleep. The depletion phase may also cause ketones to build up in your bloodstream—intermediate products of fat combustion that can clog up and permanently damage your kidneys. Depletion, therefore, is particularly dangerous for diabetics, people with kidney or liver trouble, and, just as a general precaution, anyone over forty years old. The loading phase may release myoglobin, the muscle pigment, which also clogs the kidneys. It also swells each muscle fiber, including heart muscle fiber. If you don't burn off the glycogen or if you overstuff the fibers, they may rupture. People with heart problems are at particular risk. Besides, those stiff, overstuffed muscles are uncomfortable and may slow you down at the beginning of a race. Because of all of these dangers, even the people who swear by carbo loading only do it once a year.

Ironically, too, the whole process can backfire. Carbohydrate loading makes your muscles prefer glycogen to fat. Since you must rely on fats to exercise efficiently throughout the rest of the year, this once-a-year fiddling with your metabolism could foul up your training for months afterward.

Stockpiling

If you want to play it safe but still increase the amount of glycogen that your muscles store, simply eat a higher proportion of carbohydrates beginning four days before your event. Instead of storing up about 4 grams of muscle glycogen per 100 grams of body weight, as you might with carbohydrate loading, says Nathan Smith, M.D., author of *Food for Sport*, you'll stockpile about 3.5 grams per 100 grams of body weight—not a significant difference for most people. Just make sure you don't pig out and put on a few pounds that could slow you down considerably on the big day. Drink extra water to accompany the extra carbohydrates, because your muscles draw extra water out of your blood in order to store the extra glycogen; if you don't replace this water, your blood becomes too concentrated for your kidneys to process normally.

Eating During Competition

Sprinters, weight lifters, and wrestlers neither eat nor drink during a match or race; they are too busy. It doesn't matter. The duration of their event is too short for water or food to get into their systems in time. This is true for athletes in middle-range events too. However, for endurance athletes, including swimmers, water during the race is essential, and many people find they get an energy boost from drinking a half cup of fruit juice diluted in one cup of water over the course of an hour, each and every hour.

The old practice of eating sugar or drinking sugar or honey dissolved in water before exercise has been abandoned. The sugar didn't improve the amount of energy you had; it actually decreased your endurance by about 19 percent, by spiking your blood sugar so high it triggered the release of extra insulin to process it. In getting rid of the new sugar, the extra insulin also got rid of some of the precious blood sugar you had before you drank the sugar water, so you wound up in worse shape than before, and less able to mobilize fat for fuel.

Sugar before or during a race has another disadvantage: It ties up some of the water you need for sweating and cooling during heat waves. Thus, for most people, it's best to stick to water and save the carbohydrate replenishing for afterward. However, some people do get a late pick-up from diluted fruit juices during a race, after the fructose has been converted into glucose in the liver. Others swear by defizzed cola soft drinks, tea and honey, or commercial glucose replacement drinks. If it's a cool day or if you handle heat well, experiment. Otherwise, you are probably safer to stick with plain cold water, about one cup every fifteen minutes.

For ultra-long-distance events, or for noncompetitive exercise such as bicycle touring or cross-country skiing lasting more than two or three hours, you must eat as well as drink to keep going. If you are working at top effort, bananas (rich in fructose and potassium), white bread, cookies, and other easily digested carbohydrates are probably all that your body will tolerate. For submaximal prolonged effort, eat anything that appeals to you, although you will probably find that sandwiches, fruits, juices, trail mix or gorp (nuts, raisins, and M&M candies), and other easily digested carbohydrates will revive you with a minimum of gastric distress. Save your day's protein intake for dinner, after the workout is over. Don't forget juices, water, or—in cold weather—bouillon or tea to replenish your bodily fluids.

The Post-Competition Meal

This is probably the most ignored meal of the nutritional game plan. Immediately after exercising, drink all the liquid you can stand. Fruit juice is particularly revitalizing. A loss of more than a pound or two of weight indicates both water and salt depletion, as do any signs of heat weakness (see chapter 10). In these cases, drink bouillon or broth instead of plain water. Otherwise, the usual amount of salt in your food will replace what you lost. If you are keyed up, exhilarated, or disappointed, you may not feel like eating right after the event. That's fine. Wait an hour or so until your appetite returns, but be sure to replace the fuel you burned within a few hours by eating a meal containing carbohydrates, as well as at least half a day's protein allotment.

ERGOGENICS

Athletes are always looking for an edge—vitamins, secret foods, even the horrendous practice of injecting air into the intestines of swimmers for additional buoyancy. Anything that gives you extra energy is called an ergogenic. Ergogenics come and go; the turnover is swift because very few work. And yet the urge to try the latest one is irresistible if you think it may shave seconds off your time or add pounds to your dead lifts or miles to your pedaling.

Caffeine

For endurance athletes, plain old caffeine from coffee may increase your ability to do work by about 16 percent, says David Costill, Ph.D., director of the Human Performance Laboratory at Ball State University in Muncie, Indiana. "Caffeine stimulates the process of mobilizing fat for fuel," he says, "and also reduces the amount of carbohydrate you burn."

For dosage, figure about 2 milligrams of caffeine per pound of body weight. A cup of drip coffee has 150 milligrams of caffeine, a cup of percolated coffee has 100 mg, a cup of instant coffee has 85 to 100 mg, one No-Doz tablet has 100 mg, eight ounces of cola soft drink has 40 to 60 mg, one Excedrin tablet has 66 mg, one Anacin or Midol tablet has 32 mg, and a cup of tea has 60 to 75 mg of theophylline, a very close cousin of caffeine with almost identical effects. (In contrast, a cup of decaffeinated coffee has 2 to 4 mg of caffeine.) Take your caffeine about an hour before you start exercising.

Caffeine has the advantage of being a known commodity. Tests have proved that it works as an ergogenic, and people have been drinking caffeine beverages for centuries. However, the FDA has stated that caffeine is a powerful drug and is reviewing its safety. It passes the brain-blood barrier as quickly as alcohol—that's why it gives such an immediate buzz. Regular consumption reduces the amount of iron your body can absorb, raises the resting heart rate, and irritates the heart muscle. It probably aggravates high blood pressure and may cause heart attacks (especially if you smoke), birth defects, miscarriages, and cancer of the bladder, pancreas, or breast. It increases the stomach's output of acid (harmful to people with ulcers), and mimics the action of uric acid by causing joint pain in gout sufferers. It makes some people anxious or depressed when they drink it or when they stop drinking it. Caffeine and its relatives in tea and chocolate can cause breast pain and cysts.

Ironically, using caffeine as an ergogenic will encourage you to stop drinking coffee or tea on a regular basis. Habitual caffeine users build up a tolerance to the chemical. The only way to get a real boost from those couple of cups of coffee before a race is to abstain from it during the rest of the week.

If you do take a dose of coffee or tea before a race, remember it is a diuretic (a promoter of urine flow). There is nothing more annoying than having to stop several times during a race to run behind a bush. (Male bicycle riders are said to pee *while* they pedal, an anatomical advantage they have over women.) This diuretic effect may dehydrate you on a hot day. Caffeine also upsets the stomach and can give you the runs or make you too jittery to perform at your best.

Vitamin B₁₅ (Pangamic Acid, or DMG)

One of the hottest ergogenics of the early eighties, this compound is said to increase an elite athlete's maximal oxygen uptake by over 25 percent and increase the time to exhaustion by more than 20 percent, according to Thomas V. Piper, Ph.D., of the Institute for Human Fitness in Escondido, California. It supposedly works for all sports—anaerobic, combined, and aerobic—a lure the coaches of several nationally ranked college track and field teams and professional baseball and football teams have been unable to resist.

Neither a vitamin nor pangamic acid, this compound (N, N-dimethyl glycine, or DMG) has been used by Soviet athletes for the last few years. The few tests performed in the United States have been done on men. In a small group of volunteer physical-education students at the University of Southern California School of Medicine in Los Angeles, DMG lowered lactic acid levels and made it easier for the body to recycle chemical products of energy metabolism into new fuel, according to Jerzy W. Meduski, M.D., chief of the Nutritional Research Laboratory there.

No one knows yet what the proper dosage of DMG is. It does appear, however, that your body comes to need bigger and bigger doses of the chemical in order to get results. For this reason, athletes who take DMG build up the dosage gradually by taking one tablet more every week or every other week until they are up to four; then they reverse the process and gradually decrease the dosage down to nothing; abstain for a few weeks; and then start the cycle all over again.

No safety studies have been done on DMG in the United States, and no one knows the effects of prolonged continuous use. For this reason, it is illegal to sell DMG as a drug, food additive, or vitamin. However, manufacturers are selling substances labeled Vitamin B₁₅ or pangamic acid as a food, because the FDA doesn't regulate foods. Without legal controls or definition, bottlers can and do sell just about anything they want as "B₁₅." (The exercise physiology tests were done only on laboratory-quality DMG.)

Dr. Victor Herbert, chief of the Hematology and Nutrition Laboratory at New York Downstate Medical Center in Brooklyn, says tests in his laboratory showed that DMG mixed with saliva has a 90 percent chance of causing cancer. DMG supporters dispute this, because DMG is a normal mid-product in the digestion of choline, a B vitamin found in many foods.

Negative Air Ions

The Israelis, who have done extensive, although not universally accepted, work on electrically charged oxygen particles in air, recently claimed that breathing negative ions will improve an athlete's cardiovascular response by 8 percent. These tiny particles are carried in the wind on a crisp clear day, or cling to the mist near a waterfall or a bathroom shower, or emanate from special negative-air-ion machines. The Israelis haven't actually tested their theory on athletes, but health food stores are doing a brisk business in little black ion boxes, some of which produce dangerous amounts of ozone as well.

The most eminent negative-air-ion researcher in the United States, Albert P. Krueger, Ph.D., professor emeritus of bacteriology at the University of California in Berkeley, has shown that plants placed in an atmosphere laden with negative ions grow more quickly than other plants, and that mice resist infections much better. However, he cautions that no reliable research has been done on humans. Another University of California scientist, anatomy professor Marian Diamond, Ph.D., wonders whether exposure to large quantities of negative air ions might not accelerate the aging process. It is possible that running or cycling in the clean air of a brisk autumn day might give you more energy than laboring along in the smog, but it's a quantum leap in logic from that to living with a black box humming away all day in your office or home.

Blood doping or boosting

In one of the more ghoulish ergogenic procedures, doctors remove one or two units (a pint or a quart) of blood from your veins, usually over a period of several days, about two months before an extremely important distance competition. This blood is frozen and stored either as whole blood or just as red blood cells. You continue to train, and your body replenishes your blood supply until it is back to normal levels in time for the big race. Then, your own stored blood is transfused back into your veins, drastically raising the number of oxygen-carrying red blood cells you have. Your maximal oxygen uptake increases by 5 percent, your endurance is markedly improved, your lactic acid accumulation is halved, and your heart rate is lowered. The effect lasts six or seven days. This procedure does nothing for anaerobic, short-term, stop-start athletics.

At first glance, blood doping looks like the solution to the woman athlete's low red-blood-cell count. If you have more red blood cells for an important race, you have more oxygen available and thus more stamina. However, during the two months your body is replacing that quart of blood, you are training, and perhaps even racing, with fewer red blood cells than ever before. The chances are you are already borderline anemic. Why would you want to heighten that effect?

Leave the vampire antics to the exercise physiologists, who use blood doping as a valuable research tool for learning how the body works under stress. Instead, boost your blood for the most important race of your career by training at altitudes above 5,000 feet. The body responds to any lack of oxygen, including the thin air at high elevations, by producing more red blood cells. Train for two to four weeks at high altitude, and you will grow new red blood cells to carry more oxygen. Return to sea level and race within forty-eight hours of your descent, and you will enjoy most of the benefits of blood boosting. If you stay in the mountains more than four weeks, or if you race after a couple of days back at sea level, your body readjusts and you lose your advantage.

Altitude Simulators

If you can't get away, try an altitude simulator. These expensive gadgets imitate at sea level the effects of altitude training and look like the self-contained breathing apparatuses firemen sometimes wear when battling chemical fires—a face mask covering both mouth and nose, connected by hoses to milk-bottle-sized canisters strapped to the back. Carbon dioxide stored in the canisters dilutes the oxygen you inhale from the outside air from the usual 21 percent to 16. This mimics the oxygen level of 7,500 feet above sea level, thought to be the best endurance-training altitude. (Sea level is best for building strength.)

Although they cost between $200 and $300, altitude simulators are certainly cheaper than the cost of a four-week mountain vacation, and they permit you to break your workout into high- and low-altitude sessions so that you don't become acclimated to altitude and lose your advantage. Furthermore, your muscles keep their sea-level strength. (In real altitude training, your muscles don't contract as forcefully, so you lose strength you need when you return to sea level.)

On the other hand, these devices take the fun out of each workout because it is hard to breathe and exercise with a four-pound pack strapped against your back. And you look mighty odd running around as if there's been an acid spill in the neighborhood. Not everyone is ready for that kind of attention.

Drugs

You have to be pretty desperate to resort to drugs. Not only do they have some dire side effects—"Speed Kills"—but there is good evidence that they don't increase your endurance or speed or strength in the first place. The scientifically based research on the subject is woefully inadequate, which is odd, since drugs in athletics are a favorite topic of athletes, trainers, and television sportscasters. Amphetamines ("speed" or "uppers"), including the ephedrine and pseudoephedrine available in cold medicines, don't actually give you more energy; they just make you *feel* as if you have more energy. They give you the will to go on, to be more aggressive. But they also slow down your reaction time and raise your pain threshold, so that you are more likely to hurt yourself. They also increase your pulse, something an athlete doesn't need. No matter what some ex-jock down the block tells you, good training, adequate rest, and self-confidence will do everything the stimulants do without the nasty side effects.

Many weight lifters and shot-putters of both sexes use anabolic steroids to build more muscle faster; former world champion German swimmer Renate Vogel has charged that her broad shoulders and heavily muscled body were the result of steroids fed to her from the age of ten by her East German coaches.

Anabolic steroids are tissue-building male hormones, and most studies agree that they do increase the amount of muscle you can grow (a few theorize that the steroids make you more aggressive, so that you work harder and that's what builds the muscle). All scientists agree, however, that these hormones turn you into a half man. They deepen your voice; make you grow a beard and chest hair and cause baldness, menstrual irregularities, and clitoral enlargement; damage your reproductive abilities; and cause temporary or permanent liver damage and maybe even liver cancer.

Who needs that? It's best to avoid all drugs. They rarely give you speed or strength, but they do damage you for life.

4 / **Weight Control**

Are you looking for a foolproof way to lose weight—one that doesn't require incredible willpower or starvation diets, boring menus, or tedious calorie counting? One that is fun, invigorating, and builds self-confidence? One that keeps your weight where you want it *for life?* There is one plan, and one plan only, that does all this and more. It's called the Exercise Plus or Minus Diet Plan. With it, you lose weight, change your metabolism, and diminish your appetite. You customize it to your own body chemistry, your own personality, and your own needs, so that it is tailor-made for you and you alone. It is very easy to follow, and you feel stronger, more vibrant, and more supple while you are on it—none of the weakness, depression, and frustration you get from fad diets.

Why a "Plus or Minus" diet? Because you choose whether or not you want to diet at all. Exercise is so much more effective than diet alone as a weight-losing tool that you don't have to diet if you don't want to. As long as you exercise properly—and that means aerobically—you will continue to lose fat as long as you have fat to lose. However, this loss is gradual—about a pound a week. If you are carrying around a lot of extra fat, you may get impatient with that pace and decide to combine diet with your exercise for faster weight loss.

As a general rule, you don't need to diet if you are less than 10 percent overfat. For example, if you weigh 110 pounds and only want to lose 10 pounds, or if you weigh 135 and only want to lose 15, exercise alone should do the job. If you are more than 10 percent overfat, you can either speed up the process with the Plus diet or eliminate the diet, lose the weight more slowly, and luxuriate in the fact that you are eating normally.

Sound too good to be true? Far from it. Obesity, says Michael Pollock of Mount Sinai Medical Center in Milwaukee, citing a study at

FAT AND SPORTS

Extra fat poses particular problems for women in sports. In addition to aggravating rheumatoid arthritis of the knees, encouraging high blood pressure, making you more resistant to your own insulin (encouraging diabetes if you have that tendency), and setting you up for kidney trouble, cirrhosis of the liver, and gall-bladder disease, fat makes you much less efficient at using oxygen, so it slows you down and decreases your endurance. Fat also slows you down because you are carrying around dead weight—as if you were exercising while carrying a 15- or 30-pound suitcase. According to Kenneth J. Cureton and colleagues at the University of Georgia's Human Performance Laboratory, 5 percent extra fat can make you 3.9 percent slower, 10 percent extra fat can make you 5.8 percent slower, and 15 percent extra fat can make you 8.6 percent slower. Fat rubs between the muscle fibers, acting as a friction brake on the smooth motion of your muscles and thus the speed and power of your movements. Finally, a thick layer of fat insulates you. In cold weather that's fine, but in hot weather you can't cool yourself, and you risk heat exhaustion or heatstroke.

the University of California at Irvine, is due more to inactivity than overeating. In the early seventies, Grant Gwinup, M.D., showed that overweight women who made no change in their eating habits but who walked briskly at least thirty minutes every day lost an average of twenty-two pounds per year, or half a pound per week, and the women who lost the most weight were the ones who walked the longest each day.

When you do aerobic exercise, at least five things happen:

1. *The exercise itself uses up calories.*   The "average" woman uses 215 calories if she walks briskly for an hour. If this were the only physiological result from exercise—and it's not—she would burn almost 3,500 calories in sixteen days, without reducing the amount of food she eats. There are 3,500 calories in a pound of body fat, so every sixteen days, she would lose one pound of body fat. In a year, she would lose twenty-three pounds without dieting.

2. *The exercise speeds up the metabolism of your muscle cells.* That's why you burn more fat and calories when you move than when you sit still. But this elevated metabolic rate doesn't crash back to normal the moment you stop exercising. It slows down very gradually. Your muscles continue to use calories at a faster rate for as long as six hours after you stop exercising. Therefore, you burn more calories watching television or typing *after* exercising than you do before.

3. *The exercise burns fat for fuel.*   In contrast, dieting triggers a

starvation reflex, and your body burns muscle for fuel instead of fat. (It is saving your fat for your heart—that organ won't use anything else.) As long as you diet, you continue to lose weight, but most of that weight loss is muscle mass. Only a little fat is lost. As soon as you go off your diet, your body must replace the essential tissue it lost, and you put on 5 or 10 pounds in the first few weeks. There is no way to prevent this rebound. When you exercise, with or without dieting, your body shifts into its fat-burning phase and draws fat from every depot it can find—ugly saddlebag, thick waist, double chin, enormous buttocks. That fat stays off because the body doesn't need it. You'll put it back on only if you *stop* exercising or overeat.

4. The exercise builds muscle. Muscle burns calories. (Fat doesn't burn calories; it just sits there.) Therefore, the more muscle you have, the more calories you burn each day. You raise your Basal Energy Requirement, the number of calories you need each day just to stay alive. A higher BER means that you can either eat the same amount of food and lose weight or eat more food and still maintain the same weight.

5. The exercise brings your appetite into scale with your energy consumption. Most people become less hungry when they exercise regularly. The few whose appetite stays the same or increases are hungry because they need more food, not because they have the urge to overeat.

When you are sedentary, your appetite regulator, the hypothalamus, doesn't get the chemical cues it needs; it gets stuck in the "on" position and tells you that you are hungry when you're not. When you become active, this mechanism resets itself. You no longer crave a doughnut two hours after you ate breakfast.

Exercise also controls your appetite by releasing fat into your bloodstream. This fat keeps your blood-sugar level high. When your blood-sugar level is high, you feel full. When your blood-sugar level falls, you get hungry again. The new muscle fibers you grow help you use more oxygen and, therefore, burn more fat. This further maintains your blood-sugar level.

IDEAL PERCENTAGE OF FAT AND IDEAL WEIGHT

In chapter 1, you estimated your percentage of body fat by measuring skin folds. When you know how much of you is fat, you can calculate how much your bones, muscles, and other lean mass weigh and what your total weight should be. Every woman is different. The amount of fat one athlete totes around to play at her peak may be too much or too little for another. "I feel that the body weight which *feels* healthiest to a female is probably her healthiest weight," says Victor Katch, Ph.D., professor of physical education at the University of Michigan.

CALF SIZE

Complaining that their boots won't zip up, many women try hard to reduce the size of their calves, but neither exercise nor diet slims down these muscles.

The size of your calves is determined by heredity and is related to the number of fast-twitch and slow-twitch fibers you have. Fast-twitch fibers are thicker than slow-twitch and therefore bulge more. If you have a high proportion of fast-twitchers in your calf muscles, your legs will be large. Furthermore, since you use your calf muscles all the time, they are among the best developed muscles in your whole body, and strong muscles have thick fibers.

The only way to reduce the size of your calves is to lie in bed all day and let your muscles atrophy. Isn't it better to take pride in your well-developed musculature and hope that fashion and the boot manufacturers catch up with you?

The amount of fat *you* need depends partially on your sport. If you are a swimmer, you can permit yourself to be a little fatter than most other athletes because that extra fat buoys you up and insulates you. A downhill skier can also use a little extra fat for insulation against the cold and for the added momentum it gives her. A cross-country skier, on the other hand, doesn't need the insulation because she generates heat of her own, and might prefer to be as lean as a runner or other dry-land endurance athlete. A gymnast or ballet dancer aims for low body fat not only because she is graded on her lean look but also because any extra fat shifts her center of gravity and makes it more difficult to perform vaults, lifts, leaps, and other required movements.

It's very hard for an adult woman to drop below 17 percent body fat. Estrogen and other female hormones encourage the conversion of food into fat to insulate and fuel you and to support and protect a fetus during a pregnancy. The fat in your breasts, buttocks, inner thighs, and genitalia makes up 10 to 12 very hard-to-lose percentage points. Your brain and spinal cord hold another 3 percent. Albert R. Behnke, M.D., a pioneer in body fat research, warns that a woman who drops below 13 percent may endanger her health. (The average male is 14 to 19 percent body fat, and male athletes get down to 6 to 8.)

Somewhere between 20 and 23 percent of body fat works for most women, but you must determine what gives *you* the best appearance, the most energy, and the best athletic peformance. Remember that

---

THERE'S NO SUCH THING AS SPOT REDUCING

If you want to get rid of flabby thighs, fat buttocks, or a beer belly, exercise . . . any part of your body. That's right. There's no such thing as spot reducing. Specific exercises for specific parts of the body do not selectively burn away fat in just those areas. When you exercise any part of your body, your body draws fat from storage depots in an inherited order that has nothing to do with which muscles you move.

Frank I. Katch, Ed.D., of the University of Massachusetts at Amherst (and Victor Katch's older brother), took fat biopsies from the abdomen, buttocks, and shoulder areas of twenty-one people (including himself) before and after twenty-seven days of progressive sit-ups. At the end of the experiment, they had all lost a small amount of fat from their midriffs—*and* from their butts and backs. In other words, the abdominal exercise drew fat from all over.

---

some women are built chunky. Not everyone can look like Nadia Comaneci.

Once you have chosen your own ideal percentage of body fat, calculate your ideal body weight, based not on the statistical generalities of height-weight charts but on the certitudes of your own frame size and needs. Your frame size is called lean body weight. Find it by subtracting the weight of your fat from your total body weight. Then add your lean body weight to your ideal fat weight.

> Weight of current fat = total body weight × percentage fat
> Lean body weight = total body weight − weight of current fat
> Ideal weight of fat = desired percent fat/current percent fat × weight of current fat
> Ideal weight = lean body weight + ideal fat weight

Let's say you weigh 125 pounds and measure 27 percent body fat. You want to have only 22 percent fat. In round figures:

> Your fat weighs 125 pounds × 27% = 34 pounds
> Your ideal fat weighs 22% ÷ 27% (or 0.8) ×
> 34 pounds = 27 pounds
> Your ideal weight = 91 pounds + 27 pounds = 118 pounds

Use your own ideal weight to calculate your daily caloric expenditure and intake if you follow the Plus Diet along with your exercise. Ideal weight is also a quick reference point whenever you step on a scale. However, to see precisely whether you are losing fat and becoming fitter, you will have to rely on skin folds. Nothing beats skin-fold measurements to calculate your percentage of body fat and keep an accurate record of your progress. Take new measurements every six to eight weeks as long as you are on the Plan, and every six to twelve months thereafter, and record them on the fitness profile at the end of chapter 1.

YOUR EXERCISE PLAN

In order to lose fat, you must exercise aerobically at your target pulse rate a minimum of three times a week for at least thirty minutes at a time. During each session, you must do an activity that burns at least 300 calories. Table V lists the energy costs of sports and daily activities per hour for an "average" 150-pound woman. If you are smaller, you will use fewer calories. Subtract 13 percent for every 20 pounds under 150. If you are larger, add 12 percent for every 20 pounds above 150.

You can go above these minimums, but you can't go below them and still lose fat, says Michael Pollock. If you try to cut the number of days you exercise by increasing the number of calories you burn each time, you won't lose body weight or fat because you won't grow new capillaries and muscle fibers or burn fat more efficiently. You must exercise three, four, five, or even six times a week in order to trigger the necessary metabolic changes.

Most women start losing fat immediately, but a few don't lose significant amounts for a few weeks because they are too out of shape to move nonstop for thirty minutes at a 300-calorie pace. As soon as these women can work at their target pulse rates for thirty minutes, they start losing fat normally.

After about a year, you become so efficient at your sport that you actually burn fewer calories. If you are still exercising in order to lose weight, you will reach a point of equilibrium. At this point, you have two choices. You can accept this balance as a sign that you have reached the percentage of body fat most comfortable for you, and continue with the same program just to maintain your weight. Or you can increase the intensity, duration, or frequency of your exercise and lose more fat. (If you can't reasonably increase the intensity or duration, perhaps you have outgrown this sport and should switch to something more challenging.)

How efficient you are affects your choice of exercises. If you are in good shape, only the most aerobic activities will elicit a weight-loss effect—bicycling at thirteen miles per hour, running at ten miles per hour, skiing cross-country at ten miles per hour, or swimming at one and a half miles per hour. If you are in only moderate shape, you may burn your 300 calories per half hour in one of the less intense exercises—hiking uphill, swimming at a quarter-mile-per-hour pace, roller skating at a fast clip, or practicing some of the Asian martial arts. If

TABLE V: ENERGY EXPENDITURES FOR THE "AVERAGE" WOMAN°

Daily Activities	*Calories Per Hour*
Cooking	80
Ditch digging	300
Dressing	80
Driving car	50
Dusting	80
Eating	30
Gardening	135
Ironing (sitting)	35
Ironing (standing)	45
Kissing (depends on intensity)	6–9 per kiss
Making beds	130
Marketing	80
Mowing lawn (hand mower)	185
Office work	75
Sawing or chopping wood	300
Sexual intercourse (depends on intensity)	125–300 per session
Sitting or doing quiet seated work	30
Standing	40
Washing floors	130

Sports and Exercise	
Aerobic dancing (low intensity)	215
Aerobic dancing (high intensity)	485
Asian martial arts	370
Badminton (polite game)	255
Badminton (power game)	485
Basketball (full court)	380
Bicycling (5½ miles per hour)	185
Bicycling (9 miles per hour)	320
Bicycling (13 miles per hour)	540
Bowling	180
Calisthenics (not circuit training)	150
Canoeing (2½ miles per hour)	185
Canoeing (vigorously)	350
Circuit training	410
Dancing, ballet (no figures, but considered equivalent to running 10 miles per hour)	750
Dancing, ballroom	275
Dancing, belly	230
Dancing, disco	400
Dancing, modern	240
Dancing, square	255
Field hockey	490
Fencing	210
Football	450

° Adapted from *Exercise and Weight Control*, President's Council on Physical Fitness and Sports, and other sources.

Sports and Exercise (*cont.*)

Golf (walking, carrying clubs)	165
Gymnastics, light	240
Gymnastics, heavy	455
Handball	485
Hiking (20-pound pack, 2 miles per hour)	150
Hiking (20-pound pack, 4 miles per hour)	235
Horseback riding (trotting)	255
Horseback riding (galloping)	315
Ice hockey (no reliable figures, considered about as strenuous as soccer)	500
Ice skating (figure)	255
Kayaking (leisure paddling)	150
Kayaking (vigorous paddling)	350
Lacrosse (estimate)	550
Mountain climbing	450
Race walking	415
Racquetball	485
Roller skating	400
Rope jumping	540
Rowing (two oars, 2½ miles per hour)	210
Rowing (scull, racing)	695
Running (7 miles per hour)	485
Running (10 miles per hour)	750
Running, cross country	600
Running up stairs	900
Running up *and* down stairs	540
Skiing, cross-country (10 miles per hour)	485
Skiing, downhill	270
Soccer	500
Speed skating (ice or roller)	770
Squash	485
Stair stepping	400
Surfing	(no information available)
Swimming (¼ mile per hour)	210
Swimming (1½ miles per hour)	460
Swimming, fast crawl	570
Table tennis (ping pong)	270
Tennis, singles (recreational)	205
Tennis, singles (competitive)	315
Tennis, doubles (recreational)	140
Tennis, doubles (competitive)	205
Volleyball (competitive)	255
Walking (2½ miles per hour)	130
Walking (3¾ miles per hour)	215
Walking uphill (100 feet per hour)	385
Water polo	600
Water skiing	375
Weight training with machines (Universal, Nautilus, etc.)	520
White-water rafting	400
Yoga	115

you are just beginning to exercise, walking, hiking, or playing basketball will work. If the activity you choose doesn't burn 300 calories in a half hour, extend your session for however long it takes to use up those calories. Remember that Table V lists energy expenditures for one hour, so divide each figure by half.

Whatever sport you choose, it must be continuous. A half hour of tennis, for example, includes several rests, walking after out-of-bounds balls, and standing around waiting for your opponent to serve, so it doesn't qualify. (Why not play tennis *in addition* to your aerobic exercise?) Downhill skiing can be stop-start or continuous, depending on how long the runs are and whether you stop in mid-run to socialize. However, even the longest run isn't going to last thirty minutes. Breaking the exercise into three or four parts doesn't work. Three ten-minute ski runs divided by rides up the chair lift doesn't equal thirty minutes of continuous aerobic exercise. If you choose volleyball or basketball as your sport, don't decide you've exercised enough if you just stand on the court while everyone else is running around you. You must keep moving the whole time. (Overweight people tend to move much less than normal-weight people. A 1964 analysis of films taken of overweight and normal-weight teenage girls showed that the overweight girls stood in the background and let the leaner girls do all the work.)

You don't need a chart of calorie expenditures to know whether you are burning 300 calories every half hour. Your pulse will tell you (see chapter 2). If you are working at the upper limits of your target pulse rate, you are probably burning your 300 calories. (Don't go above 80 percent or you will switch into anaerobic metabolism and won't burn nearly as much fat.)

Weight lifting is not listed on Table V. Weight lifting by itself is not an aerobic exercise and does not help you lose weight. However, weight lifting does build muscle fiber and decrease body fat, according to Michael Pollock. If you are overfat by 10 percent or less, weight lifting will reduce your body fat while it trims your figure, and you will appear to be thinner although you will actually weigh the same. Heavy weights with fewer reps are more effective for this than light weights with more reps. Circuit training, on the other hand (see chapter 6), will bring both weight and fat loss as long as you work at your target pulse rate. When you become so adept that you can't get your heart rate high enough, you'll have to add rope skipping, running, or some other aerobic sport to your routine.

For optimal weight loss, remember the minimums:

- target pulse rate
- three times a week
- thirty minutes each session
- 300 calories each session

You may exceed these basic figures, but don't go below them.

YOUR PLUS DIET

If you want to lose more than ten pounds, or if you want to lose the weight more quickly, add the Plus Diet to your exercise plan. Although you don't have to count every calorie on this diet, you must learn your daily caloric needs and expenditures so that you can coordinate the diet with the amount of exercise you are doing.

Calculate your daily needs according to your ideal weight, not your current weight. First find your Basal Energy Requirement (BER), the number of calories you need each day to operate your heart, lungs, and brain, rebuild your cells, and stay warm, even if you lie in bed day and night and don't move your fingers. (Your brain alone uses about one fifth of your BER calories.) As a rough estimate—and you can't get much more precise without going to the doctor for a basal metabolic rate test—figure that you need one calorie per hour for every 2.2 pounds (or one kilogram) of body weight. In other words, your Basal Energy Requirement equals your ideal weight in pounds divided by 2.2 (to convert it to kilograms), multiplied by one calorie per hour multiplied by twenty-four hours in a day, or:

$$\text{BER} = \text{ideal weight (lbs)} \div 2.2 \times 1 \text{ calorie/hr} \times 24 \text{ hours/day}$$

or

$$\text{BER} = \text{ideal weight (kilograms)} \times 1 \text{ calorie/hour} \times 24 \text{ hours/day}$$

In the following simplified formula, twenty-four hours has been divided by a factor of 2.2 to eliminate all those repetitious steps:

$$\text{BER in calories per day} = \text{ideal weight (lbs)} \times 10.9$$

For example, if your ideal weight is 115 pounds:

$$\text{BER} = 115 \times 10.9 = 1{,}254$$

To find the total number of calories you use each day, add your BER to your activity calories as given in Table V. Total Energy Consumption (TEC) equals the sum of your Basal Energy Requirement and your daily activity calories.

$$\text{TEC} = \text{BER} + \text{activity calories}$$

For example, if you are a typist in an office, your activity calories might go something like this:

Seven-and-a-half hours of typing	225 calories
One-half hour shopping	40
One-and-a-half hours eating	45
One-and-a-half hours cooking and washing dishes	120

Three hours watching television	90
Twenty minutes (⅓ hour) dressing	27
Forty minutes (⅔ hour) driving	33
One half hour jumping rope	370
Eight hours sleeping (already figured into your BER)	
Total	950 calories

(The hours don't add up to twenty-four. I can't know what you do with every minute of your day. . . .)

Therefore, if your ideal weight is 115 pounds, your Total Energy Consumption is:

TEC = 1254 + 950 = 2,204 calories per day

Now you know the number of calories you burn each day when you weigh your ideal weight. If you already weigh your ideal weight, and you eat the same number of calories as you expend in your TEC, you will maintain that weight. If you eat more, you'll gain, and if you eat less, you'll lose. If you weigh more than your ideal weight, but the amount of food you eat matches your TEC, you will lose weight gradually.

It takes 3,500 calories to make a pound of fat. If you eat 200 calories a day over your TEC, you will gain a pound of fat every seventeen-and-a-half days. If you eat 900 extra calories a day, you will gain a pound every four days. Conversely, if you eat 200 fewer calories a day, you will *lose* a pound of fat every seventeen-and-a-half days. You can also lose weight by burning off extra calories. If you add another half hour of rope jumping, you will burn up a pound of fat every nine or ten days. If you become less active and avoid, say, the half hour of jumping rope, you will gain a pound of fat in nine or ten days—unless you also decrease the amount of food you eat.

Here's the beauty of the Exercise Plus or Minus Plan. You can create a calorie deficit by combining exercise and diet. If you want to create a deficit of 500 calories a day, you can exercise away 300 of them and deny yourself only 200 calories' worth of food. If you want to create a 1,000-calorie-a-day deficit, you can exercise away 300 or 500 calories and diet away the rest. Just make sure that your exercise amounts to *at least* 300 calories each day.

Do *not* fast. Fasting triggers starvation and water-loss reactions. If you fast, you may become too weak to exercise, become faint, or suffer heatstroke from lack of water as well as nourishment.

Do *not* eat fewer than 1,000 calories a day. When your diet falls below 1,000 calories, a starvation reflex is triggered and your body starts breaking down muscle for fuel instead of tapping your storage fat. (You can tell you are burning protein if your sweat smells like ammonia. The odor comes from urea, an end product in protein breakdown.) Feeding off your own muscle is not only extremely unhealthy, it is futile; as soon as you raise your diet above the starvation level, your body replaces that muscle tissue and you gain weight. (Some very skinny athletes who try in vain to gain weight may, in fact, be burning the protein in their muscles to fuel each workout. No matter what their total calories are, their proportional carbohydrate intake is insufficient to supply enough glycogen for fuel. Increasing the ratio of carbohydrates to fat and protein often adds a few welcome pounds of muscle to their frames, bringing with it an increase in strength and stamina.)

Furthermore, such extreme diets throw off the balance of potassium, sodium, and other mineral salts in and between your cells. As a result, your tissues give up their intercellular water. (This is the reason you urinate so frequently the first few days of a fad diet, and lose five or ten pounds in two days.) If you exercise while your water level is low, you may suffer a heatstroke. As soon as you start eating a balanced diet again, your minerals are replaced and so is the water—and you gain the weight back.

SWEAT SUITS

Sweat suits do not help you lose weight, they help you lose water. If you exercise while wearing a sweat suit, you may suffer serious dehydration and even heatstroke, because you don't have enough water left to cool your skin. Besides, the moment you drink water, you gain all your weight back. Body builders sometimes use sweat suits immediately before a competition to sharpen the definition of their muscles. Without the normal intercellular water, each bulge and ripple stands out in striking relief. Jockeys use sweat suits too—and saunas—to eliminate a few pounds before their weigh-in. Just because both practices are common doesn't make them safe.

Try to lose only one pound a week—two at the most. At this rate, the weight you lose will be entirely fat. To lose one pound, or 3,500 calories, a week, you need a calorie deficit of only 500 calories a day, well within the reach of most people. To lose two pounds a week, however, you need a calorie deficit of 1,000 calories a day. If you are small, this may be too drastic for you and force you to eat less than 1,000 calories a day. If you are tall, however, you may be able to sustain a two-pound-per-week weight loss and stay perfectly healthy.

The actual diet is simply an adjusted version of your basic diet (described in chapter 3 as 15 to 20 percent protein, 20 to 30 percent fats, and 50 to 65 percent complex carbohydrates). On the Plus diet, you eat

- 20 to 25 percent of your total calories as protein
- 20 percent as fats
- 55 to 60 percent as carbohydrates

This is a slightly higher *proportion* of protein, in order to give you the same absolute *amount*. To replace cells and build tissue, you must consume 0.28 gram (0.01 ounce) of usable protein for every pound of body weight. That means a 105-pound person needs only 29.4 grams (about 1 ounce) of usable protein, and a 128-pound person needs 35.8 grams (or 1.28 ounces) of usable protein each day. The key word is *usable*. Not only are there many other nutrients in protein foods, but the amino acids (protein building blocks) don't always balance to make perfect protein, so you must eat much more than 1.28 ounces of protein food to *absorb* 1.28 ounces: about 7 ounces of meat, or 8 ounces of fish, or 5 cups of milk, or 6 eggs, or 13 ounces of dried beans, or 12 ounces of nuts, for example.

Your body demands no less than 0.28 gram per pound of protein each day. There's no way to fiddle with this number. If you reduce the amount of total calories you eat each day but still follow the same proportions, your protein intake remains at 15 or 20 percent but the actual quantity, or number of grams, goes down. (If you consume 2,000 calories each day, your 15 or 20 percent protein allowance amounts to 300 or 400 calories. If you reduce your daily caloric intake to 1,500 calories, 15 or 20 percent equals only 225 or 300 calories.) If you eat vegetable protein for some of your 20 to 25 percent protein allowance, you combine protein and carbohydrate in the same food and ensure you eat enough carbohydrate for energy for exercise.

More than half your fat allowance should come from vegetable sources. You may be tempted to reduce your fat intake below 20 percent to speed weight loss. Don't. Dietary fat is necessary for powering every metabolic process. You also need fat in order to process the high amounts of carbohydrates you eat. Tom Bassler, M.D., a pathologist at Centinela Hospital in Inglewood, California, believes that an extremely low-fat diet may cause some of the sudden deaths that occur in very fit runners who have no history of heart disease by triggering a metabolic imbalance that sets off a disruption in the heartbeat pattern. Fifteen percent is probably okay, but keep your fat intake at 20 percent just to be on the safe side. Besides, when you eat fat, it slows down your digestion, so you feel full longer.

When you first begin the Plus diet you will constantly use a chart of the nutrients found in each food. Once you get used to eating this way, you'll need neither nutrient charts nor calorie counters. You'll know—almost by instinct—how to balance your meals. And you'll have more energy and good spirits than you ever thought possible while you were dieting.

SOME DIETER'S TRICKS

Every naturally thin person and successful dieter has special ways of keeping her weight low. Some of these may work for you.

Work out in the cold.   Several reports have shown that thin people burn more calories as heat and give off more heat than fat people. This is something that is genetically programmed within the individual. However, some physiologists suggest that moderately overweight people who do aerobic exercise in cold water or cold weather burn extra fat, and this fat stays off even when the weather turns warm.

Drink plenty of water.   When you become dehydrated after prolonged exercise in hot weather, your hypothalamus confuses thirst and hunger. You become famished when you are actually thirsty. Drinking water while you exercise not only prevents heat exhaustion but also forestalls this inappropriate hunger.

Eat several small meals daily.   Eat two meals a day instead of three, but supplement them with low-calorie snacks. This keeps your blood-sugar level up, and you don't feel hungry or tired. Alternatively, eat six small meals a day. Whatever you do, don't eat just one meal a day. If you starve yourself all day, your body reacts as if it is in a real famine. When you finally eat, enzymes are overprimed and convert as many calories as possible into ugly storage fat to protect you against the next deprivation. Moreover, you will be so hungry when you finally sit down to dinner that you are likely to overeat.

Eat dinner early.   Don't eat after seven or eight o'clock in the evening. Although physiologically it doesn't matter whether you eat immediately before bedtime as long as you don't exceed your TEC, psychologically it can make a big difference. If you eat early in the evening, you still have time to exercise away some of your dinner calories. In addition, this rule will break that fattening habit of snacking while you watch television.

Avoid becoming overtired.   Whether from overtraining or overwork, extreme fatigue stimulates your appetite. This is another reason to increase your training load gradually. If you overtrain, you'll overeat.

Splurge occasionally.   Once in a while, if you are dying for some rich, gooey dessert, indulge yourself. Just don't eat dinner before it. Splurges are good for the soul—nobody can be self-controlled all the time—but skipping dinner and going straight to the hot fudge sundae means you'll increase your daily calorie intake by only, say, 300 calories, instead of the 800 or so if you tacked dessert onto a full dinner.

Don't eat little tastes.   Whenever you eat, be it snack or full meal, sit down and have a measurable portion, not a spoonful. Those dribs and drabs you don't remember eating add up.

Eat high-fiber foods.   Whole grains, raw fruits, raw vegetables, beans, and nuts will make you feel full sooner than processed or low-fiber foods, including meat. Only plants produce roughage or cellulose. (Even a chewy steak is a low-fiber food.) The feeling of fullness lasts longer too because your stomach and intestines spend a long time trying to break down the indigestible cellulose. This means you will feel satisfied on fewer calories.

Give up saturated fats and sugar.   No more butter on your toast or baked potato, no more sugar in your coffee, no more candies, cookies, or cakes. (Don't worry. You're still eating the fat and sugar nature put into its raw ingredients.) This may sound extreme, but it doesn't seem such a sacrifice when you know you can eat just about everything else. But be prepared for withdrawal symptoms when you give up sugar. If you are a sugar junkie, it will take you about a week to stop craving your sugar fix, and you will feel edgy and quite nervous. Vigorous exercise helps reduce the symptoms. If you are a chocoholic, you may actually become depressed during your first week without chocolate. Chocolate, it turns out, is loaded with phenylethylamine, the same amphetamine-like chemical your brain produces when you are in love or in a wonderfully happy mood. When you fall out of love, your phenylethylamine level plunges. It also drops during the worst of your premenstrual tension. That's why you crave chocolate at the end of a love affair or immediately before your period. Does it help to know that your depression is biochemical? Maybe. At least you're not imagining things. And you can take solace in the fact that a week of exercise will probably raise your spirits again.

II / SPORTS AND EXERCISES

I bicycle in a hilly park for an hour late every afternoon. When I start out, I'm beaten down after seven hours in the office. My back aches from tension, and it takes about ten minutes—an eternity—for me to get my wind. Then, like clockwork, at twelve minutes I catch my breath and start to relax. The fresh air is glorious, the trees smell sweet, and the flowers sparkle. At forty-five minutes I'm drunk with the splendor of the wind through my hair and the magical feeling of my body moving, and by the end of my ride I'm exhilarated, refreshed, and full of energy.

—A forty-six-year-old gynecologist

5 / Five Basic Sports

Walking, swimming, bicycling, running, and jumping rope. Every woman has tried most of them at some time in her life. These five are the natural exercises. You don't need lessons to walk, run, or jump, and you need only the most rudimentary swimming or cycling lessons before you can start paddling or pedaling around on your own. In contrast, it takes months before you can rally in tennis, ski down a mountain, apply an arm bar in judo, or develop even an elementary degree of competence in most other sports.

The basic five are lifetime activities, and they require very little special equipment or cash outlay. You can walk in any pair of comfortable shoes, you can run a year or two in one well-fitted pair of running shoes, you can jump with almost any rope lying around the house, and you can ride on a borrowed child's bicycle with as much joy as you get on the shiniest new ten-speed. Even swimming is cheap if you join the local Y instead of a health spa or country club. Every one of these sports can be done any time of the year in cities, suburbs, or open countryside. (If you live in an area with severe winters, you can't bicycle when snow and ice are on the ground, but you *can* pedal a stationary exercise bicycle indoors.)

These five are the building blocks (every other sport either runs, jumps, walks, kicks, or moves the arms against some kind of resistance), and every one gives your heart, lungs, and muscles a healthy workout.

The basic five make greater demands on your body as you ascend the list. Walking, the mildest, is one of the best ways for senior citizens, obese women, and cardiac patients to get back into shape. Add a backpack and a mountain trail, though, and you've got a real challenge. Swimming is variable. It may be as undemanding as a slow walk or as strenuous as a marathon run, but it is easier on the joints than either because the water supports your body. Bicycling demands more muscular strength in your legs than the first two, but it also adjusts from smooth easy pedaling to a thorough aerobic workout. Running, which stresses the legs and builds up your heart and lungs, requires a moderate level of conditioning before you start. Jumping rope is the most strenuous of all because you can't start out gently—the rope simply won't go over your head if you turn it too slowly.

Sports Bras

It would be nice if exercising without a bra would firm up your breasts the way pulling in your tummy without a girdle tones up your abdominal muscles. Unfortunately, it doesn't work that way. All that bouncing up and down only encourages your breasts to sag and droop. Your breasts, you see, are supported by skin and a few ligaments—no muscle—and the bouncing motions of most sports stretch that skin. When you run without a good bra, says Christine Haycock, M.D., associate professor of surgery at New Jersey Medical School, your breasts slap against your chest with a force as large as seventy pounds of pressure. "If you spend your life without a bra," she says, "you end up with your breasts hanging down to your navel." In addition, exercising without a bra hurts women who wear a B cup or larger or who have fibrocystic breasts. All that bouncing and slapping causes anything from a dull ache to a sharp pain in the breasts themselves or the chest wall behind them either during or after your workout. This pain will probably be worse immediately before your periods if your breasts swell or become tender. Even if you are small-breasted, you should wear a bra, or wrap your breasts in an Ace bandage wound across your chest and around your back, or coat your nipples with Vaseline, or tape bandages over them. Otherwise your clothes will rub your bare nipples raw and bloody.

It is often easier to find a good sports bra in a sporting goods store than in the lingerie section of a local department store. A saleswoman in a sporting goods store is likely to understand your needs and to have tested each bra style personally. Be sure to try on several models to find the one most comfortable for your figure. Jump up and down in each bra to simulate the movements of your sport.

A properly fitted, supportive sports bra has the following features:

- It keeps your breasts steady. They don't bounce or swing.
- No breast tissue oozes out of the sides of the bra. If it does, it will rub against the inside of your arms or against the edges of the bra and cause a painful rash.
- The straps are wide and made of nonelasticized material to prevent bouncing. They stay firmly on your shoulders without being pulled so tight that they cut into your skin.

- The bra lifts from below, so the straps are not your breasts' sole support.
- The back of the bra does not ride up when you move.
- The fabric of the bra is at least 55 percent cotton so that it will absorb perspiration. Synthetic fabrics can cause allergic reactions, particularly when you perspire. The bra should feel soft, like a T-shirt, so that it can't irritate your skin.
- The bra has no elastic except around the rib cage to allow the fabric to stretch as you breathe. If there is elastic in contact with the sweating parts of your body, make sure it is covered with nonallergenic fabric to prevent rashes. (Some women chafe wherever elastic meets the skin, because elastic stretches and contracts more quickly than the chest and shoulder muscles do. As it moves against the skin, it rubs and scratches.)
- Any plastic or metal fasteners are covered with fabric so that they can't scrape or press into your skin.
- Seams are padded or placed away from underarms and nipples so that they can't rub you raw.
- The bra has no decorative lace, exposed metal hooks or eyelets, or front closures to scrape your skin during strenuous exercise.

If you wear an A cup, just about any minimally supporting bra will do. You may enjoy the soft seamless bras sold in dancewear stores for use under leotards. You may also find the Jogbra (see Appendix B) very soft and comfortable. Its seams are external so they can't rub your skin, and its straps meet in the back like a swimmer's racing suit, so there is no binding at the shoulders. It flattens the breasts close to the body, like a very firm T-shirt, and compresses rather than supports the breasts.

If you wear a B or C cup, you will need a bra with real cups and support from the bottom as well as the strapes. Just pressing the breast tissue flat to the rib cage, says Dorothy Harris, isn't enough. "There is still movement," she says, "even when the breasts are close to the chest wall."

The Lady Duke, made by a leading manufacturer of men's athletic supporters, is smooth, very soft, and made of an absorbent cotton and polyester blend. It has a minimum of elastic and a maximum of support and has pockets for the protective pads used in fencing, soccer, ice hockey, and some other contact sports. Playtops by International Playtex also provide support without excessive movement (see Appendix II).

"Heavily endowed women, especially women who wear D, DD, or E cups," says Harris, "may not be able to find a sports bra to fit them because the cups of sports bras seem to be smaller than the cups of standard bras. I know one woman who wears two and sometimes even three bras when she runs." Maternity bras and the special support bras sold at surgical supply houses may work if you have very large breasts.

WALKING

Conduct a survey of America's sports attitudes, as Louis Harris Associates did for Perrier in 1978, and you will discover that walking is America's number-one athletic pursuit. Twenty-two percent of American adults, or 34.1 million people, call themselves walkers. Walking is an endurance conditioner as effective as jogging, cycling, swimming, or other continuous exercise—as long as you walk long enough and hard enough. If you doubt that walking is good exercise, just take a three-week vacation to New York, London, Hong Kong, or any other good walking town. After a couple of days of sightseeing on foot, your calves and shins ache. By the end of the trip, your step is lighter, your leg and abdominal muscles firmer, and your clothes looser, even if you nibble local pastries along the way.

Evaluation

Vigorous walking strengthens your heart, raises your HDL level (see chapter 3), and improves the oxygen-carrying capacity of your lungs and circulatory system. You move smoothly, with none of the jarring and pounding that runners endure. Walking injuries are very rare. While runners sit at home nursing their blisters and shin splints, walkers march undaunted through parks, city streets, and rural woods.

Like other endurance exercises, walking firms your muscles and burns calories. It just takes a little longer. Whereas a runner or swimmer can burn 300 calories in thirty minutes, a walker must exercise at least forty to achieve the same results. If you are in good physical condition, you'll get a cardiovascular training effect by walking several miles a day nonstop, or walking up and down hills or stairs, or carrying a pack on your back. If you have heart or lung disease, diabetes, or arthritis, or if you are recuperating from major surgery, walk slowly on level ground and get back into shape—with your doctor's approval.

Walking is a lifetime addiction, and only nature's angriest weather discourages the intrepid walker. With boots, slicker, or umbrella, walkers stand up to sleet, snow, and even black of night if necessary. Since walking is part of daily life, it is easier to walk each day than it is to take an hour off to bicycle, swim, or run. You can walk to work, walk to the supermarket, walk around the park with friends, walk up the stairs of the Eiffel Tower, or walk the dog.

Walking provides experiences no other exercise can match: tours of cities, hikes along mountain streams, strolls through autumnal woods or along miles of deserted beaches. As you walk, you taste each new season, learn the personality of every house in the neighborhood, feel the texture of the air. Your senses become sharper, your observation more acute. A vigorous walk will start the creative juices flowing, without leaving you so sweaty that you have to shower and change clothes before you go back to work. For centuries, poets, playwrights, and physicists have taken walks to clear their heads and have gone back, refreshed, to their papers.

Equipment

Walking is cheap. If you already own a pair of stout, comfortable shoes, you don't have to spend a cent to get started. Running shoes are fine; so are well-made oxfords with flat heels, nonskid cushioned soles, and arch supports. The shoe should grip your heel firmly but bend across your instep. You should be able to wiggle your toes easily inside the toe box. Ventilated nylon uppers allow air to circulate around your feet in hot weather, but leather uppers protect against rain and snow. (Wet feet get blisters.) A flexible lugged sole grips any terrain. Don't wear hiking boots except for hiking—they are heavier than shoes, unyielding, and take longer to break in. Socks should be absorbent and cushiony, made of wool or cotton.

If you add backpacking at the intermediate level, you'll need a pair of lightweight hiking boots with traction or lugged soles and a steel shank built into each arch and heel area. The stiff shank absorbs the impact of sharp rocks and lets you edge along steep, angled trails. Firm heel counters (tapered thermoplastic or molded nylon cups) hug the heel to prevent blisters and twisted ankles. (Most ankle injuries are caused by turning the bones below the ankle.) Reinforced toe caps of rubber or leather keep you from stubbing your toes. For serious backpacking, carrying heavy loads, or for mountaineering or cold-weather hiking, you'll need expensive rugged, insulated, and waterproofed leather uppers, but they'll make the shoe very heavy (upwards of three pounds per boot). For trail and weekend backpacking, nylon uppers are lighter and let your feet breathe, while Gore-Tex uppers are tougher, waterproof, equally as light (weighing as little as one pound), and reasonably priced. Gore-Tex and nylon boots must be reinforced with leather at stress points, but the leather should not be stitched in place because the needle holes destroy the boot's waterproofing even if the stitches are smeared with sealant at the factory. While all leather boots may feel a little stiff when you first try them on, they should still feel comfortable. If they aren't, they never will be. Lightweight boots with fabric uppers need no breaking in at all and should have shock-absorbing molded foam insoles, cushioned heel wedges, and knit fabric linings. Leave enough room between your toes and the end of the shoe so that your toes don't jam into the toe cap when you walk downhill.

Safety and protection.   If you walk at night on country roads, walk facing the traffic, except when you are walking uphill. Wear light-colored clothes marked front and back with reflecting tape, or wear reflecting suits or backpacks. Carry a flashlight to illuminate the road and warn approaching cars.

Relative cost.   Nothing, if you already have a good pair of shoes; $50 or more if you must buy them.

Precautions

Although walking places little stress on the heart, lungs, muscles, and joints, it may be too strenuous if you are seriously ill.

Goals for Fitness

According to Michael Pollock, Ph.D., director of the cardiac rehabilitation and human performance laboratory at Mount Sinai Medical Center in Milwaukee, you must walk at least forty minutes, four times a week, at 60 percent or more of your maximum heart rate in order to get a training effect. Either count your pulse or use the talk/sing test (see chapter 2), walking as fast as you can as long as you can still talk or sing. If you are in good or excellent condition, you will have to add hills or carry a six-pound backpack to increase your workload.

Training

The universal warm-ups in chapter 2 are sufficient. Pollock says you should stretch the backs of your legs before and after every walk. To warm up your heart, the first five or ten minutes of the walk should be slow. Cool down the last five or ten minutes by walking slowly, and then stretch.

Beginner's Level

Start out easy and build up, advises Pollock. If you haven't exercised for a while, go slow the first day, even if it seems easy. "When you first start out," says Pollock, "you don't feel sore while you are actually walking. But you are giving your muscles a pretty good workout, and you feel it later. If it turns out that the pace was too easy, you can speed up the second day." He suggests that a healthy twenty-five-year-old woman should walk a little over two miles in forty minutes, or a 17-minute-per-mile pace. A normal healthy middle-aged woman should walk for forty minutes at a 20-minute-per-mile pace, or two miles: one mile out and one mile back. A woman with short legs may find a 20-minute mile (3 miles per hour) a moderate pace, and a 15-minute mile (4 miles per hour) quite fast, whereas a very tall woman may find a 17-minute mile a beginner's crawl, and 11- or 12-minute miles (5 to 5½ miles per hour) fast but not impossible. Height and leg length are more important in walking than in most other sports. In running, there is a moment in every stride when both feet leave the ground at the same time. The length of your stride is controlled by the springiness of your step as well as the reach of your legs. In cycling, the pedals, gears, and wheels are great levelers; in swimming, the length of your legs barely affects the power of your kick. But in walking, one foot stays on the ground while the other reaches out. There is a limit to how far you can reach with that other leg.

Walk briskly. Point your feet straight ahead. Put your heel down first, feeling your weight distribute itself evenly along the outside of your foot as you rock forward onto the ball of your foot and then your big toe. (Check your shoes. If you are wearing down the outside of your heel and the inward side of your sole, you're walking wrong.)

Stretch out with your stride and swing your arms in a natural rhythm with your feet, right arm forward as the left foot steps forward, left arm out as the right foot moves ahead. Slightly bend your arms and swing them loosely from the shoulders. Relax your hands so that your wrists flap slightly with each motion and your fingers are gently curled. Do not move your hands across your body.

As you walk, hold your head high, with good but not stiff posture. Walk in straight, purposeful, rhythmic, evenly paced, relaxed strides. When you hit your stride, you will feel weightless—it will take no effort to keep moving. Good posture strengthens your abdominal and back muscles as you walk. Suck in your gut to tighten these muscles even more. If you run errands as you walk, carry your packages in a knapsack on your back rather than in your arms. Packages in one or both arms throw off your balance and force you to use one leg more than the other.

Table VI (page 102) outlines a schedule for walking. If it is too fast for you, slow it down. If it is too slow, speed up.

Intermediate Level

You are in good condition if you are thirty years old or less and walk 4½ miles in an hour, at least four times a week; you are between thirty

TABLE VI: WALKING PROGRAM

Week	Miles	Time	Miles Per Hour
(first day)	1–2 (maximum)	40 minutes	3
1	1–3	1 hour	2½–3
2	1–3	1 hour	2½–3
3	3	1 hour	3
4	3–3½	1 hour	3–3½
5	3½	1 hour	3½
6	4	1 hour	4
7	4	1 hour	4
8°	4½	1 hour	4½
9°	4½	1 hour	4½
10°	5	1 hour	5
11°	5	1 hour	5

° Even if you are in good shape, this pace may be too fast for you if you have short legs.

and sixty years old and walk a little over 4 miles an hour, at least four times a week; you are over sixty years old, and you walk 3½ miles in an hour at least four times a week.

From now on, intensify your effort. Lengthen some of your walks to two hours. Add impediments: a 6-pound or heavier backpack, or ankle weights. Walk up every flight of stairs you can find, and add hills to your route. Take day-long hikes on weekends.

Go backpacking as much as possible. You can't go backpacking at least four days a week every single week, so it doesn't qualify as a basic fitness activity, but it is a reward for good physical condition. You can't enjoy the peace and power of a hiking trip if you are out of shape.

BEAR WARNING

Bears are attracted to menstruating women and move in when they smell their odor or the scent of a discarded tampon or sanitary napkin, say researchers with the Border Grizzly Study Project at the University of Montana. They postulate that human menstrual odors resemble the sexual attractants female bears give off to draw a mate. This phenomenon may explain the increasing frequency of bear attacks on women hikers in the last few years. The solution: Stay out of bear country during your menstrual periods.

For backpacking, condition your hamstrings and quadriceps (back and front thigh muscles) by walking up and down stadium stairs and steep hills while wearing your backpack and hiking boots or ankle weights. Also do squats or kiddie kicks and run-'em-out-of-gym-class sprints. If your quadriceps are weak, your knees may give out on long downhill treks. To carry your backpack, strengthen your abdominal muscles with killer sit-ups and your back muscles with locusts. To prevent back strain, keep your back and neck flexible with knee-nose touches or king of Siam kowtows and plows. (See chapter 6 for a complete discussion of exercises suggested here.)

Advanced Level

None. When you reach this level of fitness, graduate to one of the other basic sports.

Injuries

Walking injuries are rare. If the muscles down the back of your leg or in your shins ache, warm up longer. Check your stride—you should rock from heel to toe. If you have muscle aches and your shoes indicate uneven wear, you may need orthotics: podiatrist-prescribed shoe inserts that redistribute your weight along your foot. If you get sharp pains, cramps, or numbness in your calf muscles when walking up inclines of more than 20 degrees, you are out of shape and are building up lactic acid wastes. Gradually add stair stepping to your routine to improve your circulation—either climb and descend a flight of stairs in your house or march up and down the stairs of a nearby stadium, starting with one short flight at an easy pace and working yourself up to fifteen continuous minutes of brisk treading.

Pollock warns that heat and cold may be particular problems for walkers. "In extremely cold or extremely hot weather," he advises, "start off gradually. If it's hot, drink plenty of water, and then test yourself. Go out for a half mile and come back for a half mile. If you are comfortable with that, take your regular walk. In cold weather, bundle up in layers. Layers are warmer than one heavy garment and can be peeled off as you warm up. It is always colder going into the wind. Walk into the wind at the beginning of your walk so that your back is to the wind when you are coming home tired and sweaty."

SWIMMING

Women are better distance swimmers than men. In distances over two miles, women are 15 percent more efficient, says Paul Hutinger, P.E.D., professor of physical education at Western Illinois University. A woman's high proportion of body fat not only provides more fuel to burn in long races but insulates her and buoys her up in the water. A man has to work harder just to stay afloat. "Women are tough in endurance swimming," he says, "but they don't know it yet. As programs develop, I think we're going to see lots of sensational performances by the women."

Swimming is the second most popular sport among adults in the United States. Seventeen percent—26.4 million people—swim on a regular basis each year. (Only 11 percent run, and 9 percent play tennis.)

"Don't you dare recommend swimming," threatened one woman who swims a mile every day. "There aren't enough pools around as it is." In some cities pools are so scarce that swimmers have to reserve their swimming time a few days in advance. "No one is more obsessive," wrote Sol Stern in the *New York Times Magazine*, "than a swimmer fighting for his or her precious lane space. Indeed, the only serious risk of injury that swimmers now face is the increased chance of a head-on collision in an overcrowded lap lane."

Learning to swim is very easy. In a few lessons, you can pick up the basics from a friend or a certified instructor, but you'll spend the rest of your life perfecting your skills. If you can't find a teacher, you can even learn to swim by following the excellent step-by-step instructions in Cuthbertson and Cole's *I Can Swim, You Can Swim*. Swimming is a lifelong sport. Infants as young as six weeks can learn the rudiments of water play and swimming; you can continue to swim no matter how old you become.

ANOTHER OLD WIVES' TALE BITES THE DUST

Don't swim within an hour of eating or you'll get a stomach cramp and drown. Right?

Wrong. Strenuous exercise or breathing, especially in cold water, *may* cause a stitch in your diaphragm or a cramp in your leg or arm muscles. The cramp will hurt, but it won't kill you.

If you swim within two hours of a meal, however, you will feel heavier and more sluggish and might even come down with the exercise-induced diarrhea that may afflict anyone who exercises too soon after eating.

Swimming is infinitely adaptable. You can swim laps in a pool. You can swim in oceans, lakes, or rivers—rough or open water, as swimmers call it. In mass ocean swims in Hawaii and California, over a thousand people may show up to swim through ten or more miles of pulling tides and swirling currents. You can swim lonely open-water marathons of twenty, fifty, or even a hundred miles with only a coach in a pace rowboat for company. You can play water polo, one of the most demanding sports in the world, or skin-dive, for the most spectacular and ethereal experience of your life. You can dance, do calisthenics, or lift and submerge inflatable "weights" or flying disks (such as Frisbee) to tone your body faster than the same exercises would on land. (Whenever you move through water, the water resists you, or pushes you back. Therefore, you have to work harder in order to run or dance through water than you would on dry land.) The resistance and the buoyancy of water together make it possible for post-surgical patients, arthritis sufferers, and even people confined to wheelchairs to do strengthening exercises and get an aerobic workout—under the watchful eye of a physical therapist, of course.

For an extremely strenuous, all-around sport, try synchronized swimming. Forget those films of Esther Williams shimmering through a pool of flowers as twenty sweet young things form themselves into a kaleidoscopic daisy chain. Today's synchronized swimming is a demanding sport, to be contested for the first time at the 1984 Olympic Games in Los Angeles. In compulsory figures and freestyle events, synchronized swimming requires power as well as grace. If you don't believe it, just try doing an upside-down corkscrew spin in slow motion with your head down in the water and your legs and hips entirely above it. It takes a great deal of strength and stamina just to hold any part of your body out of the water. Because power, flexibility, and stamina are necessary for good performance, competitive synchronized swimmers reach their peaks later than most other swimmers—in their early twenties rather than their middle teens.

If you are interested in competitive racing, there are junior, scholastic, open, and masters programs all over the country. Swim meets include 100-, 200-, and 400-yard races in each of the four competitive strokes (freestyle, backstroke, butterfly, and breaststroke), medleys, and long events of 1,650 yards (1,500 meters). Every event is graded—you swim only against people within five years of your own age. Says one sixty-eight-year-old, "I never thought I'd look forward to turning seventy, but now I can't wait. I'm fast enough to beat every one of those old ladies in the seventy to seventy-four age bracket, and when I move up I'm going to collect me a pile of first prizes."

Evaluation

"When you swim," says Ransom J. Arthur, M.D., founder of the masters swimmers program and dean of the University of Oregon School of Medicine, "you exercise all the skeletal muscles of the body, and, if you push it with any vigor, you improve your cardiovascular tone and develop a training effect." Swimming makes you more flexible, especially in your shoulders and ankles, and swimming sprints improves the power in your arms and shoulders. The prone and supine positions used in swimming permit a higher cardiac output than cycling or running, so that swimmers can work longer and harder, in any weather, than runners or cyclists. No wonder the President's Council on Physical Fitness declared that only running compares with swimming for building cardiovascular and muscular endurance.

Because the water supports some of your body weight, you can become very efficient in the water even if you are overweight. Furthermore, swimming an hour or so a day is virtually injury-free. There is no pounding or impact shock to the legs and feet, as in running or jumping rope, and shoulder problems generally don't occur unless you swim five or six hours at a time. This makes swimming particularly attractive to people with back or circulatory problems or arthritis. The head-back, outstretched position of the backstroke alleviates many sorts of back pain, according to Paul Hutinger, and may prevent or at least stop the progress of kyphosis, the humpbacked head-thrust-forward posture of some older people.

Swimming is excellent exercise for all children but is a special boon for pre-teens and teenagers who are too stocky or too short to play basketball, football, or other competitive sports. "Size is not as important in swimming," says Harold M. Sexton, a recently retired Honolulu pediatrician. "Small kids are 'more equal' in the water, so they can do as well as larger ones. Or they can become divers. And they are not going to get hurt or injure their knees the way they might in football."

Equipment

Any swimsuit is fine as long as it doesn't rub or cut your shoulders, underarms, back, or thighs.

At first, swim in a pool rather than open water. Pools have smooth water and a preset distance so you can pace yourself. Competition pools are twenty-five yards long, but a twenty-yard pool is acceptable. If you swim in shorter pools, you spend more time turning and pushing off from the sides than swimming, and it's very hard to get any training effect. (June Krauser, the editor of *Swim-Master*, began her masters swimming career by swimming in her mother's ten-yard pool. "I got to where I did a mile in that little pool," she says, "and my neck got sore from turning, so I went to a larger pool.") A water temperature of 78 to 80 degrees is ideal. Colder, and you become too chilled to swim your full workout. Warmer, and you become enervated and listless. Swim in a pool organized for lap swimming, with lane markers to keep people from hogging the whole pool and some system to regulate the flow of traffic.

When you reach the intermediate and advanced levels, use some sort of training device to strengthen your stroke or your kick and to vary your workout. Kickboards, hand paddles, thigh floats, pull tubes (to immobilize your ankles), swimsuits with pockets (or a baggy second suit worn over your regular one) to increase your resistance in the water, all force you to work harder.

If your eyesight is so bad that you must wear contact lenses in the pool, wear a pair of the new lightweight goggles with plastic lenses. They are airtight, so you won't lose your lenses, and their new lenses don't distort your vision. You can also order goggle lenses with your correction from opticians throughout the country.

Safety precautions and protection.   Because the water is smooth, and there are sides and lap ropes to cling to in emergencies, pools are much safer than open water. Don't swim in lakes or oceans until you are a strong swimmer, and even then work out inside a demarcated area, within view of a lifeguard. Swim parallel to the shore, rather than away from it, and always make sure someone is watching you.

Do not hyperventilate when you dive or race. When you inhale normally, oxygen is used by the muscles. The muscles give off carbon dioxide as a waste product, and it is the buildup of carbon dioxide in your blood that tells your lungs to take another breath. When you hyperventilate by inhaling several times without completely exhaling, says James H. Flippen, M.D., of Palo Alto, California, you blow off more than the normal amount of carbon dioxide and remove your chemical stimulus to breathe. If you are underwater when your oxygen runs out, you have no urge to breathe and will pass out and drown.

Relative cost.   Tank suits cost $7 and up. Access to pools ranges from a nominal towel fee of 50 cents for the use of high school and municipal plunges to $400 or more for membership in exclusive urban swimming and health clubs. Balance this cost against the annual cost of buying and repairing shoes, bicycles, rackets, or other sports equipment, and the expenditure looks smaller. Then figure in the annual doctor bills of runners and other athletes, and the cost of injury-free swimming doesn't seem so high after all.

Precautions

Because swimming is an infinitely adjustable sport, like a rheostat on a lamp, there are very few people who can't participate, provided they know how to swim. However, if you have serious ear problems, such as a perforated eardrum, your doctor may not permit you to swim without custom-fitted latex earplugs.

Goals for Fitness

For a training effect, you should swim more than three times a week for at least thirty minutes at 70 to 85 percent of your maximum heart rate. (As a swimmer, you can work harder than athletes doing land sports because your heart holds 10 to 20 percent more blood when it is horizontal than when it is vertical. Therefore, it can pump more blood with less effort during each contraction.) Since swimming is less demanding and less jarring than other sports, it's better to swim five times a week than three, and to check your pulse every few laps to make sure you're working hard enough. Most swimmers prefer the carotid pulse, but do whatever is comfortable. (Any pool for serious swimmers has a very large pacer clock prominently displayed on one wall.)

Training

In addition to the universal warm-ups in chapter 2, stretch your arms, shoulders, and chest with two or three birds (described in chapter 6). If you can't grasp your hands behind your back, try holding onto two ends of a towel or broomstick. Move your hands closer together as you become more limber.

To warm up your heart, swim a few laps slowly, gradually increasing your speed. Cool down by swimming slowly.

Beginner's Level

June Krauser offers the very gradual program for beginners shown in Table VII. If you have swum before, the pace may be too gentle. If so, progress to each new stage as soon as the last becomes easy.

Swim in a straight line. Don't weave all over the pool. Any of the standard competitive strokes (freestyle or crawl, breaststroke, backstroke, or butterfly), alone or in combination, tones your muscles and your heart as long as you do it vigorously. Don't scissors kick with the crawl, and don't use the sidestroke except during your cool-down. If there are more than two people in your lane, stay to the right and remain in your half of the lane. If there are three or more people in your lane, always stay to the right, down and back, and pass only in the middle. If you are a slow swimmer, use the outside lanes. (In competition, the middle lane, lane four, is reserved for the top-seeded—fastest—swimmers.) To vary your workout, substitute pulls or kicks for one quarter to one third of your repeats. Pulls strengthen your arms because your legs are immobilized by floats or pull tubes. Kicks performed while your hands hold onto a kickboard will strengthen your legs and ankles. *Or* use hand paddles to make each stroke more difficult.

TABLE VII: SWIMMING PROGRAM

Week	Intervals	Total Distance
1 and 2	4 × 25 yards°	100 yards
3–5	2 × 100 yards	200 yards
6–15	4 × 100 yards	400 yards
16–23	3 × 200 yards	600 yards
24–31	4 × 200 yards or 2 × 400 yards	800 yards
32	8 × 100 yards or 4 × 200 yards or 2 × 400 yards or straight 800 yards 1 × 800 yards	800 yards

° Swim 25 yards, one length of the pool, stop and catch your breath, then swim the next, for a total of four repeats.

When you can swim the 800 yards nonstop, work yourself up to 1,000 yards in thirty minutes. Then try to cut down your time rather than increasing your mileage.

Helpful hints:

- In the crawl, alternate breathing sides, coming up for a breath one time on your left side and the next time on your right. This helps you hold to a straighter course.
- In the crawl, exhale in the water before you raise your head to take a new breath. Let the air trickle from both the mouth and nose at first, but blow out explosively when you start to tilt your head toward the surface. This gets rid of any air left in your lungs as well as clears the water away from your mouth so that you can inhale unimpeded. Most distance swimmers breathe once for every pair of strokes (one right-arm stroke and one left).
- In the crawl and the butterfly, keep your elbows high. The arm pull begins with the elbow almost straight, but about halfway through the stroke, the elbow should be bent a little more than 90 degrees in order to push the water back most forcefully.
- Keep your body as straight and flat as possible. Lightly point your toes, submerge your face to your hairline, and keep your legs high for streamlining. Don't bring your feet to the surface, however, or you'll be kicking air.
- Don't wiggle or roll from side to side or you'll cut your smooth, streamlined contour.

LONG STEADY DISTANCE (LSD)

If you want your workout to be fun, with almost no injuries, try LSD— the training method, not the psychedelic drug. With LSD, you work at a *moderate* pace—a target pulse rate of 60 to 80 percent—for thirty minutes or more. You work through the first inevitably uncomfortable ten minutes of exercise to arrive at that warm plateau where you feel like a smoothly functioning rhythmic machine. LSD gives you the time to enjoy yourself. If you have fun, you'll stick with it and get the maximum training effect with the minimum injury. For most sports, LSD takes at least thirty minutes nonstop. For bicycling and swimming, it takes an hour.

Intermediate Level

You have graduated to the intermediate level if: you are under thirty-five years old and can swim 100 yards in less than two minutes and 1,000 yards in less than twenty-two minutes; you are middle-aged and can swim 100 yards in two and a half minutes and 1,000 yards in less than twenty-five minutes; you are over sixty years old and can swim 100 yards in three minutes and 1,000 yards in twenty-seven to thirty-two minutes, depending on how much over sixty you are. (You lose about one percent of your speed each year after your sixtieth birthday.)

To progress beyond this point, work up to one hour or one mile, whichever comes first, five days a week. Many women find this nonstop long steady distance swimming their favorite kind of workout. "Sometimes I sing songs to myself in my head," says one fifteen-year-old, "but most of the time I just concentrate on the way my arms and body feel when they're moving through the water. You're not part of the regular world. You're in a dream state, floating and all alone. It's incredibly peaceful."

When you become an efficient swimmer, you won't be able to get your heart rate up with just long steady distance, so add a little fartlek (the Swedish word for speed-play) to your workouts two or three times a week. Speed up and slow down every few minutes. For example, begin with a slow speed for five minutes, then swim 400 yards at a very fast pace, then slow down to a moderate pace for another five minutes, then swim at top speed for a length or two, then swim at a leisurely pace for five minutes, and so on for an hour. Never swim so fast that you have to stop swimming to catch your breath.

If you can swim a mile easily and are interested in racing, add some interval training to your workouts.

Intervals *must* be timed. First, test yourself by swimming fast enough for 100 yards to bring your heart rate up to 80 or 90 percent of your maximum, depending on your age and health. Note your time. Immediately check the time it takes for your pulse to drop to two thirds of that heart rate. This is your "rest time." (Your recovery usually amounts to half of your 100-yard "swim time.") Set up a program of 100-yard sets, matching or slightly improving your swim time and resting between each set of your established rest time. Swim, rest, swim, rest, until you have swum between half a mile and a mile. As your condition improves, shorten your rests until you are only resting ten or fifteen seconds between each repeat. If building speed is important to you, swim a few fast intervals, sprinting at top speed for one or two lengths, then resting a little longer than the sprint itself, or until you have completely caught your breath, before swimming another fast repeat. Swim your intervals with one stroke, a medley, or even with kickboards or paddles.

Swimmers' intervals differ from runners and cyclists' intervals. A dry-land athlete needs much longer rest periods to dissipate the heat she generates during all-out effort. As a swimmer, you are cooled by the water, so you don't need long rest stops. Furthermore, the non-weight-bearing nature of swimming makes your recovery quicker than a runner's and also permits you to work harder. Because a runner's or cyclist's rest period is much longer, she must keep moving slowly while she rests. You, on the other hand, stop moving completely and hold onto the side of the pool or do light stretches.

Advanced Level

If you can swim 3,500 yards, or two miles, nonstop you are an advanced swimmer.

INTERVALS

Intervals are a series of repeated intense efforts over the same distance at the same speed, allowing yourself only a partial rest between them. The greatest stimulation to the heart is said to come during this incomplete rest period, when the volume of blood pumped by the heart per beat is the largest. Many coaches believe that intervals bring the fastest improvement *to an already fit* athlete of any training regimen. They are also extremely hard work. Because intervals dramatically overload your muscles, they have the same effect as weight training. They tear down muscle fiber so that the body can rebuild it larger and stronger than before. Therefore, like weight training, practice intervals a maximum of three times a week and never on two consecutive days. On your other days, work long steady distance.

At this point, you might want to add some weight-training exercises to your regimen. The average woman swimmer should strengthen her abdominal muscles, the triceps in the backs of her arms, the latissimus dorsi (running underneath her arms and down the sides of her body), and the pectorals, across the top of the chest. Swimming movements are so specific that ordinary resistance exercises can't precisely duplicate the way your muscles move in the water. Nonetheless, chinups work the lats and biceps, pull-ups work the lats and triceps, push-ups work the chest, shoulders, and triceps, and killer sit-ups strengthen the trunk flexors. Stretch very conscientiously before and after doing any weight exercises, or they will shorten your muscles and decrease your flexibility. In addition, practice your strokes on dry land while holding dumbbells, and your kick while wearing ankle weights.

If you have any questions about style or technique, now is the time to find a coach. Phone your local Y or write the Masters Swimming Program (see Appendix A) to find a reputable coach in your area.

Injuries

If you swim an hour or so a day, five or six days a week, the chances of hurting yourself are almost nil. An elite swimmer in training sometimes swims ten to twenty *thousand* meters a day. If she swims 10,000 meters a day, each of her arms goes through at least 10,800 freestyle, backstroke, and butterfly strokes each week. Frayed muscles and tendinitis of the shoulder ("swimmer's shoulder") becomes a real possibility. (See chapter 10 for treatment and prevention.)

Sometimes the latissimus dorsi become tight and sore. These muscles, running from your underarms down your sides, are the muscles you use most in swimming. They must be stretched out before and after each workout with door leans.

A full-blown cramp in your lats during or after swimming is the equivalent of a cramp in your calf when you walk or run. Stretch your arm straight above your shoulder to its full length and flex your hand.

Occasionally, breaststrokers hurt their knees because the frog kick stresses the ligaments or tendons stabilizing the knees. Stretching and strengthening your hamstrings and quads may steady your knee. Stretch with gravity toe touches and storks, and strengthen with squats (or kiddie kicks if the squats hurt your knees), hamsters, and run-'em-out-of-gym-class sprints (described in chapter 6). Make these changes in your technique: Do not put the full snap into your kick until you are thoroughly warmed up, and straighten your legs later during the backward thrust of your feet.

Irritated, burning, red eyes are caused by chlorine disinfectants or high acidity in the pool water. Goggles prevent most of the irritation,

---

DOOR LEANS

Stand about two or three feet from a high ledge of some sort—mantel, tall fence, or very sturdy shower curtain pole. Place your hands shoulder width apart on the ledge and bend forward enough to put most of your weight on your hands. (Your head will come forward between your arms.) Bend your left knee and cross your right leg as far as you can reach behind it. This stretches your whole right side. Hold for thirty seconds and then reverse the position of your legs to stretch your left side.

---

and nonprescription eyedrops or a mild over-the-counter sterile saline solution soothes your eyes. The irritation goes away by itself after one or two hours. (For full discussion, see chapter 10)

Burning, itching skin is probably due to a chlorine allergy. Open-water swimming is your only recourse.

To prevent recurring painful sinuses, sinus headaches, and sinus infections, wear nose clips.

Swimmer's ear—oozing, itch, and pain intensified when you tug on your earlobe—is caused by a continuously damp ear canal. (See chapter 10.)

If you have tinted, permanented, or easily tangled hair, apply the merest touch of baby oil to your hair before putting on your bathing cap. This prevents tangles and repels chlorine. Wear a cap with a Velcro band for an almost leakproof seal. Afterward, wash the chlorine out of your hair with plain soda water or tap water as soon as you leave the pool. Most shampoos remove any chlorine residue.

Although the water cools your body, you still sweat in the water and can suffer heat exhaustion from dehydration. Drink as much water as you can stand before and after each workout. (See chapter 10 for full discussion of heat exhaustion.)

Colds are the bane of swimmers during the winter. If you don't want to lose a couple of weeks of precious swim time, dry your hair before you go outside and, to be safe, cover your head with a hat or scarf.

BICYCLING

Women's cycling will finally become an Olympic event in 1984. It's about time. Cycling is the fourth most popular adult sport in the United States—20.2 million people (or 13 percent) cycle regularly to stay in shape. That's pretty impressive, but it's not the whole story. The number of bicycles in this country jumped from 25 million in 1960 to 95 million in 1980. What happened to those extra 70 million bikes? Many of them went to children, who are rarely counted in physical fitness surveys, maybe because the pollsters assume that children exercise instinctively anyway and can't be called athletes until they reach majority. The rest of the bicycles went to people who use them as cheap transportation to commute to work or ride to the supermarket. To these people, cycling isn't a sport; it's a necessity.

But cycling is a sport too, one of the best in the world. As a total aerobic exercise it strengthens your heart, lungs, and leg muscles, although it does nothing for your trunk, arms, or shoulders. It is complementary to speed skating and downhill skiing because it strengthens the leg muscles in the same ratios. Thus, you can cycle in the summer to stay in condition for skating and skiing in the winter (1980 women's world cycling champion and Olympic bronze medalist speed skater Beth Heiden says that cycling and speed skating share the same restricted and unnatural breathing position). Runners and tennis and racquetball players have discovered that cycling increases their stamina and the endurance in their leg muscles.

Your choices in cycling are boundless. Ride laps around the block, counting them off until you have ridden the requisite number for your workout. Or take thirty-minute to one-hour rides through city streets or down country roads. Once you are in shape, take cycle touring trips alone or with organized groups. Clubs all over the country organize day-long local outings or two-month European sightseeing tours. On tours, you ride fifty miles or so by day and bed down in comfortable hotels by night. (Touring isn't a sport just for young people; some clubs cater only to people over the age of fifty.) Or cycle-camp and sleep under the stars. Cyclecross, "off-road," or cross-country cycling uses a specially equipped bike to carry you over any terrain. Kids love bicycle motocross because maneuverable BMXes can do wheelies, cut sharp corners, and stay upright in mud and rain. Bicycle polo, once very popular in Great Britain and the United States, follows most of the rules of traditional horse polo.

Bicycle racing is making a comeback in this country after a hiatus of some forty years. (During the Depression, six-day 2,600-mile nonstop bicycle track races were as popular an entertainment as marathon dances.) Local bicycle competitions are held several times a year in most cities, although racing doesn't yet enjoy the popularity here that it does worldwide, where road racing and track racing combined make up the second most popular spectator sport, just behind soccer.

There are several kinds of cycling events. Outdoors, time trials take place on a measured flat course, "criteriums" of several laps run through a route set up along city streets, and road races of sixty miles or so speed over varied terrain, most of it mountainous. Combined, these are called tours, giros, or stage races. Outdoors or indoors, track races circle 336-meter banked oval circuits.

Evaluation

"Cycling is an excellent cardiovascular conditioner," says Allan J. Ryan, M.D., editor of *The Physician and Sportsmedicine*. "Some of the largest heart sizes measured in athletes are found in cyclists. They're right up there with cross-country skiers and oarsmen." Elite cyclists also have very high maximal oxygen uptake and lower heart rates.

According to cardiovascular physiologist William L. Haskell at Stanford University School of Medicine, cycling is "very useful" for weight reduction, raises the amount of high-density lipoproteins and lowers the amount of low-density lipoproteins (cholesterol) in your blood. It "improves the biochemical status of the body" so that there is less chance you will develop glucose intolerance or adult-onset diabetes. It doesn't prevent diabetes, but it can minimize its effects.

Cycling strengthens your thighs, your hips, and, to a much lesser extent, your calves. It has no effect on how flexible you are. It is much easier on the foot, knee, and hip than the jarring and bouncing of running and jumping sports, and so is more comfortable for many big-busted or overweight women.

Equipment

Before you run out and buy a nifty 26-pound ten-speed with a chrome molybdenum frame, alloy cranksets, and 240-gram skinny tires, ask yourself how you will use the bike. If you are going to ride around the neighborhood on flat terrain, just long enough to get a training effect, a no-speed, three-speed, or, at most, five-speed bike will serve amply. No-speed balloon-tired bikes use foot (or coaster) brakes and handlebars that let you sit upright as you pedal. While they are heavy and difficult to ride up and down hills, they force you into good condition on level ground because they provide resistance to each pedal stroke. They are sturdy but unfashionable, making them unattractive to bike thieves.

Three- and five-speed bikes use hand instead of foot brakes but have the no-speed's flat steer-horn handlebars. They are proportioned so that you can touch your feet to the ground while sitting on the seat. Thus it's easier to stop suddenly without falling off. The frames are lighter than the balloon-tired bombers, but they still have enough weight to give you a good workout.

If you ride more than thirty miles nonstop, or pedal up and down hills, you need a ten-speed. A ten-speed is an elegantly designed piece of machinery whose drive mechanism is 95 percent efficient. It gives you precision control over the terrain and over your effort to conquer it. A ten-speed, however, is hard to learn to ride. The position of the ram's horn (or "drop") handlebars, the hand brakes, and the seat and pedals force you to ride hunched over, the most aerodynamically efficient position. Until you get used to it, this position is murder on your back. These same proportions mean that you can't get off without rolling your bike halfway over onto its side. Many accidents happen when a cyclist must stop suddenly but can't steady herself with her feet or get off the bike in time. (Racers say that ten-speeds are meant to go, not to stop. Apparently they don't ride on city streets.) The skinny tires on a ten-speed make balancing difficult, and it takes savvy and experience to use your gears properly. Nonetheless, as one woman says, "They eat up the hills, and they're a gas to ride. On one of these things, you don't feel like an engine pushing a pair of wheels. You feel as though you *are* the bicycle."

Unless you are interested in racing, you'll want a touring bicycle. It has fenders to protect you from splattered mud; frames for carriers; heavier tires, rims, and wheels than racing cycles; and a wide range

---

SAFETY LEVERS

When you first ride long distances, the classic racer's crouch hurts your back, and you can't see the surrounding traffic, so you compensate by riding upright and holding the handlebars on top instead of down on the drops. This hand position moves your hands dangerously far from the brakes unless you install safety (or "assist" or "cheater") levers running from your main brake levers across the front of the handlebars. Unfortunately, these safety levers are anything but safe at high speeds, because they can cause your brakes to stick or can break off in your hands when you suddenly grab them forcefully for an emergency stop.

If you plan to tour and want to sit upright on a ten-speed, either tilt your handlebars up and move the brakes closer to your hands or buy a set of flat-bar hand-lever brakes that fit ten-speeds but operate like the hand brakes on three-speeds. They cost more to buy and install and are hard to find, but they do exist.

Mafac and Weinmann make brake levers for people with small hands (see Appendix B). If you have very small hands, buy children's levers.

between the low and high gears to carry you across any sort of landscape. Its sturdy frame and heavier tires make for a softer ride.

A road racing bicycle has a light frame, hard thin tires, and close gear ratios with ten- or twelve-speed derailleurs (the mechanism which disengages the chain and moves it from gear to gear). A track racing bicycle has no brakes or gearshifts at all. The racer adjusts the gears to suit the track before a race begins, and stops by pedaling backward while rubbing the front wheel with a gloved hand. Its steering is the most responsive of all bicycles. Cyclocross, bicycle motocross, or cross-country racing bicycles have heavier frames, wheels, and gear changers than other ten-speeds to keep them steady and upright in rough country. Some cyclocross bikes have handles so the racers can portage across creeks, ditches, or fences.

If you simply can't learn to balance on a two-wheeler, try one of the new adult tricycles. They are lightweight, streamlined, and have ten-speed gearshifts.

Bicycle frames come in three styles: men's, women's, and mixte (pronounced "meexed" in France and "mixty" in the United States). The woman's frame's low-slung crossbar permits you to mount while wearing a skirt but is weaker than the man's frame. The man's high crossbar, parallel to the ground, reinforces the frame but is difficult to mount. If you are short or plan to pedal in a skirt, try the mixte. It has a crossbar for reinforcement like a man's bike, but the bar comes down from the steering column at a diagonal instead of straight across.

To estimate the proper frame size, measure the inseam of your pants or the distance from your crotch to your ankle, and subtract 11 inches, for a rough approximation of the height of your bicycle. Bicycles are measured from the point where the seat post slides into the frame to the center of the crank, where your pedals attach to the axle. If you wear pants with a 33-inch inseam, you want a frame that's about 22 inches high. (Adult bikes are no longer measured by wheel size. Most general-purpose bikes have 27-inch wheels.)

Each brand is proportioned differently, so the best way to choose the right size is to stand straddling a man's bike. When you stand flat-footed, the crossbar should come as close as possible to your crotch without actually touching it. If you want a woman's or mixte style, measure yourself on a man's bike first and then get the same size in the other frame. Bicycle dealers usually steer you toward the correct size, if only because they must adjust the bicycle to your physique before you ride it out of the store. An under- or over-sized bike is almost impossible to adjust properly. Buy your bicycle only from a dealer who promises to readjust it free at least once during the first three months or 1,000 miles, so that you can customize it as you become more familiar with it.

When you are seated on the saddle (or seat), your knee should be slightly bent when your foot is at the bottom of the pedal stroke. If your knee is bent too much, your thigh muscles have to work too hard in order to get maximum drive power; if your leg is straight at the bottom of the stroke, you strain your knee. You should be able to touch the ground with both toes while sitting on the seat.

These specifications work for the average person. But what if you're not average? If you are short, you may have to lower the seat of even the smallest adult ten-speed to be able to touch the ground at all. If you do, however, the conventional geometry of bicycle design will leave you sitting on this lowered saddle with knees bent more than the prescribed "slight" angle. The added stability in start-stop riding more than compensates for the additional stress on your thigh muscles. When you take long uninterrupted rides, raise the seat back up for more power as you pedal. If you have particularly long legs, especially in the thigh, move your saddle back so that its nose lies directly above a point as much as three or four inches behind the hanger (where your pedals turn around).

The seats on no-speeds and three-speeds are wide, flat, and springy for a soft ride. The springiness, however, absorbs some of the push of your pedaling. The seats on touring and racing ten-speeds are narrow, to support only a portion of your weight; your arms on the handlebars support the rest. The narrow design also keeps your legs close together in an efficient pedaling position. Buy a woman's saddle, with its short nose and wide padded rear end indented to accommodate your curves. A leather saddle is the best investment. You have to break it in, like a pair of shoes, but once it conforms to your backside, you'll never give it up. Even when you buy a new bicycle, you'll put your old saddle on it. A plastic saddle conforms quickly to your anatomy, does not bleed dyes onto your clothes, and doesn't lose its shape when it gets wet. But it wears out faster, feels hot, and makes you sweat on hot days. Whatever saddle you buy, any edges that touch your legs should be smooth and padded to avoid chafing.

The tilt of the seat affects the comfort of your ride. The "average" person goes for a level saddle, but many people tilt the nose of the seat upward slightly, to put the weight on their buttocks, or downward, as many women prefer, to take the pressure off the crotch. Tilt the saddle down too much, however, and your arms and legs will have to work too hard to keep you straight on the bike. Sliding the seat forward may also take the pressure off your crotch. A forward position gives you power for sprints; a seat slid back of center gives you a comfortable touring position.

Gearshift levers are placed on the gooseneck (the stem holding your handlebars), or on the down tube (the lower diagonal tube of the

BREAKING IN A BICYCLE SADDLE

Even a so-called preconditioned stretched leather saddle may still feel rock-hard after 1,000 miles unless you beat it around. When you first buy a seat, sit on it for a general idea of the shape and then take it off and leave it in the sun for about a half hour, or until it feels soft. Rub neat's-foot oil, mink oil, or saddle dressing on the underside. (Don't oil the top.) Tighten a belt or strap around the center of the saddle to turn under the edges where your thighs rub. Let the saddle sit out in the sun for a day, and in a warm (not hot) place for a night. Next day, rub the top of the saddle with saddle soap and beat it lightly and rhythmically with a ball pean hammer or a heavy dowel. Concentrate on the rear and top, corners, and any other area that felt uncomfortable. When you've softened the seat (stubborn saddles may take several days of heating and beating—but not oiling), wipe off the oil and residues, tighten the tension nut at the front of the saddle, and put it back on the bike. The oil will continue to ooze through the leather for a few weeks—or months—so wear dark pants.

frame), or in the ends of the handlebars. Levers on the gooseneck are easiest for a beginner—and anyone who rides upright—because you don't have to move your hands far in order to reach them and they are accessible for repairs. Racers prefer their levers on the down tube because, they say, the action is direct, and it is easier to move a hand from the drops to the down tube if you ride in a crouched position. Tip shifters, in the ends of the handlebar, sit close to your hands in the classic racing crouch but are not responsive, because every movement of the lever must travel through a long length of cable inside the handlebar and then down the central stem before it can signal the derailleurs to shift. If the model you choose has its shift levers in the wrong place, your dealer will move them, free of charge, when you buy the bike.

Until you start riding more than thirty miles a day, wear any comfortable hard-soled shoe. Soft shoes, such as running or crepe-soled shoes, absorb too much of the force of each push on the pedals. For long mileage, stiff cycling shoes, with or without a steel shank along the arch, transmit the maximum force to your pedals.

Toe clips add a huge measure of efficiency to each pedaling stroke. These little cages for the front half of your foot bolt onto your metal rat-trap pedals. By using the clips to pull up on one pedal while you push down on the other, you double the power of each stroke. Toe clips keep your feet straight on the pedals so you don't apply side pressure on your knees. They also keep your feet from slipping off the pedals, the most common cause of bicycle accidents.

Safety and protection.   Bicycle riding is the most dangerous recreational activity in the country, according to the National Electronic Injury Surveillance System. In 1980, 537,100 people were hospitalized from bicycle accidents, as compared with 438,860 for baseball, 425,300 for football, and 319,850 for basketball. Sixty-two percent of all those injured in bicycling accidents are children between the ages of five and fourteen years. Bicycling deaths have risen by more than 25 percent since 1967 because bicyclists now ride in the streets instead of on the sidewalks. Cars hitting bikes—and bikes hitting cars—cause 20 percent of all accidents but 90 percent of all deaths.

The face and head are injured more frequently than any other part of the body. If you wear a cycling helmet, you reduce your chances of a disfiguring or fatal accident by up to 50 percent. In helmets, you get what you pay for: The expensive helmets give you more protection and are less confining than bargain-basement models. A good helmet is light, well ventilated, and doesn't obstruct your forward or peripheral vision. It has a high-impact shell outside and snug foam cell cushions inside. Leather racing "hairnets" don't provide much protection at all. The Mirrycle, a motorcycle-style mirror available in bicycle shops, attaches to the brake lever assembly on your handlebar to provide an excellent rear view at near eye level.

Riding at night is extremely dangerous because you can't see hazards on the street and car drivers can't see you. The reflectors required by most states on the front and rear ends of your bike, the sides of your wheels, and your pedals help, but not all of them are effective enough. Bicycle reflectors vary. Replace yours with three-inch red reflectors sold in auto parts stores.

Studies show that drivers don't react to spots of light unless they figure out what they mean. To look like a person on a bicycle, wear reflectorized slacks and a windbreaker. Reflectorized backpacks and reflectorized tape liberally stuck all over your clothes are less expensive but far from ideal alternatives. However, the all-over reflectorized material these suits, backpacks, and patches are made of do not reflect light well when the rider is under streetlights or in two-way traffic. They only work when a car's headlight beams hit you in pitch blackness at an optimal angle. Until these technical problems are solved, you must augment your passive reflector system with an active light source. Attach a battery-operated or generator-powered headlight to the handlebars of your bicycle and wear a battery-operated light on your arm or your leg, or both.

Observe the following fifteen rules for safe bicycling:

1. Obey all traffic signals, street signs, and one-way streets. Consider your bicycle a road machine just like a car, motorcycle, or truck. Your state's vehicle code does, and you are subject to citations and fines

for going the wrong way on one-way streets, running stop signs, and riding two abreast.

2. Ride with the prevailing flow of traffic. On a two-way street, ride in the right lane, but don't hug the curb or the row of parked cars. Ride at least three feet out into the lane, clear of suddenly opening car doors and cars pulling out of the parking lane. Force the car behind you to pull out fully into the next lane to pass you. (If you ride close to parked cars, a car may try to squeeze past you by pulling out only slightly into the next lane. Oncoming traffic may force the car back into your lane to pin you against the parked cars.) Don't duck into spaces between parked cars or at intersections. You are invisible tucked into each curbside niche, and a car coming up on your flank may sideswipe you as you try to pull back into the traffic lane. Don't ride abreast of a car's right rear quarter—that's the driver's blind spot. If you are riding at slower than prevailing speed, pull over into long empty curbside spaces occasionally to let cars pass. On a one-way street, ride on the side with fewer hazards.

3. Use the conventional motorist's hand signals to tell automobile drivers you are stopping or turning. However, make eye contact with each driver to make sure he or she understands your signal.

4. Watch for opening car doors and cars pulling into traffic.

5. If traffic is very heavy, do not attempt a left turn from the left lane. Instead, get off your bike and cross at the crosswalk as a pedestrian. Most car/bike accidents happen at intersections.

6. Ride defensively, watching not only the car immediately in front of you but the car in front of that. Stay a few bike lengths behind a car so that you have enough time to stop or swerve.

7. Whenever possible, ride in bike lanes instead of congested streets.

8. Do not ride on sidewalks—you become a menace to pedestrians as well as yourself.

9. Watch for potholes, gravel in the street, soft shoulders, drain grates, cattle guards, railroad tracks, and other road surface hazards. Even on clean streets, loose sand and gravel may accumulate at corners.

10. Keep your brakes in perfect working order and all moving parts clean and oiled. Keep your tires properly inflated, so that the bicycle will steer responsively. Make sure your bicycle fits you, and check pedals, lights, reflectors, shifting mechanisms, tires, spokes, saddle, handlebars, sounding devices, and all nuts and bolts regularly.

11. Don't carry passengers, especially if they interfere with your vision. A second person throws off your balance.

12. Don't carry packages in front of your handlebars if they interfere with your vision. Put baggage in panniers or other carriers designed for bicycles and properly installed.

13. Never hitch a ride on a truck, car, motorcycle, or other vehicle.

14. Wear a helmet.

15. Don't ride at night unless it is absolutely essential. If you must, wear lights and reflective clothing.

Relative cost.   Until you know exactly what kind of bicycle you want, ride a borrowed one if you can find it. They are free. Otherwise, used bicycles, often in very good condition, begin at $5. New three-, five-, and ten-speeds start at $100; superduper racing machines cost more than $1,200. Good-quality helmets cost upwards of $25, and shoes begin around $15.

Precautions

Bicycling is an infinitely adaptable sport. You can ride slowly with easy gears on a flat street or ride at high speeds in stiffer gears over hills and mountains. Thus it is safe for just about anyone except a person with very serious heart disease.

Goals for Fitness

"Cyclists," says Allan Ryan, "should allow at least thirty minutes of nonstop riding at least three times a week at a heart rate of 60 percent." Riding at a higher rate is exhausting and may wear out your thigh muscles before you get a thorough workout. You get a training effect just by keeping your legs constantly pedaling for thirty minutes. Ride in a medium gear to feel a moderate amount of resistance on flat terrain. (If you live in the city, you may have trouble finding a relatively flat area free of stop signs or traffic lights to ride nonstop.)

Use the talk/sing test or count your carotid pulse at first. You may lose control of your bicycle if you try the contortions necessary to take your radial pulse while steering.

Training

Perform the universal warm-ups, concentrating on the quads, hamstring, and calf muscles. Trunk and arm warm-ups will prevent cramps after holding the same cycling position for a half hour. For your cardiovascular warm-up, either jog around slowly for a few minutes or ride very slowly. At the end of a hard ride of hill climbing or sprints, cool down by riding slowly and leisurely for five minutes and then repeat the warm-ups to relax your muscles. After a long but not arduous ride, just the five minutes of lazy cycling is enough.

TABLE VIII: BICYCLING PROGRAM

Week	Miles	Time	Miles Per Hour
1	1	at your ease	
2	2	at your ease	
3	3	18 minutes	10
4	4	24 minutes	10
5	4	20 minutes	12
6	4	18 minutes	13.5
7	4	16 minutes	15
8	5	30 minutes	10
9	5	25 minutes	12
10	5	22 minutes	13.5
11	5	20 minutes	15
12	6	36 minutes	10
13	6	30 minutes	12
14	6	27 minutes	13.5
15	6	24 minutes	15
16	7	42 minutes	10
17	7	35 minutes	12
18	7	31 minutes	13.5
19	7	28 minutes	15
20	8	48 minutes	10
21	8	40 minutes	12
22	8	35 minutes	13.5
23	8	32 minutes	15

Beginner's level

To teach yourself to ride a bike, temporarily lower the seat so that your feet scoot along the ground. Push yourself off with your feet, lift your feet from the ground, and try to balance. Once you can balance, start pedaling. This will add a little speed, which actually makes balancing easier, not harder. Once you can balance, raise the seat back to its adult height.

It takes longer to build up your ability to cycle over a distance than to run over a distance. It may take you only four months to learn to run for thirty minutes nonstop at a decent pace, but it will take you six months to be able to cycle for the same length of time. If you have never ridden before, cycle only a half mile the first day and work up to a mile by the end of the first week. Then, following the schedule in Table VIII, alternate weeks of adding miles with weeks of increasing your speed. If this schedule progresses too quickly for you, spend two weeks at each stage. If it moves too slowly, eliminate the 10-mile-per-hour weeks and never ride slower than 12 miles per hour, even when you add new mileage.

Continue riding eight miles in thirty to thirty-two minutes until it feels too easy. Then gradually increase your mileage until you are riding an hour a day at least three days a week. Because bicycles are such efficient machines, they do much of the work once you are in condition. To stay in good shape, you'll probably have to ride for an hour instead of thirty minutes.

SPEED AND WIND RESISTANCE

If you are in moderate shape, your cruising speed is 10 miles per hour. At this speed, you are expending one third of your energy just to push away the air in front of you. If you are in good condition, you cruise and tour at 15 mph and sprint at 20 mph. At 20 mph you expend half your effort just to push the air, and at a racing speed of 30 mph you use 90 percent of your energy to push away the air.

Intermediate Level

If you can ride comfortably for at least an hour at a speed of 10 to 15 miles per hour, you have reached the intermediate level. In addition, you should be able to ride in a straight line without wobbling or swerving, shift without taking your eyes off the road, lean into turns, make tight turns, and steer around potholes or broken glass by aiming your front wheel to one side of the obstacle and your back wheel to the other. You should also know the rudiments of repairing and adjusting your own bike so that you don't suffer week-long layoffs while your bike is in the shop for some minor malfunction. (*Bicycling* magazine and *Anybody's Bike Book* have step-by-step instructions; see Selected Reading.)

Now you're ready for tours and races. Add some fartlek, or speed-play (see "Running"), to your workouts for the anaerobic capacity you need on hills, fast starts, and sprints for the finish line. Once or twice a week, ride a course of alternately hard and easy legs. Either ride briskly over a flat course interspersed with steep hills or sprint to breathlessness for ten minutes, coast until you're rested, and then sprint again—hard, easy, hard, easy—until your hour is up. Because fartlek and other kinds of interval training stress your muscles the way weight training does, never practice them more than three times a week and never on two consecutive days.

Once you reach an intermediate level, little elements of style make a big difference in your performance. For example, pedal on your toes and the ball of your foot rather than the arch or flat of your foot. "Keep the ball of your foot centered over the axle of your pedal," says Keith Kingbay of Excelsior Fitness Equipment Company, a division of Schwinn Company, "and use a lot of ankle motion. Extend your ankle

---

CADENCE

Pedaling cadence makes the difference between an exhausted rider and one who can ride for hours without aching muscles. If you know the number of times per minute you are comfortable pedaling, you can synchronize your gears so that you always hover around that cadence.

To find your normal cadence, ride up and down a mile-long road in whatever gear feels most comfortable and count the number of times per minute your right foot reaches the bottom of its stroke. A recreational rider or cycle tourist usually has a cadence between 60 and 80 revolutions per minute. A racer works at about 90.

However, very skillful cyclists spin. They ride in an easy gear at a cadence of about 120 rpms in order to ride for long distances without tiring. Although they move their legs faster, they do less work. It takes practice to spin. At first, your feet seem to whirl around the pedals and you feel as if you are speeding out of control. Ease into spinning. Ride in the lowest gear you can stand, and step down to lower gears as you become more adept. Once you can spin, you'll be able to ride farther with less effort and more pleasure.

---

on the down part of your stroke, and flex it by dropping your heel on the upstroke so that you can lift and pull the toe clips."

Moving your seat forward or back can also improve your efficiency. "The saddle should be behind the place where the pedals turn around," says Kingbay. "We call that the hanger. If the cranks of your bike are parallel to the ground, and your foot is on the pedal, a plumb line dropped from the knob of your knee should fall about three quarters of an inch behind the pedal." If your saddle is too far forward, you can't move your ankles freely.

Hand position makes a 14 percent difference in your effectiveness, according to a study done at California State University at Sacramento. If you rest your hands on the tops of the bars, you are only 86 percent as efficient as if you rested them on the drops the way racers do. However, using the drops and the racer's crouch for touring long distances is very uncomfortable. To compromise, tilt your handlebars so that the tops are parallel to the ground, the drops are angled up a bit (more like a living ram's horns), and the brakes are moved closer to your hands.

Advanced Level

If you can ride for two hours at an 18- or 19-mile-per-hour pace, you are an advanced cyclist. If you want to tour, you need progress no further.

If you want to race, however, you must improve your anaerobic capacity, build up your speed, and increase your endurance. If you work on only one of these skills, you train only some of your fibers.

Interval training imitates the fast-slow, uphill-downhill nature of most road races. To improve your power, ride for short bursts at 90 to 95 percent effort, coast until your pulse comes down to the 60 or 70 percent level, then lay on the steam again. Ride slowly even during your rest periods because, as in swimming, much of the training effect comes during these incomplete rests. If you ride in hilly countryside, where short steep uphills alternate with equally short steep downhills, you have built-in intervals. If you ride a flat course, sprint at top speed for one minute, then coast or soft-pedal for one minute, then sprint again, for a total of ten to fifteen intervals per workout. You can get the same effect by alternating high and low gears. To cap off this exhausting workout, do two or three longer intervals, pedaling all-out for two or three minutes, then pedaling at your 60 or 70 percent rate for an equal amount of time in order to recover. Practice intervals no more than three days a week, and never two days in a row.

Speed distance training requires a 70 percent effort over a minimum of an hour to condition your muscles to ride at a fast pace for a sustained period. Once a week, ride a 10- to 25-mile course as fast as you can. Try to improve your time each week.

Long Steady Distance training for a racer involves at least 60 miles (about 100 kilometers) in two and a half hours pedaling at 80 to 100 revolutions per minute at least once a week to build your endurance. Ride a total of 150 miles each week. If you enter 30-mile (48-kilometer) races, however, you don't need this advanced sort of LSD. Forty-five to 90 miles a week are enough.

Stationary bicycles.   Can't cycle in winter? Desperate for exercise while you're recovering from tennis elbow? Want exercise but don't want to leave the house? Try a stationary bicycle.

A stationary bicycle (or Exercycle, ergometer, or exercise bike) gives you the same muscular and cardiovascular workout as cycling in the same length of time. Because you move your muscles through different angles and at different tensions than in other sports, you can often cycle when you can't play your usual sport, so you stay in shape and get the high of a good workout without pain. And you can ride LSD on an ergometer while reading a magazine set on a music rack or watching television.

A good exercise bike is very stable. (Test it in the store by standing up during your ride.) It has an adjustable tension device so that you can adjust the resistance by moving a dial or lever on or very near the handlebars while the pedals are moving. The wheel spokes are covered, the pedals have straps to keep your feet in place, and the gauges record revolutions per minute, speed, and distance.

The training principles are the same as for outdoor cycling. You must work at least thirty minutes—one hour is optimal—at 60 percent of your target pulse rate at least three times a week. However, the speedometer is not as good a pacer as a miles-per-hour gauge is for outdoor bikes. Indoors, you have no wind resistance pushing against you, so you may pedal at a rate of 30 miles per hour and not get your pulse above 55 percent of maximum. Warm up your muscles with universal warm-ups, and then warm up your heart by pedaling for the first five minutes with the tension set at an easy mark. Next, increase the tension a bit until you are breathing heavily. When you get your second wind, increase the tension slightly again to maintain your target heart rate. Pedal, huffing and puffing and dripping sweat, until your thirty minutes are up. Cool down with a light-tension cruise for five minutes, and you're done.

If you want to train for summer riding with some fartlek or intervals, your exercise bicycle will oblige, but first it needs a few modifications. You must proportion it to resemble a real bike so that you are exercising the same muscles in the proper ratios. Change the slippery rubber pedals and vinyl foot straps to rat-trap pedals and toe clips. (If standard pedals don't fit, try BMX pedals.) Replace the wide cushiony seat with a ten-speed-style saddle. Angle it and move it up and down, forward or backward, until its position feels comfortable and familiar. If you like, replace the flat handlebars with a pair of drops. Thus equipped, you can alternate bursts of hard and easy riding, changing the tension when you would shift gears, for a complete workout.

Injuries

Cycling is easier on the foot, knee, and hip than running or jumping sports. If your knees ache, check the size of your bicycle and the position of your seat—your bicycle is probably too big or your seat too low. If you get neck- or backaches from the racer's crouch, you are probably rounding your back. Keep your back straight, at a 45-degree angle to your hips. Leg cramps over distances or on hills may disappear with adequate training, although they may be caused by overuse of one leg or the other, a common habit of cyclists. Saddle sores and bruises fade away when you break in your saddle. If your hands get numb on long rides, pad the handlebars with special foam tubing available at bike shops, tilt your handlebars so that the tops are parallel to the ground or the drops are 15 degrees or more below horizontal.

Heat is always a problem for cyclists. Drink plenty of water before and during any ride. Keep the water in your water bottle tolerably cool by wrapping it in a water-soaked sock or other fabric tube. Evaporation off the sock lowers the temperature of the bottle. Take the usual precautions to prevent heatstroke.

Even if the weather seems merely brisk, you become very cold bicycling because you move through the air quickly enough to create your own wind-chill factor. (Just as you feel colder on a windy 10-degree winter day than a calm 10-degree day, you feel colder riding 15 miles per hour than walking 4 miles per hour or running 8 miles per hour.) For example, if it is 45 degrees outside, and you are riding at 15 miles per hour, while the wind is blowing at 10 miles per hour, your combined windspeed is 25 miles per hour, and the temperature feels like 23 degrees. (See Table XIV in chapter 10.) Therefore, you must dress for 23-degree weather, not 45. Temperatures of 50 degrees or more don't feel cold unless you get wet. If it rains on you in the middle of your ride, however, you increase your heat loss twenty-five fold. Dress in layers, with cotton or polypropylene fishnet closest to your skin to carry moisture away from your body while trapping heat in its air holes, and wool in your outside layer to carry away moisture and still keep you warm. Layers leave air pockets for insulation and permit you to strip if you get too hot. Wear a hat; you lose at least 30 percent of your body heat through your head. For rain gear, avoid long raincoats or ponchos because they can get caught in your chain or wheels. Instead, wear a waterproof jacket and waterproof pants made out of a breathable laminate. If you've ever exercised in an ordinary impermeable plastic rain suit, you know you can get as drenched from your own sweat inside the suit as you can in the rain. Gore-Tex and other breathable waterproofs are well worth the investment.

If your feet get cold, wear fleece-lined boots or shoes or put Baggies over your shoes as Keith Kingbay does. Remove the baggies if your feet sweat, because perspiration will eventually make you colder.

RUNNING

Running has been overplayed. Although it is only the sixth most popular sport in the country (17.1 million adults, or 11 percent), it gets more ink in newspapers and magazines than any other sport. Much of this publicity focuses on the metaphysics of running and the religious and emotional highs of distance work. And that's too bad, because such talk turns off many people who would enjoy running simply to condition their hearts and lungs and get out in the fresh air.

Running is one of the best cardiovascular conditioners there is. It trains you faster than all other sports—with the exception of rowing and cross-country skiing—and promotes fat loss best. However, it strengthens only the backs of the legs and it decreases your flexibility.

Running is an easy, natural, instinctive sport. You need no lessons at all to get out on the road, although once you're hooked you'll spend the rest of your life adjusting and perfecting your stride. You can run in almost any kind of weather—even rain or snow if you are dedicated enough—and, in fact, may discover that cold and inclement weather is the best time because you have the roads to yourself and can't get overheated.

Running gets you out of the office or house and onto a running path or your neighborhood streets. Since running is such a visible sport, it's easy to find partners to keep you company and keep you honest. ("What do you mean you want to quit now? We've only run two blocks.") You can run almost anywhere, wherever you work, live, or travel, so you can work out daily no matter what you're doing. A sales rep who travels regularly runs up and down hotel corridors and stairways when she is afraid to go out into the surrounding neighborhood. A New York woman who can only run at night runs twenty-three-lap miles around her terrace, reversing direction halfway through to develop both legs equally.

Running is an entirely personal experience. You can run Long Steady Distance for an hour just for the thrill of moving and the pleasure of smelling the flowers, or you can challenge yourself to improve steadily by recording your time and distance in a daily diary. (Don't overdo the speed, however. You get a better aerobic effect from running a moderate pace for a half hour than from running as fast as you can for fifteen minutes.)

Running began as a private passion, but somewhere along the line an unfortunate shift in emphasis took place. You aren't a runner if you're not a racer, said the gurus. Come off it. If you run every day, several days a week, month in and month out, you're a runner. If you dislike all competitive sports, or if you prefer to vent your killer instincts on the handball court or hockey rink and save your running for conditioning and relaxation, you are still a runner.

If racing intrigues you, however, the contests scheduled in almost every city in the country give you a chance to see how you compare with other runners of your age and experience. It's addictive—that prickly excitement you feel the first time you finish a marathon or ultramarathon—because you have conquered two challengers: the opponent and yourself. There are so many races—on tracks, roads, and over the countryside, ranging from 440 yards and one-milers through 10Ks (6.2 miles) and marathons (26 miles, 385 yards) to ultramarathons of 100 miles—that you can, with a little experimentation, find the race best suited to your body type and run it all year long. Don't expect to reach your peak of experience or endurance for several years. Even in championship-level racing, the top runners in middle- and long-distance events are in their late twenties or early thirties. It takes time to develop your racing potential.

Orienteering combines the thrill of a cross-country race with the beauty of wilderness hiking and the intellectual challenge of planning routes and developing strategies. A Swedish import introduced into the United States by the Boy Scouts at Indiana Dunes Park in 1946, orienteering is the road runner's equivalent of an automobile road rally. Runners navigate a preordained cross-country course by means of compass and map in search of several hidden station markers, or "controls." At each station, the orienteer perforates her card with a distinctive punch. But whereas a car rallyer tries to arrive at each station—and at the finish line—at a specified hour, the orienteer tries to navigate across the terrain in the shortest possible time. Running speed is important, but so is map-reading skill and judgment. The only equipment you need besides your running shoes is a liquid needle compass, available for $3 to $10 and often loaned to entrants at meets. Because every meet has several courses, graded for difficulty, novices and elite orienteers may compete together in this "thinking runner's sport."

Evaluation

Running is an aerobic exercise, pure and simple. It does wonders for your heart, increases the oxygen capacity of your lungs and circulatory system, and burns calories faster than most endurance sports, but it does nothing for your flexibility. In fact, it tightens you up if you're not careful. It strengthens only the backs of your legs (the hamstrings and calves), while it weakens the quadriceps in the fronts of your thighs. If you are looking for the maximum amount of cardiac conditioning in the minimum amount of time, running is for you. If you want all-around strength and flexibility too, you will have to augment your running with swimming or rowing or weight lifting for upper body strength and concentrated flexibility exercises for limberness.

Equipment

All you need is shoes, but the choice can be overwhelming. Rival running magazines publish ratings of the "best" and the "worst" shoes of each year, but all too often the best shoes on one list are rated poorest on another. Shoe buyers must choose among racing flats, trainers, and shoes with all sorts of special claims for stability, lightness, flexibility, sturdiness . . .

What you want, first and foremost, is protection for your foot. Running may be natural, but tell that to your feet. If you run for long distances, especially on concrete, you are likely to get blisters, blackened toes, perhaps even shin splints or runner's knee, particularly if you fall for one of those streamlined, elegant pairs of racing flats which provide little support or shock absorption. Well-fitting shoes, designed for your type of foot, eliminate most of these problems.

Women's sizes are cut narrow, so if you have wide feet, you may be happier at the men's rack. Choose a shoe with a cushiony sole for shock absorption. If you weigh under, say, 105 pounds, and if you run on dirt paths or grass, you can probably get away with a super-light training shoe. Otherwise, look for some spring to the shoe when you try it on. Although the sole should be flexible under the balls of the feet to allow the foot to bend through each running step, it should have a solid shank (or arch) to keep your foot from over-pronating. Place the shoes on a flat surface and view them from eye level. Neither heels nor soles nor toe boxes should tilt inward or outward. Otherwise, they will force your feet to tilt inward or outward.

The toe box should feel roomy, and there should be about an inch between the end of your toes and the end of the shoe. You should be able to wiggle and spread your toes a bit, but the heel should fit snugly. The heel cup should be shaped like a shallow bowl, not a flat plate, because your heel is rounded on the bottom. The heel counter should be padded where it hits the Achilles tendon. The heel should be about an inch high.

Good cross-country and orienteering shoes have spikes or rubber studs on the soles, with some clustered near the front of the toe so you can drive off at the end of each stride. Studs and strong, heavy construction support you over muddy and rough terrain and steep downhill runs.

These are merely generalized hints. If you are flat-footed or have high arches, or if you turn your ankles in when you run, or if your feet

---

RUNNING BAREFOOT

Running barefoot is one of the most transcendent experiences in athletics. Your toes stretch out and grab the grass or sand, and your feet seem to skim the ground. The soles of your feet are almost as sensitive to touch as your hands. Smooth beaches and rippling meadows conceal textures of the finest silks and velvets. Unfortunately, there are also hidden rocks, prickles, thorns, chuckholes, and squooshy places.

Unless your feet are calloused from walking barefooted on concrete or through woods, and your ankles are very strong, don't run barefooted in meadows or woodlands. If you want to run on the beach, run along the edge of the water where the sand is firm and smooth. The extra work you do to push off the sand will add power to your stride and strength to your legs. Mounded dry sand is too soft and allows your heels to sink so far that it stresses your Achilles tendons or twists your ankles.

are particularly wide or especially narrow, you need specially designed shoes, all available at any well-stocked running-shoe store. As much as possible, road-test your shoes in the store. Jump up and down in them or run in place. Many serious running-shoe stores even have a hall or runway for testing. Don't count on breaking in a pair of shoes. If they don't fit in the store, they never will.

Dress for the weather. If it is hot, wear loose-fitting shorts and a sleeveless T-shirt made of natural fibers to allow your perspiration to evaporate and cool air to enter. If it is cold, dress in layers so that you can peel off the excess. Wear a hat in cold weather, to avoid heat loss through your scalp.

Relative cost.   A pair of running shoes costs from $30 to $70. If you can find a genuinely comfortable shoe at the lower end of the scale, buy it, but if you have an odd foot structure demanding an expensive pair of shoes, indulge yourself. You will never enjoy running if your feet hurt all the time.

Precautions

Although you can run fast or slow, depending on your condition, running is a strenuous sport. Don't start a running program if you have heart disease, high blood pressure, or high serum cholesterol levels unless your doctor approves. (Since running is prescribed for people recovering from heart attacks and open heart surgery, the odds are that it will be okay.)

Running is extremely jarring. During each running stride, there is a moment when both feet are off the ground and the body is floating in air. When one foot lands again, it absorbs up to five times the body's weight—over 600 pounds of pressure for a 125-pound woman—so that with each footfall you squash your spine up like an accordion, tighten your Achilles tendons, shins, calves, and hamstrings, and throw your knees out of whack. If you already have knee or lower back problems, running may aggravate them. If you are overweight, all that pounding may hurt your knees. In these cases, swimming, cycling, or walking may be more suitable.

Goals for Fitness

You can improve your cardiovascular tone with as little as fifteen minutes of actual running at your target pulse rate three times a week, but if you want to lose weight too, work up to at least thirty minutes. It is not speed but distance that burns calories. If you sprint through your day's run, you enter a partially anaerobic phase and actually burn fewer calories than you do at slower speeds.

When you first begin running, monitor your heart rate. Take your pulse while you're running and clock your recovery rate as soon as you finish. Then, once you get the rhythm of running, use the talk/sing test instead.

Training

"Your range of motion in running," says Fred Kasch, "is even less than that of walking. You don't move your shoulders or your upper trunk. The longer you run the more you use your lower back muscles, buttocks, hamstrings, calves, and Achilles tendons—all your posterior muscles—until they tighten and ache." Stretch out these muscles before and after each workout. In addition, strengthen their antagonists, for you can't run very fast if one set of muscles is short and tight while their opposite numbers are long and weak.

The universal warm-ups will serve you well until you join the four- or five-mile-a-day set. Then add squats or kiddie kicks to strengthen your quads (the muscles in the front of your thigh) and strengthen your shins by doing a variation on kiddie kicks: Instead of raising your lower leg, just flex your ankle. Your killer sit-ups and knee-nose touches will protect your back. If your hamstrings, Achilles tendons, and groin feel very stiff, add towel stretches and wall splits (see chapter 6).

Running ten miles or more a day shortens your hamstrings and may send the muscles along your vertebral spine into spasm. Under these conditions, doing a rounded back gravity toe touch by bending from the waist can hurt your back and even herniate a disk if you are susceptible. If gravity toe touches put a strain on your back even when you keep your back straight and bend from the hips, eliminate them and do towel stretches or runner's starts (see chapter 6). Or try barre hamstring stretches.

Warm up your heart before moving into your full run with a brisk walk or slow jog, and cool it down the same way. (The word "jogger" is to a runner as "duffer" is to a golfer. Jogging has been demoted, as of late, to slow warm-up and cool-down shuffles.)

BARRE HAMSTRING STRETCHES

Stand up and prop one leg on a table, ironing board, or ballet barre. Holding your back straight and flat, lean forward slowly from the hips, reaching for your toes with your hands. Hold, release by bending both knees, and repeat with the other leg.

Beginner's Level

You must walk before you can run. At first, walk during most of your session. As your wind and muscular endurance improve, increase the ratio of running to walking until you are running the entire time. Your goal is time (thirty minutes) rather than distance or speed. Even after you can run nonstop for thirty minutes, you needn't worry about distance or speed, for as you become a more efficient runner, you naturally pick up speed and thus go farther in the same thirty minutes.

Don't begin the run/walk program in Table IX until you can comfortably walk three miles in forty-five minutes. If the schedule moves too quickly, spend two weeks on each run/walk interval. If it is too slow, skip a week. Until your muscles stop aching, run only three days a week, and never two days in a row.

TABLE IX: RUN/WALK PROGRAM

Week	Run Interval	Walk Interval	Repeats
1	one minute	two minutes°	10
2	1½ minutes	two minutes	9
3	two minutes	two minutes	8
4	three minutes	two minutes	6
5	three minutes	two minutes	4
	five minutes	two minutes	1
6	five minutes	three minutes	4
7	five minutes	two minutes	4
8	six minutes	three minutes	1
	five minutes	two minutes	3
9	six minutes	two minutes	4
10	eight minutes	three minutes	1
	six minutes	two minutes	2
11	eight minutes	two minutes	3
12	ten minutes	three minutes	1
	eight minutes	two minutes	1
	five minutes	three minutes	1
13	ten minutes	four minutes	2
14	ten minutes	three minutes	2
	five minutes	none	1
15	ten minutes	two minutes	2
	six minutes	none	1
16	ten minutes	one minute	3
17	thirty minutes nonstop		

° If this recovery interval is too short, walk until you have caught your breath and stay at this level until you can comfortably continue with the schedule.

After you finish each run, jog for five or ten minutes, until you have caught your breath. Don't just collapse on the ground in an exhausted heap. Stretch again, after you have caught your breath, and then collapse.

In the beginning, your stride will be relatively short, and that's fine. It will lengthen naturally as your muscles become stronger. Keep your steps close to the ground but don't shuffle. Bouncing is just a waste of energy. You want to go forward, not up.

Don't look at your feet when you run because it throws your posture out of line and makes it harder to breath properly. Breathe deeply with your mouth open, trying to fill your abdomen as well as your lungs with air. If you ever become so winded you can't catch your breath by normal means, get down on all fours, drop your head between your arms, and pant like a dog.

Bend your elbows so that your forearms are more or less parallel to the ground. Keep your arms loose and hold your elbows very slightly away from your body. Keep your hands gently cupped, and swing your arms freely in natural opposition to your legs—your right arm forward with your left leg, and vice versa. Your wrists break (or flop) naturally with each swing. Your arm motion balances your leg movements and keeps your trunk from twisting. The pumping motion helps drive you forward, pushes your body up hills, and sets the tempo for your stride. Occasionally, shake out your arms and let them dangle to keep your shoulders relaxed.

Run in a straight line and keep your feet under your body. Don't swivel your legs out to the sides and run knock-kneed. All rumors to the contrary, your wide female pelvis does *not* predestine you to run "like a girl." It's just a bad habit, and if you don't break it, you'll be not only an inefficient runner but an inefficient runner with bad knees.

Vary your route to keep your runs interesting. Run around the neighborhood. Run around the park. Run with friends. Run alone (but only in daylight in very well-populated areas). Once in a while, run on the high school track. Running around and around in a circle (it's actually an oval) is the most boring running there is, unless it's a novelty. However, if you run on a premeasured track once every few months, you learn how many miles you can run in your half hour. Enter this distance in a logbook, and compare it with the distance you ran six months earlier.

No matter how advanced you become, don't run more than five or six days a week. You need one or two days off to let your muscles recover and to prevent overtraining.

Once you can run thirty minutes nonstop at least three days a week, you have a fitness program to last you a lifetime. For health, weight control, and mental diversion, thirty minutes a day is plenty. Your distance will increase as your stride becomes stronger and faster, but from now on the only reason to run longer than a half hour is for the fun of it.

DOG'S BEST FRIEND?

It's a beautiful sunny day, perfect weather for a run—or a bike ride—with your dog. You begin together, but after about a mile your dog starts to pant heavily and lag behind. You whistle and he leaps up again and off you go. A minute or so later, he's lagging much farther behind and limping, with his tail dragging and his head down, gasping for air. Whistle, and he tries to catch up but can't. Instead, he stumbles and falls, and dies of heat prostration in your arms.

Many a thoughtless distance runner has run her dog into heat prostration. Because dogs are naively loyal and instinctively obey the commands of their pack leader (you), they run when you tell them to run even when they are in great pain. They try to keep up because they're afraid of being left behind in strange territory.

Dogs have no sweat glands. They cool themselves by panting, not a terribly efficient method of lowering body temperature. Bulldogs, boxers, and other dogs with square, flattened faces handle heat particularly badly. So do overweight or aging dogs.

They must be trained to heat and distance, the way humans are, with a walk/jog/run program over weeks or months. If your dog isn't already an athlete, leave him at home when you go out for your usual run. Even if your dog is in very good shape, make sure he drinks a lot of water before, during, and after his exercise. If you notice that he looks exhausted, lags behind, just lets his tongue hang limply from the side of his mouth, pants, coughs, and, in the last stages, actually stumbles and falls, lay him in the shade immediately, wet him down with water, and cool his head. Then call the nearest veterinarian.

Intermediate Level

You are an intermediate runner if you can run 3½ miles in thirty minutes (or 8½-minute miles) three or four times a week. If you want to increase your distance, gradually work yourself up to an hour of non-stop running. First, add one more day to your weekly schedule but run your usual thirty minutes. This adds another 3 miles to your body's weekly workload. If your body accepts the added stress with good grace and continued vigor, gradually increase your mileage. Apply the hard/easy principle. Add fifteen minutes to two of your weekly workouts, but stay with your usual thirty minutes for the alternating days. After at least four weeks of this, when you no longer feel particularly tired after your forty-five-minute runs, run for forty-five minutes straight on all four days. Again, give your body at least four weeks to adjust to this new stress, and then add another fifteen minutes to two of the workouts, so that now you are running one hour on, say, Monday and Wednesday, and forty-five minutes on your Tuesday and Thursday runs. Allow another four-week adjustment period. When the sixty-minute runs no longer leave you tired the next day, add fifteen minutes to your easy days, so that now you are running for an hour each time you go out. Your age, your physical condition, your diet, whether your smoke or drink—all these affect how long it will take to train your body to a one-hour workload. There's no rush.

If you reach a plateau and can't seem to run beyond it, you may discover, on analysis, that boredom, not exhaustion, is holding you back. When you're bored, you feel every ache and twitch, and your pain tolerance is lower. Vary your routine, or join a running club, or run with friends you enjoy talking to. If you aren't bored, you may be running too fast. Remember the talk/sing test. Or you may be running with your shoulders tight and hunched up around your ears. Your swinging arms actually help propel you forward, but if you hold them tightly, you swing your whole trunk instead of just your arms and that's hard work. Relax your shoulders and arms. If that doesn't help, try running through a couple of laps of the upper body exercises in the strength circuit in chapter 6, every other day.

If none of this helps, examine your stride. Perhaps it's too long. "Women, especially women with short legs," says Harmon Brown, M.D., director of student health services at California State University in Hayward, "try to increase the distance they cover by lengthening their strides. They bound too high and float in the air." If you want to move forward, any time you spend in the air is wasted, and so is the energy expended to launch yourself skyward. "The way to cover more ground," Brown says, "is to take medium-length strides but to take more of them." You actually do the same or less work by adding a few steps per minute to your tempo because you channel some of the vertical push into another forward stride.

However, the very act of running forces every runner to be airborne sometime during each sequence, and "biomechanical data show that a woman runner spends more time in the air and a shorter time on the ground than a man," says Kenneth E. Foreman, Ph.D., director of education and research at the Sports Medicine Clinic in Seattle.

To train your legs to push horizontally instead of vertically, and to pack more explosive energy into the push-off point in your gait, start by leaping and bounding on cushiony grass or a dirt track for thirty or forty yards—much as you did as a kid set free in the park—and then jog until you catch your breath. Together these count as one set, and six sets make a workout. Over the next few weeks, work yourself up to four or six sets of 440 yards each. When these become comfortable, graduate to hills or run up the stairs of the local football stadium.

Box jumping, the next step after stadiums, is reserved for competitive sprinters, jumpers, and card-carrying masochists. Set up two boxes of the same height—12 inches at first; 36 inches at your peak—and jump down from one box, up onto the next, back and forth, up and down, until you're breathless. Do these exercises a maximum of three times a week, and never two days in a row.

Advanced Level

You are an advanced runner if you regularly run an hour nonstop four or five times a week. This means you are running at least 25 miles per week.

If you want to add even more miles, increase your distance by no more than 10 percent each week and only on one or two days—hard days. Run your usual time the other—easy—days.

If you want to race, experiment with different distances to find the one you like. To improve your speed and stamina, add some fartlek three times a week.

FARTLEK

Fartlek, the Swedish word for "speed-play," is a kind of interval training in which you do bursts of speed whenever you get the urge and then slow down to your usual LSD pace to rest. The bursts of speed train your fast-twitch muscle fibers and improve your lactic acid tolerance, while the moving partial-recovery periods hasten the training effect for your heart. Eight or ten times during your run, sprint 100 to 300 yards as fast as you can and then slow down—but keep running—while you catch your breath. Like cyclists, runners who go up and down hills have built-in fartlek bursts and rests. For painless fartlek, try a nonstop game of soccer or field hockey or tag with your kids.

For intensified speed training, run intervals instead of fartlek on some hard days. Time yourself. Add five or ten seconds to your fastest half-mile pace and then run four half-miles at that pace, with quarter-mile jogs in between. This is even more draining than fartlek. Because any kind of interval training is grueling and breaks down muscle fiber, allow yourself at least two days between fartlek or interval runs, and never do them more than two or three times a week. The other days, run easy LSD. And never do any speed work if your legs already hurt.

Now is the time to add a three-time-per-week weight-training program to your schedule. "You don't just run with your legs," says Harmon Brown, who is also women's track and field coach at Cal State Hayward. "You run with your whole body. Your shoulders stabilize your free-swinging rib cage and get very tired when you breathe hard. Strong trunk and abdominal muscles keep your pelvis from tilting forward and prevent low back pain and knee strain." Strong arms increase the lift during your pumping motion.

Use weights that are just a little too heavy to lift comfortably more than ten times, moving to heftier weights when these become easy. Following the instructions in chapter 6, start with ten reps per set and do three or four sets per workout, building to five sets of fifteen reps each. Lift quickly, because your running movements are quick. Do these exercises a maximum of three days a week, and never two days in a row. The program includes shoulder shrugs, push-ups, arm sprints, dips, killer sit-ups, twisting sit-ups, dumbbell pullovers, locusts, run-'em-out-of-gym-class sprints, and, for the truly dedicated, squats, chin-ups, and pull-ups.

INDOOR TREADMILLS

Indoor treadmills for running in place come in two types, nonmotorized and motorized. In the nonmotorized version, your step drives the belt. They are much less expensive than the motorized types, but they can irritate your feet. A good model has adjustable speed and incline controls so that you can jog (to warm up and cool down) and walk or run against a resistance (as if you were going uphill) during the exertion phase of your workout. They cost $70 and up. The motorized versions are much larger, impossible to store or hide between workouts, and very expensive (several hundred dollars for a middle-range model). However, they are excellent for aerobic conditioning as long as you get one with adjustable speed and incline controls. Whichever you buy, run according to your target rate. The presence of the belt's resistance and the absence of wind resistance make it difficult to equate outdoor and indoor distances.

When you are training for a race, run two to three times the total distance of the race each week during the last two months before the race. For example, if you plan to run a 10K (6.2 mile) race in two months, you should now be running 12 to 18 miles a week without any pain at all. Six weeks before the race, make one of your weekly runs last two thirds to three quarters of the race distance. If you are in good shape, you should feel fresh enough after each of these to enjoy a normal LSD run the next day.

It takes at least two years of training and running shorter races to prepare for a marathon. You must be able to run 80 miles a week without any pain. As you develop this capacity, you also train your body to tolerate heat, a serious problem at most marathons.

Two weeks before a marathon race, rest your body by running

only two thirds of your maximum weekly mileage. Don't do speed work. The last week before the race, rest by running only one third of your maximum weekly mileage. This is called tapering. On the two days before the marathon, run two or three miles so that you don't get stale from inactivity.

On race day, eat a light breakfast four hours before starting time—if you can stomach it—and drink a lot of water. Warm up more carefully than usual, rub petroleum jelly on your nipples, armpits, neckline, and the insides of your thighs to prevent chafing, and powder your shoes and socks to delay blisters. (They'll sprout anyway; blisters are inevitable.) During the race, avoid puddles or water hoses. Wet shoes make wet feet, and wet feet blister easily.

FROM MARATHON TO ULTRAMARATHON

When a woman named Melpomene was barred from entering the marathon at the first modern Olympic games in 1896, founder Baron Pierre de Coubertin explained the committee's decision. "It is indecent that the spectators should be exposed to the risk of seeing the body of a woman being smashed before their very eyes. Besides, no matter how toughened a sportswoman may be, her organism is not cut out to sustain certain shocks." For the next eighty-five years, the International Olympic Committee stood by de Coubertin's position. Finally, in 1981, fourteen years after Kathrine Switzer became the first woman official-ly to enter the Boston Marathon (by registering as K. Switzer), the paternalistic International Olympic Committee bowed to an incontrovert-ible body of scientific and athletic data and accepted the running of a women's marathon event in the 1984 Los Angeles Games.

Baron de Coubertin notwithstanding, women are built for dis-tance. Fat gives them the same advantage in long-distance running as it does in long-distance swimming. Unfortunately, a marathon is barely long distance; you don't really tap your endurance fuel until a 50- or 100-mile run. In short races, a man has the advantage because he has longer bones and more lean muscle mass. At marathon distances, the differences start to even out: He has the head start of speed and pow-er, but you have the back-up fuel for the final 6 or 8 miles. At the ultramarathon distance, however, there's no comparison between the potential of female and male runners. As soon as we women catch up in our training techniques—and that's coming soon—the ultramarathon is ours. Yours.

A distance race damages your body. Expect to be sore for a few days. If possible, jog for thirty minutes the next day—it will eliminate some of your stiffness—but if you are too tired, don't run. Lay off for a week, or even two if necessary. Don't try long distances again for at least a month. Runners say it takes one or two days to recuperate for every mile you ran—one day for elite runners, two for the rest of us. If you try to run long distances before you're fully recovered, you'll pull a muscle.

Injuries

"The injury rate to the foot, ankle, and knee joints increases dramatically when runners train more than three days per week," says Michael Pollock. The strengthening and stretching exercises given earlier in this section, and in chapter 6, are essential to prevent injuries.

According to John Pagliano, D.P.M., and Douglas Jackson, M.D., in a study published in *Runner's World* in 1980, the most common injuries to runners are: plantar fasciitis, Achilles tendinitis, metatarsalgia, ankle sprains, runner's knee, shin splints, and stress fractures, most commonly in the tibia. (See chapter 10 for full descriptions.) Any change can cause an injury: running on grass after running on pavement; buying a new pair of shoes; running over hills and dales after spending your life on the flats; adding speed work; adding distance; gaining weight.

If you are sensitive to heat or humidity, don't run if the temperature is above 75 degrees and the humidity above 50 percent. Whether you are particularly sensitive to heat or not, drink plenty of water in hot weather to prevent heatstroke. Drink one to three eight-ounce glasses of water ten to fifteen minutes before you run, and drink about one cup of water every fifteen minutes throughout a long race. (See chapter 10 for a full discussion of heat injury.)

Winter running poses its own problems. Unless it's cold and windy enough to freeze your nose, or there is a hail or sleet storm outside, you can run in just about any weather. (With adequate precautions, even men and women stationed in the Antarctic run every day.) Dress for the wind-chill factor instead of the temperature on the thermometer (see Table XIV in chapter 10), with layers of long cotton or polypropylene fishnet underwear next to your skin and wool on the outside. Cotton feels soft next to your skin, but when it gets wet it feels cold. Polypropylene acts like a wick to draw moisture from your skin into the wool layer, where it can evaporate. The wool also keeps you warm even when it's wet. Add a windbreaker or a waterproof breatheable rain suit on particularly windy or wet days. Wear a hat that covers your head and ears. If it's so cold that it hurts to breathe, wear a ski mask, balaclava, or scarf over your nose, mouth, and chin. If it still hurts to inhale, it is too cold to run. For maximum warmth, wear mittens instead of gloves, and in really cold weather wear two layers of mittens—wool on the inside, leather on the outside. If the soles of your usual running shoes are smooth, buy another pair with studs or raised treads to prevent slipping on ice.

Start out running against the wind because you are dry and full of energy at the beginning of a run. At the end of your run, when you are tired and sweaty, run with the wind at your back so that you won't feel as cold. (See chapter 10 on hypothermia and frostbite.)

ROPE JUMPING

Rope jumping will never become an Olympic event. No one, not the most avid skipper, would even call it a sport. And yet it is one of the most addictive exercises there is. It combines the aerobic meditative benefits of Long Steady Distance running, the athletic prowess of high jumps and twirls and red hot peppers (double- and triple-time jumps), with the aesthetics of dance and the nostalgia of jump-rope rhymes and double Dutch. Well before the twentieth century, English boxers jumped rope to warm up their muscles, strengthen their legs, improve footwork and coordination, and develop both aerobic and anaerobic capacities. Today, boxers all over the world entertain fans at their ninety-minute training sessions with arm crossovers, high leaps, cossacklike squat-and-jump dance steps, double and triple turning, and other feats of fancy jumping. Many professional football and basketball players use the rope as much for its relaxing qualities as its training effect; as they turn the rope at a constant speed, they jump as evenly and regularly as the ticking of a clock, while the rope hits the floor at the same spot, revolution after revolution, minute after minute, for an entire hour.

Skip rope as your only form of aerobic exercise, or use it as an adjunct to other sports. When the weather is too wet or frigid for running or cycling, jump indoors. When you are traveling, jump rope if you can't take your bicycle along, or if you can't find a running path or a swimming pool. However, rope jumping is much more demanding, so you have to work at it at least twice a week or you won't be able to jump long enough to train when you can't play your other sports.

Evaluation

"Rope skipping is an excellent cardiovascular conditioner providing you develop long-term endurance—past fifteen minutes," says Richard Ruoti, Registered Physical Therapist and exercise physiologist in Pennsylvania. Whether it is the equal of running is still open to debate. Most studies show that rope jumping gives you about 90 percent of the training effect of distance running in terms of oxygen uptake and calories burned. This is an eminently respectable training effect, and there's a good chance it is even greater. Every study except Ruoti's was performed on subjects who were new to jumping, used it only as a supplementary exercise, or jumped for only five or six minutes. How can anyone compare the performance of these inexperienced jumpers after a short workout with the performance of a veteran runner after a full distance workout?

Ruoti's two-year study, done with Albert Paolone and Walter Mruk at Temple University in Philadelphia, showed that ten minutes should be the minimum test period—and fifteen minutes is better. When you first start jumping, you start at a minimum of seventy-two revolutions of the rope per minute. If you turn any slower, the rope simply won't go over your head. Therefore, you can't ease into jumping the way you do into running, by starting out gradually and increasing your speed as your heart warms up. Instead, you spike your heart rate up to your target point immediately and enter an anaerobic phase for the first three minutes. Your heart rate is also elevated by your turning arms—arm exercises raise the heart rate higher than leg exercise. A third factor raises your heart rate from the beginning of your workout: Jumping exacts thirty times more mechanical work (over a ten-minute workout) than running does.

If the first three minutes of your workout are heavily anaerobic, the equivalent of sprinting at full speed, for example, you are still in oxygen debt at the five- or six-minute mark. You haven't fully entered your aerobic phase, as any tests will show.

After countless tests on experienced runners, researchers know the precise physiological effects of distance running. No such studies have been done on LSD rope jumpers. However, Ruoti's studies suggest to him that "once you get into the aerobic phase, you can probably spike a very high heart rate and do a large amount of mechanical work and eventually increase your oxygen consumption. You *may*, in fact, be able to improve your oxygen consumption and your cardiovascular condition more quickly with rope jumping than with something that doesn't make you work as hard."

In addition to strengthening your heart and lungs and improving your circulatory system, rope jumping develops strength and endurance in your leg muscles. (Running, in contrast, only develops leg endurance.) It doesn't affect your arm muscles, however. If you want to strengthen your upper body or limber up either your upper or lower body, you'll have to supplement rope jumping with another basic sport or with circuit training (chapter 6) or weight lifting. Rope jumping also improves your grace and coordination.

Jumping rope is easy to learn. Most women, in fact, already know how to do it—they learned in schoolyards as children. It is cheap, can be done almost anywhere, indoors or outdoors, night or day, in your bedroom, your office, or your hotel room, in any kind of weather. If you are shy or self-conscious about exercising in public, you can jump at home in complete privacy. And if you have trouble finding time to exercise, you can jump rope while you watch the evening news on television or talk to friends. I usually combine my children's after-school debriefing with a half hour or hour of jumping rope. It kills two birds with one stone, and their conversation keeps me from getting bored. Other suggestions: listen to fast upbeat music, sing out loud the full score of your favorite musical comedy, practice arm crossovers and fancy steps.

Equipment

Your rope can be as simple or as elaborate as you choose. There are nylon ropes with ball-bearing handles, leather ropes with rosewood handles, ropes strung with plastic beads for weight, ropes with digital counters to record your number of jumps (actually your number of turns), and ropes with gadgets to estimate the number of calories you've expended.

The rope should be about 5/16 to 3/8 inch in diameter. Any thinner, and it will be so flabby you'll have to swing with all your might to get it over your head; any stouter, and it will be too stiff to bend easily into an arc. It should be long enough to hit the floor on each rotation while your body is straight and your hands are at hip level. To measure a jump rope, hold one end in each hand and step on the center. When you pull the rope taut, the ends should reach to your armpits. (Add extra length for handles.) I like my rope a little longer—about shoulder height—but too much excess is hard to control, and the rope tangles easily. If your rope is too long, tie knots in it at intervals, but be careful when you jump—those knots feel like rocks from a slingshot when they hit you.

To make your own jump rope—by far the cheapest way to go—buy old-fashioned cotton clothesline, cotton or hemp rope, or sash cord from the local hardware store. For handles, thread on four- or five-inch sections of rigid Lucite tubing, aluminum or plastic pipe, cannoli tubes (molds for an Italian fried pastry), or even the flocked plastic inserts used to make small candles fit large candlesticks. The tube should be wide enough so that the rope rotates freely inside it and firm enough so that it won't cave in when you grip it. Tie a large sturdy knot at each end of the rope, and you're on your way.

Shoes are a matter of personal preference. I prefer to jump bare-footed, but then I always jump on padded carpet or on hardwood floors with some give. When I wear shoes—or even socks without shoes—my toes squash together and jam against the front of the shoe, and I get blisters and bruises. Also, the rubberized sole abruptly stops my motion on the floor. Normally, I have a slight glide at the end of each jump, and this dissipates some of the stress on my shin, calves, and Achilles tendon. With shoes, I'm more likely to get shin splints.

On the other hand, running shoes cushion the balls of your feet if you jump on hard or rough surfaces—concrete or linoleum laid directly over concrete, for example. They also protect your feet from the rope. (Getting a speeding rope caught between your toes is a memorable experience).

You don't need any special clothes for jumping jope, but the exercise is so jarring that a sports bra is a must. Even women who wear an A cup say they need a bra for jumping.

Relative cost.   Sash cord and clothesline runs 15 to 35 cents a foot, 1980 prices. Ready-made ropes sell for $4 to $20. Shoes—as you will.

Precautions

Jumping rope is extremely strenuous from the first moment you begin a workout. There is no way to start slowly and regulate your pace. Because it spikes your heart to target rate or above very quickly, it isn't your sport if you have coronary heart disease or some other ailment which makes you intolerant of high heart rates.

Goals for Fitness

Jump nonstop at least fifteen minutes per session at least three times a week for an aerobic training effect. However, if you want to lose weight with this exercise, you'll have to jump thirty minutes nonstop, just as you would with any other sport.

There is a rumor that ten minutes of jumping rope is the equivalent of twenty minutes of jogging and that therefore you can jump for fifteen minutes instead of thirty and still trim away bulges and earn aerobic merit points. Alas, it's not true. The fact that you do so much more mechanical work when jumping doesn't mean that you increase your oxygen-carrying capacity or burn calories any faster than when running. It simply means you get a strong anaerobic training effect in your workout. If you want all the benefits of an aerobic workout, you must pay off your oxygen debt first, and then jump for another fifteen or twenty minutes—bringing you up to the sacred thirty-minute minimum. This, you will discover, is quite a feat.

Use the talk/sing test to keep your workload near your target heart rate. If you feel safer taking your pulse, stop and count your pulse for six seconds. Multiply by ten for your minute rate. If your pulse is hovering around your target rate, resume your jumping. If it is too high, walk around the room for a minute or two instead.

Training

According to Fred Kasch, hundreds of repetitive jumps stress and shorten the gastrocnemius and soleus muscles in your calf and shin, and the flexor hallucis longus, which extends your foot and ankle. To prevent aches and injuries, concentrate on ankle rolls, foot twisters, and calf stretches, and add heel and toes, geisha kneels, and Achilles stretches (see chapter 6).

If you are in poor shape, says Richard Ruoti, warm up your heart with some easy running in place or light jogging. In this way, you'll raise your heart rate slowly to about double your resting rate and prepare it for the sudden effort of jumping. This will also enable you to shift into the aerobic phase much earlier in your workout.

Beginner's Level

If you have never jumped over a rope before, you may feel like an uncoordinated klutz. How, you wonder, do you get the rope down near your feet when you're ready to jump over it?

Take one step at time, says rope-jumping evangelist Bobby Hinds, president of Lifeline Products. First learn to jump, then learn to turn the rope, and then, and only then, put them all together. Begin by skipping without the rope, suggests Hinds, who has demonstrated rope jumping in restaurants, supermarkets, and even in an airplane 30,000 feet in the air. Keep your arms bent easily at your sides. Step, then barely hop with your right foot; step, barely hop with your left. Step-hop, step-hop, step-hop, at the rate of about seventy-five to eighty double steps each minute. Bounce gently on the balls of your feet and push off with your toes. Don't jump flat-footed. Keep your knees very slightly bent, and skip up only a half inch or an inch off the floor. Skip in place, without any forward or backward movement. Do this until the movement feels smooth and relaxed. If you are out of shape, even these practice jumps will be exhausting. Jump until you are winded (or your heart rate is above your target rate), then walk around for a minute or two until your pulse is down to your target pace, and then jump again. (Hinds uses two-footed and jogging steps—without hops—but these are double-time steps and are too strenuous for beginners.)

Once you have mastered the basic skipping step, add the rope but don't try to jump over it yet. Instead, hold both handles in one hand and turn the rope at your side as you skip. Turn seventy-five to eighty revolutions per minute. Keep your elbows tucked close to your body and use your wrist, not your arm, to turn the rope.

When this feels comfortable, you're ready to skip over the rope. With a handle in each hand, turn the rope at the same pace as you skip. Turn with your wrists, bounce on your toes—you don't need great leaps and swings. Each foot should land in the same spot time after time. Jump just high enough to clear the rope. If it's too hard to get the two little jumps coordinated with one rope swing, jump only once on each foot in a jogging-in-place step, but this jogging step is much more strenuous than the double skip.

The schedule in Table X, recommended by Richard Ruoti, uses the walk/jump interval method to adjust your heart to the rigors of the rope. The rest stops between the short intense periods of jumping allow your heart rate to remain at a safe level. However, since you keep moving during each rest, your recovery is just incomplete enough to hasten your training effect much the way the incomplete recovery period in advanced runners' intervals stimulates the heart. If this schedule moves too quickly for you, spend three weeks at each level. If it goes so slowly you are not working up to your target rate, advance a week.

TABLE X: ROPE-JUMPING PROGRAM

	Duration (in minutes)		
Week	Jumping Interval	Walk-Rest Interval	Total Actual Jumping Time
1–2	½	2	3
3–4	1	2	3
5–6	2	2	6
7–8	2	1½	6
9–10	2	1	6
11–12	2	½	6
13–14	3	2	6
15–16	3	1	6
17–18	4	2	8
19–20°	4	1	8

°And so on, to a goal of fifteen minutes nonstop, at least three days a week.

Intermediate Level

If you can *skip* rope for fifteen minutes, nonstop, you have reached the intermediate level. To improve, you have several choices. Substitute a more strenuous step for the skip during part or all of the session. Lift your knees very high to intensify the workout and strengthen your abdominal muscles. Tap the toe or heel of the nonjumping foot to stretch the muscles of your lower leg and add a little more work to each jump. Cross the tapping foot in front of the jumping foot to improve your agility and coordination. Kick your buttocks with every jump. Cross the rope in front of you on one twirl and uncross it the next.

You may also increase the amount of time you spend skipping each day, working up to an hour per session at the end of a year. Although fancy steps and speed work (when you reach the advanced level) break the monotony of hour-long sessions, the key to this jumper's version of Long Steady Distance is an even, light double-skipping step. You want to work at 60 percent of your target heart rate for an hour, and you can't do that with any other step. Jumping LSD for an hour is exhilarating. After ten minutes, you find your second wind, and everything you see is enhanced. The colors of the trees through your window are brighter green, the shadows on your wall take on shapes and tell you stories, the colors on the television screen are vivid and sharp.

Advanced Level

If you jump for one hour nonstop at least three days a week, you have reached the advanced level. It should take you at least a year to reach this point. Rushing things will only lead to injury or frustration. There is absolutely no reason to jump for more than an hour except once in a while—just to see if you can do it.

Intensify your workout. Do some jumper's style fartlek (speed-play). Jump a jogging or two-footed step without the short hop in between. This forces you to turn 120 revolutions per minute. Jump double-time for as long as you can stand it, then return to your usual step-hop skipping step to recover. Then jump another burst of speed. As your condition improves, you'll be able to jog or two-foot jump for longer intervals, until, after another year or so, you'll be able to jump your whole hour at 120 rpms. Add double and triple turns to your speed work (bring the rope under your feet twice or three times before they hit the ground), or red hot peppers, jumping as fast as you possibly can. These are extremely strenuous techniques. Don't try them unless you're in top physical condition.

Injuries

You are not likely to be injured jumping rope, unless you have heart trouble. A few doctors have warned that theoretically jumping rope might cause stress fractures or enlargements of the metatarsal heads (the bones in the balls of your feet), but neither Ruoti nor any sports physicians I talked to have ever heard of a jumper who actually has suffered such an injury. "I haven't found any evidence that this is likely," says Ruoti, "but if you want to be on the safe side, wear canvas shoes and jump on something cushioned."

Ankle and shin pain may be caused by jumping on soft carpets or pads, or by wearing shoes with rubber soles. Bruises on the balls of the feet may be caused by hard floors. Blisters may be caused either by jumping on hard surfaces or by crowding your toes together inside shoes or socks. Prevent blisters by bandaging your feet before you jump. For a while, there was a rumor that jumping encouraged plantar warts (warts on the sole of the foot) by repeatedly bruising and scraping the balls of the feet, but this seems unlikely now. Shin splints and strains of the quadriceps (the large muscle along the front of the thigh) or in the ligaments of the knee are possible, but not as likely as they are in most other sports.

6 / The Home Circuit Training Program

Looking for an exercise program tailor-made to your own needs? One that tones and shapes every muscle in your body, flattens your stomach, shrinks your waist, firms your arms, legs, and buttocks, helps you lose fat, makes you strong and lithe, and gives you an aerobic training effect, all in one forty-five-minute workout you repeat three days a week in the privacy of your own home? Try circuit training.

WHAT IS CIRCUIT TRAINING?

Circuit training was developed at the University of Leeds in northern England after World War II to train high school, college, and elite athletes in an organized, systematic, and therefore more effective way than the hit-or-miss methods previously used. Stations were set up around a gymnasium, and one by one each athlete performed a specified number of exercises at each station while a partner monitored his or her style and helped set up the equipment. The stations included such things as rope climbs, sit-ups on incline boards, dips, and stair stepping.

Today, circuit training is an immensely popular indoor fitness entertainment for large groups of children and adults in England and the Scandinavian countries. A few times a week, during weather too forbidding for anything other than skiing, families go down to a huge gymnasium to get their winter exercise. The Swedes in particular have a well-organized program of physical fitness for their entire population, which may account in part for the fact that the average Swede lives four years longer than the average American.

The home circuit training program described in this chapter is an ultra-modern, sophisticated, scientific form of calisthenics. It combines effective calisthenic exercises with up-to-date weight and resistance training and flexibility drills by using the principles of overload, repetition, and specificity—in a format that also challenges your circulatory system as no other form of calisthenics does. Both the resistance and the aerobic exercises burn fat, which you replace with firm, tight, lean muscle. You become smaller yet more shapely as you grow new muscle fibers. (Contrary to the claims of some well-publicized stretching exercise programs, stretching will not make you trimmer or firmer; it will just make you more flexible.) What's more, you design your own program, so you do only the exercises you need. Your circuit looks like no one else's because your body works like no one else's.

This is no five-minute-a-day instant-fitness miracle. Home circuit training is hard work. If you like calisthenics—and most women do, says Fred Kasch, who has taught calisthenics classes for more than thirty years—and if you are serious about your health and don't mind the repetitious, self-challenging nature of these training exercises, then home circuit training is for you.

The program begins with warm-ups and then continues with a series, or circuit, of twelve strength exercises performed in a prescribed order. You go through the circuit three times, increasing your speed each time, executing each exercise as fast as you can without sacrificing the quality of each move. The pace, the workload, and the abbreviated rest periods between each set, or station, elevate your heart rate, increase your oxygen uptake, and give you an aerobic training effect. After your third strength circuit, you cool down with a circuit of balanced, concentrated stretches to end the session.

Each strength and flexibility exercise, or station, focuses on a particular part of your anatomy and is graded by ability because some parts of you are stronger or more limber than others. You customize the circuit by performing each exercise at your current level of expertise, advancing in each exercise individually. For example, you may have quite strong thighs and be able to carry out a credible level-three squat from the first day but be unable to do the requisite ten negative (level-one) chin-ups for two months.

You customize your workout further by fleshing out the skeleton circuits with exercises concentrating on your particular needs. If your fitness profile in chapter 1 says you have strong calves and quads but weak lower back and triceps muscles, add one or two back exercises and one or two triceps strengtheners; no need to waste time overworking your well-developed calves. Or if you want to work on a specific element for another sport—the flexibility of your lats, which are the prime movers in a swimmer's crawl, or the spring in your legs so necessary for field hockey or fencing—add sport-specific exercises listed in chapters 5 and 7. You can use your home circuit training program as your only form of exercise, as a way to train for another sport, or as a substitute for your steady outdoor sport when the weather is rotten. (When you reach the advanced stages of fitness, you'll have to augment circuit training with another aerobic sport, because your heart will be so strong you won't be able to get your pulse up to your target rate with circuit training alone. However, by that time, you'll be addicted to this total form of conditioning and will keep at it to stay in shape.)

PARCOURSE

In the 1960s, a Swiss company, the Vita Life Insurance Company, designed, constructed, and built outdoor exercise fitness trails or "life courses" throughout Switzerland. They became extremely popular throughout Europe and were introduced to the United States in 1973 by Parcourse.

Parcourse Fitness Circuits are running trails set up in public parks, corporate fitness centers, and schoolyards. You walk, jog, or sprint from station to station in a set sequence, then follow directions on the illustrated instruction board at each station to perform the exercise at your level of ability. The eighteen stations (or nine for the mini-course) provide both strength and flexibility exercises, but they are geared to people who have done no exercise at all or to people whose only exercise is running. They are not all-around programs for people interested in high levels of fitness or people who already play another, non-running sport and need supplementary exercises. The aerobic training effect comes not from the stations themselves but from the running intervals in between. (If you don't like interrupting your day's run with exercises every few minutes, either save your Parcourse for non-running days or find some other way to develop and loosen your muscles.) Many Parcourses include a separate set of signs, along the same trail, for people in wheelchairs. For more information and planning manuals for setting up a course in your community, contact Parcourse Ltd., 3701 Buchanan Street, San Francisco, California 94123.

Evaluation

Home circuit training is a total fitness and conditioning program. It strengthens just about every tendon, ligament, and muscle in your body, improves flexibility, and develops anaerobic power. In other words, it touches all bases in a scientifically balanced way. If you enlarge one set of muscles, you also enlarge their antagonists. If you stretch and lengthen another set of muscles, you also stretch and lengthen their antagonists. Because no part of the body is overstressed or underused, you can't hurt yourself doing circuit training, and you prevent injuries when you play other sports.

The amount of aerobic training effect you get from home circuit training depends on what shape you're already in. If you are just starting to exercise, it will raise your pulse to your target rate, keep it there for twenty or thirty minutes, and increase your maximal oxygen uptake by as much as 11 percent (as compared with 15 to 25 percent in running). If you are already an endurance athlete, you may not be able to get your heart rate up to your target pulse with any kind of circuit training, and what elevation you do get will be due to the vigorous movements of your arms. (Moving your arms strenuously always elicits a higher heart rate than moving your legs equally energetically.) In this case, you may show only a moderate (5 percent) improvement in maximal oxygen uptake from home circuit training alone, but this doesn't matter because you can get your aerobic workout from your endurance sport and still derive all the strength and flexibility benefits from the home program. (If, for any reason, you must substitute circuit training for your endurance sport, try adding one more lap of the circuit and performing every station as intensely as you can to get an aerobic training effect.)

Circuit training is so flexible you can even practice it when you are recuperating from a sports injury. In one test, a man with an injured leg increased the strength of that leg *inside a cast*, although he exercised only his healthy leg. You can use circuit training during the winter to stay in condition or keep your summer running or cycling muscles strong while you are skiing or skating. Circuit training is private, relaxing, and cheap. And because it sets so many tasks, it rewards you with continual satisfactions—you advance through several levels and infinite intensities for each station. Each time you graduate to a harder stage, you feel a sense of accomplishment, and when you finally conquer a particularly stubborn exercise—chin-ups, for instance—you know you are invincible.

Equipment

Mat.   You'll need some sort of mat to protect your tailbone during sit-ups and your hip bones during locusts. A well-padded carpeted floor is ideal. Otherwise, buy a one- or two-inch-thick plastic-coated exercise mat from a department or sporting goods store, or make one out of one-inch-thick foam rubber padding covered with old beach towels, bed sheets, or other fabric sewn to size.

Pole.   You'll need a chinning pole, the kind that not only sets into brackets screwed onto the sides of a doorway but also expands to squeeze against the doorjamb for additional security. Hanging from a

GOOD AND BAD EXERCISE GADGETS

Exercise devices are big business because they add variety to a workout. (Indoor exercise bicycles and treadmills were described in chapter 5; rowing machines are in chapter 7.) Gadgets are also big business because many promise miracles no one but a deity could deliver—a perfect figure or instant muscles in five effortless minutes a day. However, a few small, inexpensive, portable gyms on the market actually make good on their promises. They give you a miniaturized home version of the variable resistance workouts you get from the large Nautilus or Universal at gyms and health spas.

The Mini-Gym, a portable piece of isokinetic equipment used by high school and college athletic trainers, relies on a system of pulleys and internal mechanisms, to maintain a constant pressure throughout the exercise and may be used by people with different strengths without adjustment. Some models are designed for training for specific sports, but those meant for overall conditioning are eminently suitable for circuit weight training, although they don't allow for negative resistance.

The Exer-Genie, constructed of a rope running through a cylinder, permits you to simulate movements specific to your sport and is eminently portable.

The Lifeline Gym, small enough to fit in a briefcase, consists of a folding bar, stretchable cords, and stirrups for hands or feet and can be used for weight training, injury rehabilitation, and some sports-specific movements. When you order the gym, include your current weight, for the surgical tubing which provides the resistance comes in three thicknesses.

rafter or loft beam may work for you if your hands are big enough, but I find that the square corners of the wood cut into my palms.

Dumbbells. For about half the strength stations, you'll need dumbbells. There are two basic types, fixed and adjustable. The fixed weights are made of chrome, cast iron, or sand-filled pastel-colored vinyl. The vinyl weights are the cheapest, but if you drop one it may crack and leak sand all over your floor. The chrome dumbbells are shiny and beautiful but extremely expensive. Cast-iron dumbbells are sturdy, easy to use, inexpensive, and will last a lifetime. They come in sizes ranging from 1½ to 60 pounds each, but you will only need three sets—usually 5 pounds per dumbbell, 8 pounds, and 10 pounds. Adjustable dumbbells are not suitable for circuit training because it takes a long time to replace the plates and tighten the collar of each dumbbell with a wrench. Besides, one set of adjustable dumbbells costs about the same as the total cost of your three pairs of fixed weights.

Many exercise gadgets on the market are totally useless, and some are downright dangerous.

Any passive exerciser—"leave the driving to us"—gives you absolutely no training effect. Forget them.

The exercise wheel (a small wheel with handles instead of axles) is supposed to flatten your tummy and trim your waist. In fact, it doesn't work half as well as killer sit-ups and twisting sit-ups and forces your back into a very stressful position.

Chest pulls made of rubber tubing or steel spring cables build just a few specific arm, chest, and shoulder muscles at only a few angles of movement. Strength and circuit exercises give you more general strength.

Rope-and-pulley body trimmers build strength fairly effectively on limited parts of your body as long as you work against your own muscles at all times. However, in the time you spend lying on your back pulling those ropes with your hands and feet, you can do several strength stations and build overall strength and endurance.

Even the sturdiest of mini-trampolines are so small you can fall off or miss them entirely, and the flimsier models can topple over if you hit them along the edge.

Some of the nonmotorized joggers are nothing more than postage-stamp-sized sparsely padded boards held together with thin metal rods and drinking straws. The pads and boards are so small they can force you to use an unnatural gait to stay on them. If you miss the board entirely or slide because the pad or board wiggles, you can pull or tear a muscle or tendon.

Don't use canned goods for dumbbells, or make your own by filling water or bleach bottles with sand. Canned goods are too wide, and handles on bottles are off center. These awkward grips can cause muscle imbalances and muscle pulls. Take yourself seriously and use proper equipment.

Weights. Some exercises require ankle or foot weights. If you have a heavy pair of hiking or ski boots, these may work, as long as you can get in and out of them quickly enough. If not, invest in a pair of ankle weights. These long vinyl envelopes filled with sand weigh 2½ or 3 pounds apiece and fasten in place with Velcro fasteners. You will probably find that one 3-pound set is plenty. If you ever want to advance beyond 3 pounds per leg, either buy heavier weights or wear one weight on your ankle and another around the instep of your foot. You can also make your own ankle weights. Fill two long polyethylene bags with the appropriate amount of sand, knotting them at intervals as if you were making sausages. Knot the toe of each of two knee-length socks, leaving a tail, place the bags inside, and knot the top of each sock, also leaving extra fabric. Sew Velcro fastening strips on the toes and tops of each sock, and you're on your way. (You can also tie the weights around your ankles, but tying them, untying them, and tying them again takes too long for circuit training.) The only problem with homemade ankle weights is that they often spring leaks, and the knots sometimes press on your bones.

Relative cost.   Mats range from $10 to $55. Chinning poles cost between $7 and $12. Ankle weights run from $6 to $10. Cast-iron dumbbells cost $5 for the lightest to $15 for the heaviest you'll need.

Precautions

If you test yourself first and work at your own level, you can do circuit training no matter what your condition. However, some specific exercises may aggravate bad knees or bad backs. Obey the warnings following each exercise.

Goals for Fitness

A day's workout lasts about forty-five minutes, and during the middle twenty minutes of that time your pulse should be up at your target level. If you are not working hard enough, increase the workload (move to the next level or add more weight), increase your speed (and shorten your rest periods), or add an extra lap. If you are in such good cardiovascular condition that you still can't maintain your target pulse, add stair stepping or some other indoor or outdoor endurance exercise between the strength and flexibility circuits.

Home circuit training is a form of weight training. You are tearing down muscle fiber and must allow yourself at least a day between workouts to rebuild those muscles bigger and stronger than ever. Run the full home circuits three days a week—never on two consecutive days. Do the concentrated stretching laps every day, if you like, and play other sports on intervening days.

To build cardiovascular tone and strength throughout every inch, you must move your muscles, against the weight of a dumbbell or your own body, through their entire range of motion, from their most flexed (bent) to their most extended (straightened). When the amount of weight remains the same throughout the lift, as it does during calisthenics and free weight lifting, the exercise is called isotonic.

Although the weight or amount of resistance remains the same throughout an entire isotonic movement, the *feeling* of resistance—

how hard you work—varies with the position of your arm or leg. As you move your arm or leg, it is stronger at some angles (such as 90 degrees) and weaker at others (such as when it is almost straight.) Therefore, the exercise feels most difficult at the very beginning or the very end. Unless you are careful to keep the tension and speed even throughout the rep, you will strengthen the muscle most at its weakest point and get the least benefit at its strongest point. Counteract this tendency by moving very deliberately throughout the whole lift. Don't fling the dumbbell, or your body, into a move at the beginning, and don't speed through the end. Maintain an even tempo and intensity. In addition, resist the weight, or gravity, when you are returning to the starting position. The release is called the negative portion of a lift, and it gives at least as much training effect as the positive—you strengthen a muscle while it is contracting during the positive motion, and strengthen it while it is lengthening during the negative phase. Some weight-lifting coaches even advise you to take a little longer lowering the weight than raising it to take full advantage of the negative lift effect.

Isometrics are exercises without any movement at all. You push one set of muscles against an immovable object, creating a one-dimensional strength useful for moving, lifting, or working only at the precise angle of the isometric exercise itself. Isometrics have no place in circuit training. They stiffen you up because they force your muscles and tendons to contract and never stretch them out again. They increase muscle definition, but they don't increase your ability to move a weight through space, and that's what strength is all about. They force your heart to beat harder to handle the strain, but your static, unmoving muscles don't return the extra blood flow to the heart so you don't increase the volume of blood flowing through your veins. Furthermore, the tensed muscles squeeze down the blood vessels, so less blood can pass through and your blood pressure rises abruptly. Your heart works harder against the added resistance of your narrowed blood vessels, but without the extra oxygen it needs for all that work. The result is that people with high blood pressure or coronary artery disease risk developing irregular heart rhythms or temporary impairment of the heart's pumping capacity if they do isometrics.

Most stations in the home strength circuit set a maximum of fifteen reps at each level. (A few, as noted in the instructions, call for more.) Once those fifteen become easy, move to the next level instead of adding more reps. Somewhere between fifteen and twenty reps, you reach a point of diminishing returns where you build aerobic endurance in your muscles but don't develop and strengthen them.

Do only fifteen reps at a time and then move to another station. Because you run the circuits, you do each exercise a total of forty-five times during a workout, but your muscles have a chance to recover in between. If you did all thirty or forty-five reps of a station in one giant lump, lactic acid would accumulate in your muscle tissue, your muscles would feel very tired, and you wouldn't exercise efficiently.

Training

The workout begins with a modified version of the universal warm-ups. No other warm-ups are necessary. The concentrated stretching circuit serves as your cool-down.

Injuries

Because this program is tailored to your own abilities, it's very hard to hurt yourself. However, it is an aerobic sport, and if you practice it in hot weather, you can suffer heat injury as easily as if you were running on a hot city street. Be sure to drink plenty of water before you start, drink at the end of the last strength lap, and again at the end of the flexibility circuit. (See chapter 10 for a full discussion of heat injury.)

NO JEWELRY

WARNING

Do not wear rings or bracelets when you exercise. If a ring on your finger gets caught on an immovable object while your whole body is pulling against it, the ring will break your finger, cut off its circulation, or even rip the whole finger off. When your finger is torn off in this fashion, even the most experienced surgeons may not be able to sew it back on because the blunt ring ruptures skin, nerves, blood vessels, tendons, and bones. *No active sport is exempt from this nightmarish injury.*

CIRCUIT WEIGHT TRAINING

As the concept of circuit training became established in this country, circuit weight training was born. Here, the stations are various weight-lifting exercises with barbells, dumbbells, or, in the latest variation, formidable weight machines.

In traditional weight training, you lift the heaviest weight you can handle for twelve lifts, or reps. (You should not be able to lift it again for a thirteenth time.) You then rest your muscles for a minute—or five—before starting another set of lifts. In circuit weight training, you lift as heavy a weight as you can fifteen times in twenty or thirty seconds, and then, without resting, you immediately move to the next station for another lift, using another set of muscles. You must not become so exhausted from the first lift that you can't make your second, and then your third and subsequent lifts, through the whole circuit of ten or twelve stations.

This kind of maximal effort and minimal rest gives you an aerobic training effect as well as increasing your strength. If the exercises are done properly by moving the muscles through their full range of motion, circuit weight training maintains and perhaps even improves your flexibility. (Ordinary weight lifting shortens your muscles and stiffens you up.) However, real circuit weight training must be done in a gym because you need a spotter to set up each station. Otherwise your set-ups take so long, you catch your breath between each exercise. Circuit weight training does not work on flexibility conscientiously, consistently, and precisely.

The two best-known resistance machines are Universal and Nautilus. Using a combination of wires, pulleys, and cams, they permit you to do ballistic weight lifts for specific muscles. Both series of machines are expensive and are found in gyms, colleges, and the homes of the very wealthy. Of the two, the Universal machine costs far less. However, unless it is used properly, it doesn't keep the resistance even throughout your lift. When you first pull or push against the bars of a station, you accelerate the weight with a burst of strength, and the momentum keeps the weight moving so that you don't have to work very hard during the rest to the lift. Therefore, you only exercise the muscles at the beginning of each lift, and they develop strength only at that angle of contraction. In addition, you can bend and wiggle as you lift so that you can put your stronger back or leg muscles to work, for example, in lifts that are supposed to use only your arms or shoulders. A Universal machine can be used for circuit weight training if a spotter adjusts the machine and polices your form.

The much more expensive Nautilus machines have an irregularly shaped cam (supposedly shaped something like a spiral nautilus shell) that maintains resistance throughout the whole lift. Each machine exercises a different muscle or muscle group. You are positioned and strapped into each machine so that you fully isolate the muscle you are working on—no way of cheating here! You work at Nautilus machines with slow intense contractions. This drawn-out pace and the time it takes to strap yourself into each position makes the Nautilus unsuitable for aerobic circuit training.

Improvements in oxygen uptake and strength, says Michael Pollock, depend on the amount of work you do, not on the equipment you use. In other words, you develop your strength equally with free weights or with weight machines, provided you use them properly. With traditional heavy-weight resistance training, you need expert instruction to learn correct form. With Nautilus, the machine dictates your form. It doesn't do the work for you, but it does keep you honest. And by lifting with proper form, you isolate the prime mover muscles and develop them as efficiently and effectively as possible.

Nautilus makes smaller pectoral and pullover machines for women under five feet three inches, and a varying range of machines are available at gyms and health spas in most cities (see Appendix A).

DESIGNING YOUR OWN PROGRAM

The skeleton strength circuit covers squats, hamsters, groin squeezes, en garde, mermaid, arm sprints, and wrist curls. The skeleton concentrated stretching circuit includes towel stretches, wasp waisters, king of Siam kowtows, locusts, pigeon crawls, geisha kneels, runner's starts, hunkers, birds, and side stretches.

Every workout should include these exercises, because they work on every part of your body at least once. To flesh out the skeletons, add five exercises (seven if you have the time) to the strength circuit and three or more to the flexibility circuit. Select exercises from Tables XI and XII (see pages 162–165) according to the parts of your body you want to develop. Your fitness profile at the end of chapter 1 pinpoints your weak or stiff spots, your mirror shows you where you're flabby, and any other sport tells you what sport-specific exercises you need to practice.

When inserting exercises into the strength circuit, observe the order on Table XI. Work your leg muscles first, going from largest to smallest muscles, then move to your trunk, your shoulders, your upper arms, and, finally, your forearms. Exercise your largest muscles first and your smallest muscles last. Perform your arm exercises after your leg exercises because, in fact, you use your arms in some of the leg exercises, and if you exhaust your arms early in the circuit, you won't have them up to par for the leg exercises. If you insert an exercise from chapter 7 (for one of the sports) or from chapter 10 (for rehabilitation), be sure to slip it into its proper anatomical position.

Let's say you are a beginning fencer with weak arms and extra flab along your inner thighs. You might create the following circuit: squats, hamsters, twirling jumps, groin squeezes, side leg lifts, front leg lifts, en gardes, mermaids, pull-ups, chin-ups, arm sprints, dips, and wrist curls.

Sit-ups and locusts (for strengthening your back) are not included in the strength circuit because they aren't active or aerobic. (Sit-ups remain in the warm-ups, and locusts belong in the flexibility circuit.) If you want to add a strength exercise that doesn't move enough for an aerobic effect, add it to the stretching lap.

The flexibility circuit stretches your muscles progressively—each muscle is prepared in one exercise for greater demands to follow. To avoid hopping up and down, finish the floor exercises before you get up on your knees, and the hands-and-knees exercises before you get up on your feet. Within that plan, you can insert any stretching exercise (or any static strength exercise) from any section in this book.

Here's a sample concentrated stretching circuit for a beginning fencer who failed the knee-nose touch on the self-fitness test and has short hamstrings and little flexibility in the groin: towel stretches, plows, wasp waisters, wall splits, king of Siam kowtows, pigeon crawls, geisha kneels, runner's starts, hunkers, birds, gravity toe touches, and side stretches.

Warm-ups

Each workout begins with modified universal warm-ups. Perform them in your usual fashion, relaxing and stretching out your muscles. However, instead of doing only one killer sit-up, work yourself up to twenty. These strengthen the rectus abdominis muscles running up the center of your trunk. When this first level becomes easy—which will take quite a while—move to level two, and then onward and upward.

- Level two: Instead of folding your hands behind your head, cross them over your chest as if you were holding on to opposite collar points.
- Level three, belly busters: Perform the same killer sit-up, but with your legs bent in the air as if they were resting on an imaginary stool.
- Level four: Perform belly busters while holding a 2-pound weight behind your head. When a 2-pound weight seems reasonable—it never feels easy—switch to 3 pounds. (These are only for the most hard-core fitness buffs.)

Doing twenty killer sit-ups is hard—nay, excruciating—but do them. The abdominal muscles are usually the weakest muscles in the body, and yet they are extremely important because they help to support the lower and middle back and thus prevent backaches. The more you sit, the more you slouch when you stand, the more you run or play running games, the more exaggerated the sway in the small of your back. The operative muscles in this part of your back are the iliopsoas, which run from the inside (anterior) of the lumbar part of your spine across the pelvis to the inner part of the thigh bone (femur). The psoas work constantly because their job is to bring your thigh toward your trunk, something you do whenever you sit, run, or bend. They become

TABLE XI: <u>STRENGTH</u> CIRCUIT

	Buttocks	Inner Thigh	Outer Thigh	Front Thigh: Quadriceps	Back Thigh: Hamstring	Hip Flexors	Calves	Shins
°Squats	×			×	×		×	×
Kiddie kicks				×				
°Hamsters				×	×			
Run-'em-out-of-gym-class sprints	×			×	×	×		
°Groin squeezes		×	×					
°Split shifts	×	×	×					
Side leg lifts		×	×					
Front leg lifts with weights	×	×	×					
Swimmer's kicks	×							
°En gardes	×	×	×					
°Dumbbell lunges	×	×	×	×	×			
Heel and toes							×	×
°Mermaids	×			×				
°Dumbbell pullovers								
Twisting sit-ups								
Shoulder shrugs								
Pull-ups								
Chin-ups								
Hanging curls						×		
°Arm sprints								
°Dips								
°Wrist curls								
°Locusts (stretching circuit)	×				×			
°Killer sit-ups (universal warm-up)								
°Push-ups (universal warm-up)								

Abdominals (rectus)	Abdominals (oblique)	Upper Arm: Triceps	Upper Arm: Biceps	Shoulder: Trapezius	Shoulder and Under-arm: Lats	Shoulder: Deltoids	Chest: Pectorals	Lower Arm and Wrist	Lower Back	Middle Back
									X	
	X									
	X	X					X		X	X
X	X									
				X						
		X			X					
			X		X					
X										
		X			X	X				
		X				X	X			
								X		
X									X	
X										
		X		Ser-ratus			X			

TABLE XII: CONCENTRATED STRETCHING CIRCUIT

	Ankles and Feet	Achilles Tendon	Calves	Shins	Knees	Front of Thigh: Quadriceps	Back of Thigh: Hamstring
Foot circles	×						
Baby flexers	×		×				
°Towel stretches		×					×
Plows							×
°Wasp waisters							
Wall splits							
°King of Siam kowtows							
°Pigeon crawls							
°Geisha kneels	×			×		×	
°Runner's starts							×
°Hunkers	×	×		×	×		
Posture clasps							
Head twisters							
°Birds							
Gravity toe touches							×
°Side stretches							
Calf stretches			×				
Achilles stretches		×	×				
Storks (universal warm-ups)						×	

Groin	Hip Flexors	Hips	Waist and Sides	Lower Back	Middle Back	Upper Back	Neck	Shoulders	Chest: Pectorals	Upper Arm: Triceps	Upper Arm: Biceps	Forearm, Wrists and Hands
				×	×	×						
		×	×	×								
×												
				×	×	×	×					
												×
×	×											
×					×							
								×	×	×		
							×					
			×			×		×		×	×	
			×									

very short from all this use and force the spine to sway or arch. This is the cause of many backaches. Killer sit-ups strengthen the stomach muscles without using the psoas, so they balance the muscles and straighten the spine back into its normal S-curve. As an added bonus, firm abdominal muscles put the liquid contents of your trunk under pressure, turning this liquid into a stiff column of fluid which acts almost like a second supporting spine to take some of the pressure off the back muscles.

THE VACUUM

The vacuum, a venerable Yoga exercise, demonstrates the principles of overload and specificity while it firms your abdomen and flattens your tummy by working the upper and lower abdominal muscles.

Get down on your hands and knees. Exhale all air in your lungs, suck your abdomen in as sharply and fully as you can, and then pop your belly out, for one rep. Do twenty reps several times a day. Keep your back flat; look at something in front of you so that you don't round your spine. Overload occurs because the force of gravity is added to the weight of your own slack muscles. Specificity occurs because you are drawing in your belly more fully than you can when you sit or stand, but you are still training your muscles to hold themselves taut. If you can't suck your gut in far enough to feel as if your abdomen is touching your spine, your stomach may be full of food or your lungs may still have some air in them. Exhale again.

In your warm-ups, also work yourself up to twenty push-ups.

- Level one: Hands on a table, feet on the floor
- Level two: Hands and feet on the floor
- Level three: Killer push-ups, hands and feet on the floor
- Level four: Killer push-ups, hands on the floor, feet up on a stool
- Level five: Killer push-ups, hands on the floor, feet on the edge of a sturdy table

Strength Circuit

After your warm-ups, run through the strength circuit three times. The first lap is half speed, a slow jog; the second lap is three-quarter speed; the last lap is all out, as fast as you can go.

Speed is determined not only by how fast you do each rep but how briefly you rest between each station, and these factors vary independently of each other so that you are always working to the best of your ability without straining yourself excessively. At first, allow yourself twenty seconds of rest for every ten seconds of exercise in your full-speed lap. That means you will lift ten reps, a rep a second, and then rest for twenty seconds. (You may have to spend some of those twenty seconds setting up for the next station by putting on or taking off ankle weights or walking or jogging over to the chinning bar.) When you advance to the point that ten reps in ten seconds doesn't wipe you out, add five more reps, one per second, and reduce your rest period to fifteen seconds. When that gets easy, remain at fifteen reps but reduce your rest period to ten seconds, even shorter if you don't need setting-up time. The speed of each movement and the lack of rest periods exercise your heart. When fifteen reps and ten seconds (or less) rest is easy, it's time to increase the resistance by moving up a level or adding more weight. Every time you add resistance, you start all over with ten seconds for reps and twenty seconds for rest. (This pace is an approximation. You may find it impossible with some exercises to do one rep per second. As long as you are working as fast as possible and your heart rate reaches target pitch, you're okay.)

When you increase the pace of a circuit, experiment on the last lap only. If you try to move from, say, a 10/20 lap to a 15/15 lap in your first or half-speed lap, you may get so tired you can't complete the other two laps at their correct speeds.

TABLE XIII: CIRCUIT PACE

	Reps Per Station (one second/rep)	Rest Per Station
Beginners	10	20 seconds
Intermediate	15	15 seconds
Advanced	15	10 seconds or less

At first, you'll have to time your reps in order to maintain the proper pace. However, as soon as you learn the rhythm, you'll never have to watch the clock again. No matter how fast you have to move, don't sacrifice form for speed. Keep your movements evenly tensed throughout. Do not bend or lean into a lift to make it easier. Carry each motion out to its fullest extent and back again.

When you reach an intermediate or advanced level of conditioning, add a fourth lap of the strength circuit. At first, run your fourth lap at the three-quarter speed. In other words, run one half-speed lap, two three-quarter-speed laps, and one full-speed lap. When that becomes too easy, run one half-speed lap, one three-quarter-speed lap, and two full-speed laps. When these four laps are not enough to get your pulse rate high enough, don't add another lap of the circuit. Add fifteen to thirty minutes of an aerobic exercise such as stair stepping, rope jumping, or stationary cycling. Any extra aerobic activity should come after the last lap. You want maximal strength when you do your weight training. If you don't have the time to add aerobic exercise to the circuit program, do it on the alternating days.

Stretching Circuit

After the last strength lap (or the supplementary aerobic exercise, if you do it), start on your concentrated stretching lap. If you are very winded, walk around for a minute or two to catch your breath. Then slowly and carefully stretch out all the muscles you've shortened and tensed. You want to be looser and stronger after each session, not tighter and stiffer.

Combined Program

To sum up, then, a workout contains the following:

1. Warm-ups.
2. Half-speed strength lap. Each rep takes twice as long, each rest lasts twice as long. In a half-speed lap of a 10/20 circuit, you spend two seconds on each of ten reps, or twenty seconds per set, and rest for forty seconds between. In a half-speed 15/15, you spend thirty seconds exercising and thirty seconds resting. In a 15/10, you spend thirty seconds exercising and twenty seconds resting.
3. Three-quarter-speed lap. Each rep takes one and a half times as long as it would during the full speed. In a 10/20, you spend a second and a half on each rep, for a total of fifteen seconds exercising and thirty seconds resting; in 15/15, you spend about twenty-one seconds on fifteen reps and twenty-one seconds exercising; and in a 15/10, you spend twenty-one seconds doing fifteen reps and fifteen seconds resting.
4. Full-speed lap. A 10/20 runs ten seconds for the reps and twenty seconds for the rest period; a 15/15 lasts fifteen seconds and fifteen seconds; a 15/10 allows fifteen seconds for fifteen reps and ten seconds or less for a rest stop.
5. Concentrated stretching lap for flexibility and cool-down. (Included here are a few gradual strength exercises that would have slowed down the aerobic laps.)

CIRCUIT TRAINING EXERCISES

Strength Stations

1. Squats

First level: Stand up and hold onto a table or chair back. Keeping your back straight and your head up, bend your knees about 90 degrees, then straighten up onto tiptoes, for one rep. At first you may have to squat down on tiptoes, but squat flatfooted for good form. Do not lower your body below your knees or you may hurt them.

Second level: Squat and rise with your hands on your hips for one rep.

Third level: Squat with your hands on your hips. Straighten into a jump, for one rep.

Fourth level: Bench squats. Stand up, straddling a bench just high enough to permit you to squat three quarters of the way down. In each hand, hold a dumbbell weighing about one tenth of your body weight. Squat down until your buttocks just touch the bench and then come back up. At the lowest point, your heels may lift off the floor. Do not actually sit down or collapse onto the bench. Keep your head up and your posture erect. Don't arch your back or let your belly pop out.

Squats strengthen the quadriceps and hamstrings of the front and back thigh, and the gluteus muscles of the buttocks, as well as the muscles of the calf. If you have bad knees, squats may make them worse. Substitute kiddie kicks.

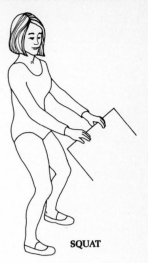

SQUAT

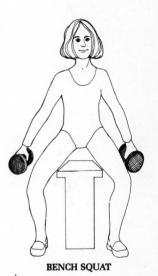

BENCH SQUAT

2. Kiddie Kicks

Sit on a high bench or on the edge of a table and let your legs dangle without touching the floor. Hang an ankle weight, a dumbbell on a belt, or an old purse filled with rocks or a dumbbell from your flexed right foot; don't put it around your ankle. Straighten your leg at the knee, then bring it back to its bent position, for one rep. Strengthens your quads and helps stabilize your knee.

3. Hamsters

First level: Lie face down on the floor, head down on one cheek, arms resting on the floor in front of your head, legs out straight behind you. Point your toes, tense your leg muscles, and bend your knees until your toes are pointing toward the ceiling, then return them to the floor,

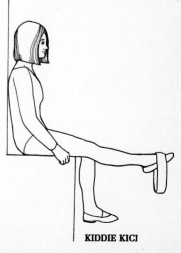

KIDDIE KICK

for one rep. Strengthens your hamstrings. If this is too easy, move immediately to level two.

Second level: Same as first level, but wear 2- or 3-pound weights around each ankle.

Third level: Get down on the floor on your hands and knees. Shifting all your weight onto your hands and right knee, straighten your left leg behind you and point your toe emphatically. Your back should be flat, your shoulders down, and your head up. Focus a short distance ahead of you to get your head in the proper position. Now,

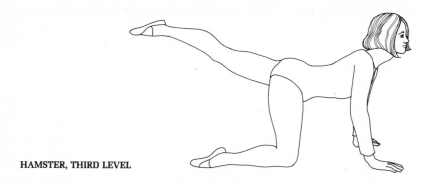

HAMSTER, THIRD LEVEL

bend your left leg to your chest, contracting your body at the same time by rounding your shoulders and looking down at your left knee, for one rep. Keep your toe pointed at all times to maintain the tension in your leg. After you complete the specified number of reps with the left leg, perform the same exercise with your right leg.

Fourth level: Add 2- or 3-pound ankle weights. These two levels strengthen both your hamstrings and your quads.

Fifth level: Stand up and dangle a dumbbell from a belt on your left ankle. The dumbbell should weigh about one tenth of your body

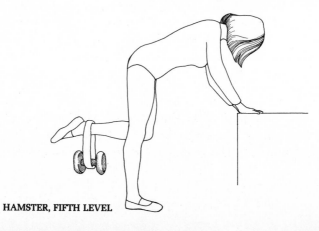

HAMSTER, FIFTH LEVEL

weight. Without moving any other part of your body, bend your left knee until your lower leg is parallel to the floor and forms a 90-degree angle to your upper leg. Lower your foot back to the floor, for one rep. You will probably have to hold onto a chair for balance. To make this even more difficult, put a book under your right foot. When you have finished the requisite number of reps with your left foot, do it with your right. Very effectively isolates and strengthens your hamstrings.

4. Run-'em-Out-of-Gym-Class Sprints

Bend down into a half hands-and-knees position, with your left leg straight out behind you and your right leg bent up close to your chest.

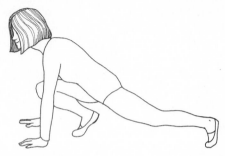

RUN-'EM-OUT-OF-GYM-CLASS SPRINT

Put your weight equally on hands and feet. Shifting your weight to your hands, bounce up high enough to reverse legs, so that your right leg is now straight out behind you and your left leg is bent up to your chest. This is one rep. Builds up your buttocks, quads, hamstrings, and the muscles used for bending your thigh toward your hip (the iliopsoas).

5. Groin Squeezes

Sit on the floor, knees apart and bent, and place one elbow inside each thigh, just above the knee. Clasp your hands and squeeze your thighs together, all the time resisting with your arms. Then push with your elbows and resist with your thighs, to return to your starting position, for one rep. Strengthens the muscles on the inside and outside of your thighs. When this becomes too easy, graduate to split shifts.

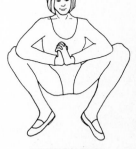

GROIN SQUEEZE

6. Split Shifts

Bend over and place your hands on the floor in front of you for good solid support. Spread your legs out to the sides to do the splits as far down as you can *comfortably* go. Your toes will probably point out-

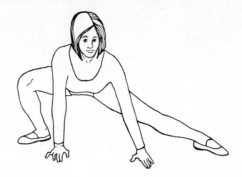

SPLIT SHIFT

ward at 45 degree angles. Leaning a bit on your hands, bend your right leg and shift your weight entirely to your right foot, leaving your left leg straight and out to the side. Now, shift your weight to your left foot, straightening your right leg, for one rep. Keep both heels firmly planted on the floor throughout the exercise. If you can't balance yourself, hold onto a chair for stability, but don't lean against it. Strengthens your groin, the muscles on the sides of your thigh, and, to some extent, your buttocks. If you have bad knees, do side leg lifts instead.

7. Side Leg Lifts

First level: Place 2- to 3-pound weights on each ankle. Lie on your right side with your right leg comfortably bent for stability and your right hand propping up your head for support. Keeping your left

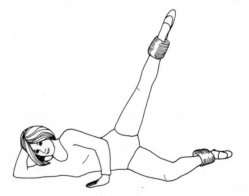

SIDE LEG LIFT

leg straight and your toes pointed, raise it as high as you can comfortably go, then lower it until your left and right thighs *almost* touch, for one rep. Don't actually rest your left leg on your right between reps. Stay on your side at all times; don't roll frontward or backward, and don't move your upper body in any way. Once you have finished the requisite number of reps on your right side, switch to your left.

Strengthens and tones the inside and outside of the thigh but doesn't work the buttocks as effectively as split shifts.

Second level: Add another set of weights on your instep.

8. Front Leg Lifts

First level: Wearing 2- or 3-pound ankle weights, lie on your right side with your right leg comfortably bent and your right hand propping up your head. Keeping your left leg straight and your toes

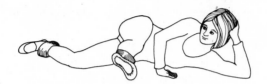

FRONT LEG LIFT

pointed, raise it as high as you can go, then bring it down across your body so that it forms a 90-degree angle with your right thigh and your toes are pointing straight ahead of you. Still keeping it straight and pointed, return it to the vertical for one rep. After reps on right side are completed, repeat on the left side. Strengthens your buttocks, inner and outer thighs, and, to a lesser extent, your hips.

Second level: Add another set of weights on your instep.

9. Swimmer's Kicks

First level: Lie face down on the floor, head on one cheek, placing your hands under your pelvic bones to cushion them and to ease the strain on your lower back. Lift both legs off the floor as high as you can and flutter-kick them once with each foot for one rep. Keep your legs straight and your toes pointed throughout. Don't touch your legs to the floor or rest them until you have finished the whole set. Strengthens your buttocks and lower back muscles. May hurt your back if you have lower or middle back problems.

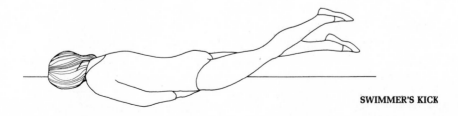

SWIMMER'S KICK

Second level: Same position. Keeping your legs straight and your toes pointed, lift both legs off the floor as high as you can, then open them as wide as you can, and bring them together for one rep. Do not lower your legs until the set is over. Strengthens your buttocks and lower back muscles. May hurt your back if you have lower or middle back problems.

10. En Gardes

Stand up, left foot aimed forward, right foot aimed to the side, and feet shoulder distance apart. Raise your left arm in an easy, bent position, and extend your right arm out to the side over your right leg, as if

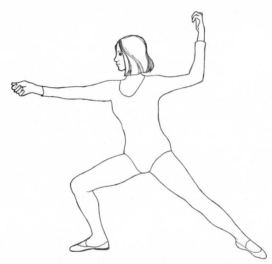

EN GARDE

you were holding a fencing foil. (Pretend you're D'Artagnan, the fourth Musketeer.) Turn your trunk and head and sight down your right arm. Balance your weight evenly on both feet. Sharply and powerfully, jump up and lunge over your right leg, stretching your right arm out as if you were about to thrust with your foil. Your left leg and arm remain loosely bent. Return to your original position for one rep. After performing the required number of reps over your right leg, reverse your position and lunge with your left. Strengthens your inner and outer thighs and your buttocks. When this becomes too easy, graduate to dumbbell lunges.

11. Dumbbell Lunges

Stand with your feet comfortably apart and hold a dumbbell weighing about one eighth of your body weight in each hand. Step forward as

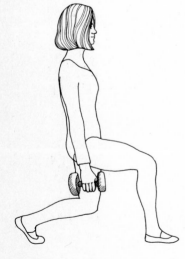

DUMBBELL LUNGE

far as you can with your right foot for your starting position. Now, lower your hips until your left knee just brushes the floor, then raise your body, for one rep. Keep the toes of both feet aimed forward. Keep your neck and back straight and look ahead of you. Don't lean forward and don't bend your right knee forward of your ankle, or you'll damage your knees. After the requisite number of reps, reverse positions and work your right leg. Strengthens your buttocks, groin, outer thigh, quads, and hamstrings.

12. Heel and Toes

First level: Place a thick book on the floor, or use a board one or two inches thick. (Start with a thick novel and graduate to a fat metropolitan telephone book.) Stand with the balls of your feet on the book and your heels hanging over the edge. Rise up on tiptoes and then lower yourself so that your heels touch the floor, for one rep. Keep your knees locked. Strengthens your calf muscles.

Second level: Perform the same exercise while holding something weighing about two pounds in each hand. Work up to weights totaling at least one fifth of your body weight.

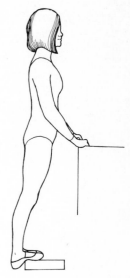

HEEL AND TOES

13. Mermaids

Sit down on the floor Japanese style, with your legs tucked under you and your buttocks resting on your feet. Clasp your hands over your head, palms facing the ceiling. Reach upward and, leading with the palms of your hands, lift yourself up onto your knees, then shift your weight so that you are leaning on the outside of your right leg, for one rep. The whole sequence should flow as one movement. Throughout the exercise, stretch your palms upward as if you could push against the ceiling. Keep your abdomen sucked in and your buttocks tight, and stretch up through your arms. Strengthens the sides of your body, the muscles around your waist and midriff, and even works your outer thighs, buttocks, and quads. When this becomes too easy, graduate to dumbbell pullovers.

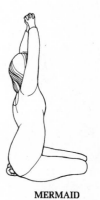

MERMAID

14. Dumbbell Pullovers

Lie on your back on a bed or long, sturdy coffee table. Your head may be on the bed or partially hanging over the edge (experiment for comfort and best effect), but either way you should be close enough to the edge that your arms go well past the end of the bed when you bring them over your head. Bend your knees up onto the bed, or put them down on the floor, but make sure that they are bent in one way or

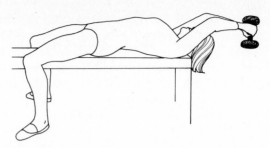

DUMBBELL PULLOVER

another to prevent straining your back. Holding one 3-pound dumbbell with both hands, raise your arms above your head until they are almost fully extended. Keep them *almost* straight and bring them back over your head and down toward the floor behind your head. At the bottom of the arc, bend them to get closer to the floor and make your triceps work harder. Return to starting position first with bent and then with almost straightened arms, for one rep. Graduate to a 5-, 8-, 10-, and 15-pound dumbbell. Stretches and strengthens your midriff, trims your waist, firms your pectorals, strengthens your back and triceps.

15. Twisting Sit-ups

First level: Lie on your back, knees bent, feet flat, hands behind your head, small of your back flattened. Tuck your chin onto your chest and curl yourself up into a full sit-up, twisting so that your right elbow touches your left knee or, if you are particularly flexible, the floor next to your left thigh. Return to starting position, for one rep. During the next rep, bring your left elbow to your right knee, and continue alternating throughout the set.

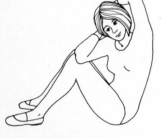

**TWISTING SIT-UP,
SECOND LEVEL**

Second level: Lie on your back with your knees bent, but with your legs in the air as if resting on an imaginary stool. Perform the same twisting sit-ups, alternating sides. These ballistic sit-ups do not work your central abdominal muscles, the rectus muscles, as effectively as killer sit-ups, but they strengthen your side, or oblique, abdominals. They also give you strength for bending and turning, something you need as much as static strength to stabilize your posture.

16. Shoulder Shrugs

First level: Sit on your hands on the floor. Keep your back straight and your legs folded comfortably in front of you. Without moving any other part of your body, shrug your shoulders up to your ears and then return them to their starting position, for one rep. Strengthens the trapezius muscles.

Second level: Stand up, posture erect, feet comfortably apart. In each hand, hold a 5-pound dumbbell. Shrug your shoulders up toward your ears and back down again, for one rep. Strengthens the trapezius muscles.

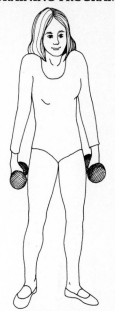

SHOULDER SHRUG, SECOND LEVEL

GRIP-STRENGTH EXERCISE

Chin-ups and pull-ups are hard for women: most women don't use their upper arms enough to have strong triceps and biceps, and few women have enough strength in their hands to hold onto the bar long enough to improve those muscles. Many exercises in this book develop your upper arm muscles, but few also strengthen your grip. Wrist curls help, but for a really solid grip, you also need a direct grip-strength exercise.

Slowly squeeze a racquetball, child's sponge ball of similar size, or a store-bought pair of hand grips which look like two or three coils of a spring with handles attached to the ends. Take three seconds to squeeze it and three seconds to release it, resisting the whole way, for one rep. One set consists of as many reps as you can do before your muscles become exhausted. Perform this exercise several times during the day, while talking on the phone, watching television, or even walking to the bus stop.

---

17. Pull-ups

First level (negative pull-up):   Stand on a chair or stool in front of your chinning bar and place your hands on the bar shoulder width apart, palms facing away from you. Your chin should be slightly higher than the bar. Holding onto the bar, step off the stool and lower yourself to a full hanging position. Stay in control; don't just drop like a stone. Climb back up on the stool for one rep. This exercise works for two reasons. First, negative lifts build muscles as effectively as positive lifts. Second, you can lower more weight than you can raise, so you are painlessly building muscle. Strengthens your triceps and your lats.

Second level (regulation pull-up):   Stand under the chinning bar, with your hands resting on the bar, shoulder width apart, palms facing away from you. The bar should be high enough that your arms are almost fully extended above your head to reach it. Pull yourself up until your chin is above the bar, then lower yourself to the floor, for one rep. Stay in control; don't just drop to the floor. These will take a long time to master, but don't despair. You can do it. Strengthens your triceps and your lats.

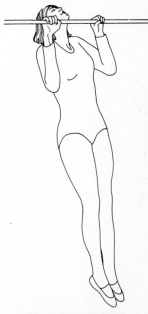

PULL-UP, SECOND LEVEL

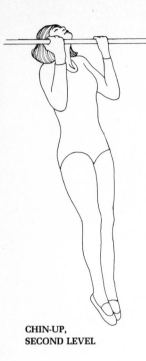

**CHIN-UP,
SECOND LEVEL**

18. Chin-ups

First level (negative chin-up):   Perform a negative pull-up, but hold onto the bar with your palms facing you. These are easier than pull-ups because your biceps are more developed than your triceps. Strengthens the biceps and lats.

Second level (regulation chin-up):   Perform a regulation pull-up, but hold onto the bar with your palms facing you. Strengthens your biceps and lats.

19. Hanging Curls

First level: Hang from the chinning bar in a chin-up position and curl your knees up to your chest, then return, for one rep. (Use a pull-up grip if you prefer, but that's harder.) When curls become easy, try hanging pikes, but only if you have a very strong back.

Second level (hanging pikes):   With your legs straight and your toes pointed, bend at the hips and bring your legs straight out in front of you at a 90-degree angle to your trunk. Lower your legs with control to their starting position, for one rep. Strengthens your lower abdominals and hip flexors.

20. Arm Sprints

Get down into a push-up position, but rest both hands on a stair or low bench. Your arms, trunk, and legs should be straight. Put your right hand on the floor, bring your left hand down to join it, then replace your right hand on the bench, and then your left, for one rep. Constantly strive to increase your speed. Strengthens your deltoids, lats, and triceps.

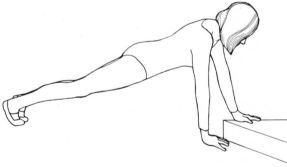

ARM SPRINT

21. Dips

First level: Place your hands behind you on the edge of a couch or an extremely steady chair. Stretch your trunk and legs out in front of you as if you were doing an inside-out push-up. Keeping your body as straight as possible, lower yourself by bending your elbows until they are bent to 90 degrees or more. Scramble back up to the starting position, for one rep. Don't bend at the hips to ease your descent. If this is too hard, start by leaning against the edge of a table. The higher your starting point, the less work you do. On the other hand, if you want to work harder, lean against something lower than a chair seat; try a stair, or even the floor. Strengthens your triceps, pectorals, and deltoids.

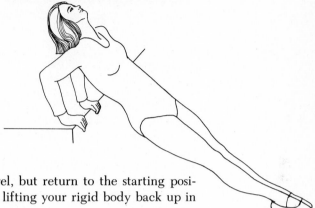

DIP, FIRST LEVEL

Second level: Same as first level, but return to the starting position by straightening your arms and lifting your rigid body back up in a kind of inside-out push-up, for one rep.

Third level: Stand up and grasp the arms of a sturdy chair. Straightening your arms to support your weight, lift your feet off the floor and bend your knees until you imitate a sitting position in the air. Bend your elbows and lower your bottom toward the seat, but don't sit down. Lift yourself by straightening your arms up to the starting position, for one rep. Do not let your feet touch the floor during the entire set. Strengthens your lower pectorals, especially if you lean forward slightly, your deltoids, your abdominals, and your triceps (if you keep your body erect).

Fourth level (regulation dip):   Stand between two sturdy tables, two waist-high cabinets, or two chair backs. These objects should be about shoulder width apart. Place your hands on the edges of the tables (they are substitutes for parallel dip bars in a gym) and straighten out your arms to lift you until they are supporting all your weight. Now bend your elbows and, with great control, lower yourself as far below the edges of the tables as you can. Return to the high straight-armed position, for one rep. You'll have to bend your legs on the dip to keep them from touching the floor. Your goal is to dip low enough to touch your shoulders to your hands—a feat that won't come easy. If the transition from third to fourth level is too drastic, perform these dips negatively for a while. Lower yourself, using only arm power, but use your legs to scramble back to the starting position. Strengthens your lower pectoral muscles, your triceps, and your deltoids.

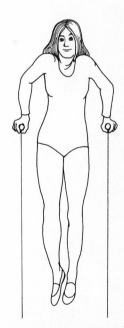

DIP, FOURTH LEVEL

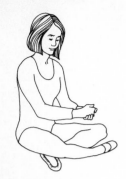

**WRIST CURLS,
FIRST LEVEL**

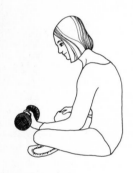

**WRIST CURLS,
SECOND LEVEL**

22. Wrist Curls

First level: Sit on the floor in any comfortable position. Rest your elbows on your thighs and place the palm of your right hand on top of the palm of your left hand, holding your hands flat and parallel to the floor rather than up and down. Keeping your hands clasped together, press down with your right hand while you resist the movement with your left. Let your right hand win, but make it work for the victory. Then push with your left hand while you resist with your right until your right hand is bent back as far as it will go, for one rep. Do not move your forearms. When you have completed the requisite number of reps, reverse the position of your hands and repeat.

Second level: Sit on the floor, legs comfortably crossed. Hold a 1½-pound dumbbell in each hand, palms downward, and rest your forearms on your thighs. Your forearms should be entirely supported, but your wrists and hands should hang free. Bend your fists up toward your body as far as you can, and then lower them as far as they go, for one rep. Do not move any part of your forearms above the wrists. After you complete the requisite number of reps, turn your fists over so that you are gripping the dumbbells with your palms facing up. Curl the dumbbells toward your body as far as you can, then lower them toward

---

USING AN EXERCISE PARTNER

If you have an exercise partner, you can turn her (or him) into a very effective variable resistance machine. Ask her to exert a force in the opposite direction you are exercising. She pushes or pulls just enough to keep you working at the same tension, adjusting her intensity as the movement reaches its easier and harder points. Don't let her push so hard that you can't move at all, or you'll be doing isometrics instead of isotonics.

The two of you can adapt almost any exercise to this technique. Your partner can hold your forearm as you raise and lower the weight during a wrist curl. She can lift you slightly as you come down from a chin-up. She can even push against your collarbone or upper chest as you do sit-ups. A partner is more effective than ankle weights during side leg lifts and front leg lifts, and can be turned into a wonderful hamstring leg curl machine: Lie on the floor, face down, with your partner kneeling beside the leg you are exercising. Your partner places one hand on the back of your ankle and one on the back of your thigh, just above your knee. As you try to bend your knee all the way up, she resists you. When you return to the starting position, she places her hands underneath your shin to provide resistance to your downward motion for one rep. This is an excellent way to strengthen your hamstrings.

the floor as far as possible, for one rep. Again, do not move any part of your forearms and do not let your elbows pop off your thighs. Increase the weight gradually up to one tenth of your body weight in each dumbbell. Strengthens your forearm flexors and extensors.

Flexibility Stations

Follow the principles of progressive static stretching. Stretch slowly until you feel a *slight* pull, then hold and stay there for ten to twenty seconds. Don't bounce. When the tension passes, reach a little farther until you feel a slight pull again and hold that without bouncing for twenty to sixty seconds more. If extreme flexibility is important to you, repeat the process a third time, and hold each stretch for the maximum count. You will find that some parts of your body are more flexible than others, and that you are looser on some days than others. That's normal.

Note: The locust, a required station here, is actually a strength exercise.

1. Foot Circles

Same as universal warm-up, but lie on your back. Extend and flex and bend each foot slowly, deliberately, as far as it will go. Stretches your ankle and calf muscles.

2. Baby Foot Flexers

Lie on your back. Bend your left knee and place your left foot flat on the floor to relieve any strain on your groin. Bring your right knee up to your chest and drastically flex your right foot, as if you were point-

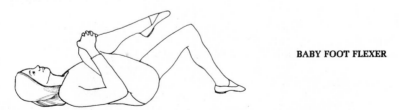

BABY FOOT FLEXER

ing forward with your heel. Smoothly extend your foot until it is aggressively pointed, for one rep. Do twenty slow, deliberate reps, and then switch legs and work on the left foot. Stretches the ankle, foot muscles, and calf.

3. Towel Stretches

First level: Lie on your back. Tilt your pelvis so that the small of your back hugs the floor. Bend your left leg to take pressure off your

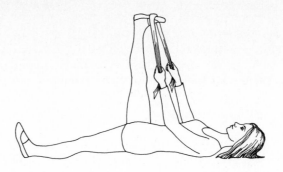

TOWEL STRETCH

back. Bring your right knee up to your chest and hook a long towel or strip of fabric around the ball of your foot. Holding onto the ends of the towel with both hands, flex your right foot, lead with your heel, and straighten your leg as much as possible, trying to point your heel toward the ceiling. Hold, then move your hands up the towel in order to pull your leg higher and closer to your face. Keep your shoulders flat on the floor at all times. Hold again, then reverse legs.

Second level: Lie on your back with your knees bent and your feet flat on the floor. Press the small of your back into the floor. Bend your right knee up to your chest and hold it there by holding the back of the thigh, just above the knee, with both hands. Without moving your knee away from your body, slowly unbend it. It won't straighten out entirely. Don't let it veer to the side. Reverse legs.

These exercises stretch your hamstrings and Achilles tendon.

4. Plows

Lie on your back, with your arms down at your sides. Slowly and deliberately, bring your legs straight over your head by bending at the hip and rolling up along your spine. Try to touch your toes to the floor above your head. If this is too difficult, support your lower back and

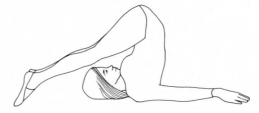

PLOW

buttocks with your hands and touch only one foot to the floor. Until you are very flexible, keep your back and legs straight. Stay in control. If you overreach and lose control, you may twist your back or neck muscles. Hold the stretch, and then roll up farther along your spine until you feel more pull in your lower back and hamstrings. The farther you roll, the higher the muscles you stretch in your back. This traditional Yoga pose stretches your lower back and hamstrings.

5. Wasp Waisters

Lie on your back and bend your left knee across your body. With your right hand, grab behind your left knee and pull until it touches the floor along your right side. Keep your left arm stretched out to your

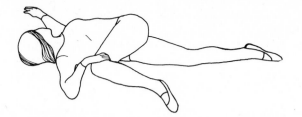

WASP WAISTER

side and turn your head to the left to sight down it to get the maximum twist in your trunk. Keep your shoulders flat on the floor. When you have held this stretch long enough, reverse legs. Stretches your waist, lower back, and sides of hips.

6. Wall Splits

Lie on your back, your legs straight up and leaning against a wall. Your bottom should be three to five inches from the wall, or as close as you can get without arching your back. Press the small of your back into the floor. Flex your feet so that your toes are pointing toward your

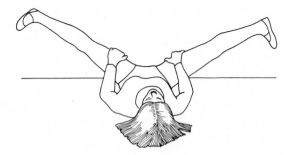

WALL SPLITS

head, then spread your legs into the splits by scraping your heels along the wall until you feel that first pull. You can use your hands to increase the pull, if you wish. Hold, spread farther, and hold again. If your feet go to sleep, roll over and shake them out, then try again. Get up slowly to avoid dizziness. Stretches your groin.

7. King of Siam Kowtows

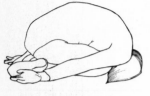

KING OF SIAM KOWTOW

Get down on your hands and knees, then lower your butt to your heels and your chest to your knees until you are curled into a fetal position. Round your spine all the way from your tailbone to the highest verte-bra in your neck. Tuck your chin onto your collarbone and touch the top of your head, not your forehead, to the floor. Drape your arms alongside your body, so that your fingers almost touch your toes. This is a very passive stretch. Just lie there, relaxing, for a minute, then get up slowly. After a few weeks, you will be loose enough to stretch your arms out in front of you. Stretches and lengthens all your back muscles.

8. Locusts

Lie face down, legs together and straight out behind you, arms along your ears and straight out in front of you. Contract your abdominal muscles and buttocks and slowly lift your head, arms, chest, and legs off the floor. Look straight ahead, sighting down your arms. Rest all

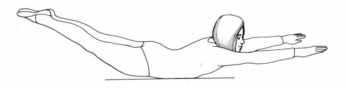

LOCUST

your weight on your rib cage and pelvis. If you lift too high, you'll block your windpipe and have to hold your breath. Don't. Hold for a ten-second count at first and work up to twenty to sixty seconds. Then, slowly and in tight control, lower yourself back down to the floor for one rep. Work up to ten reps. This sadistic Yoga pose strengthens your lower back, buttocks, rear thigh, and even abdominal muscles. If you have arthritis or lower back or neck problems, skip this station and go directly to number ten, the pigeon crawl.

9. King of Siam Kowtows

Again, to stretch out the back muscles you just shortened.

10. Pigeon Crawls

Get down on your hands and knees. Rotate your hands outward and back so that your fingers point toward your knees—as if your hands were pigeon-toed. At first, hold your arms away from your body, but as you become more flexible, bring your arms closer to your body so that your hands line up with your knees. Lean back, moving your hips toward your feet until you feel a pull in your forearms and hands. Keep the heels of your hands flat on the floor. Stretches the muscles and tendons in the heels of your hands, wrists, and forearms.

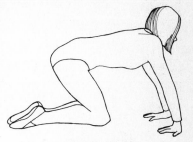

PIGEON CRAWL

11. Geisha Kneels

Kneel Japanese-style, resting your buttocks on your calves and feet and pointing your toes behind you. If you don't feel a stretch in the top of your foot (dorsum) and front ankle, lean back on your elbows and forearms. For even more stretch, lift up one knee to put the weight of that leg onto the top, or dorsum, of the foot. Hold; lower that knee, lift the other; hold again. Don't let your knees splay out; don't let your feet slip out from under your buttocks.

After holding that stretch, come back up and flex your feet under you so that your toes now support much of your weight. Sit down on your heels and lean back until you feel another stretch. Hold. Return to the first position for a final lengthening. Stretches your quads, shins, ankles, dorsum, arch, and toes. If you have a knee problem, you may want to pass this station; putting weight on bad knees when they are fully bent may stretch the ligaments stabilizing the knee and exacerbate the problem.

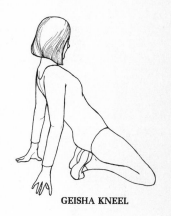

GEISHA KNEEL

12. Runner's Starts

Crouch down on your right leg while extending your left leg straight behind you. Rest your weight on your right foot and the toes of your left foot and, if necessary, your left knee too. Bend your right knee in a

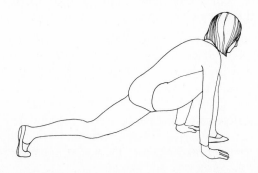

RUNNER'S START

direct line over your ankle, and keep your right foot flat on the floor at all times. Place your hands on the floor outside your legs for support. Now slowly lower your hips toward the floor, keeping both feet firmly in place but bending your left knee until you feel a stretch in the front of your left hip, right at the juncture of your thigh and abdomen. Hold. Stretch further, hold, then reverse legs. Don't lower your bottom, or your leg will bend forward of your foot and damage your knee. Stretches your iliopsoas (hip flexors), groin, and even your hamstrings.

13. Hunkers

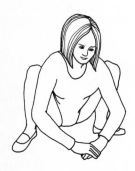

**HUNKER,
SECOND LEVEL**

First level: Hold onto a table leg or the arm of a chair and squat down with your feet flat on the floor and comfortably spaced, your toes pointed slightly outward. Keep your arms inside your legs, your shoulders forward, and your back rounded for balance. Try to get your buttocks to touch your heels. If you can't keep your balance the first few tries, practice hunkering during your bath. In the tub, the hot water loosens your joints and muscles and supports some of your weight. If this hurts your knees, don't do it.

Second level: When this position becomes familiar, hunker down without holding onto anything. Keep your arms dangling easily in front of you but between your legs so that your knees are spread wider than your shoulders. Hunkers stretch the small of your back, your groin, knees, shins, ankles, and Achilles tendons.

14. Posture Clasps

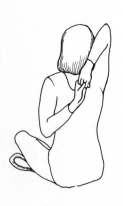

**POSTURE CLASP,
SECOND LEVEL**

First level: Sit cross-legged. Dangle a towel from your right hand over your right shoulder and down your back. Bring your left hand behind your back waist-high, palm facing out, and grab the towel as high as you can. Head up, back straight, pull up with the towel with your right hand, dragging your left arm along, and hold, then pull down with your left hand and hold. Reverse positions and repeat. Gradually move your hands closer together along the towel until you can eliminate the towel altogether.

Second level: Sit cross-legged. Bring your right hand over your right shoulder, palm down, and your left hand behind your back, from below, palm up. Clasp your hands together and pull steadily upward with your right hand for a count of twenty. (You won't actually move your left arm very much, but you will feel a good stretch.) Now, pull down with your left hand for another twenty count. Hold your back straight and your head up. Reverse positions, so that the left arm is over your left shoulder, and repeat. This traditional Yoga pose stretches both shoulders, the pectorals, and the triceps.

15. Head Twisters

Sit cross-legged. Clasp your hands behind your head, just above your neck, and pull your head down so that your chin approaches or touches your collarbone. Hold for ten to twenty seconds, or as long as you wish. (If you're tense, this feels heavenly.) Now, raise your head and cradle your chin in your right hand, with the fingers pointing toward your ear. Place your left hand on the back of your head, a little right of center. Twist your head to the right by pushing your chin up with your right hand and pulling your head down with the left. See if you can touch your left ear to your left shoulder without raising your shoulder. (Most likely you can't.) Hold, then reverse the position of your hands and twist your head to the left. Hold. Stretches the back and sides of your neck.

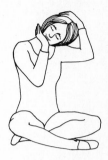

HEAD TWISTER

16. Birds

Stand up, feet comfortably apart. Clasp your hands behind your back, and then, bending from the hips, lean over as far as possible and bring your arms up over your head toward the floor in front of you. To do

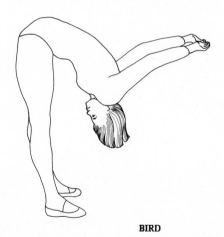

BIRD

this, you will have to turn your clasped hands inside-out after your arms reach the top of their arc. Keep your legs straight and your knees locked. Stretches the biceps, triceps, shoulders, waist, and back.

17. Gravity Toe Touches (same as universal warm-ups)

Stand with your feet comfortably close together. Bend over at the hips and try to touch your toes or the floor. Go down until you feel a stretch, then hang there, letting gravity pull you farther down, then

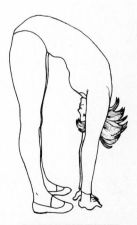

GRAVITY TOE TOUCH

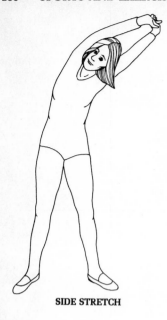

SIDE STRETCH

stretch and hold again. Don't bounce. When you release to stand up, bend your knees to prevent a strain on your lower back. Stretches your hamstrings.

18. Side Stretches

Stand up straight, legs comfortably apart. Raise your arms straight over your head and interlace your hands, palms up. With your elbows locked, lead with the heel of your left hand and slowly bend to the left at the waist. Hold. Face forward at all times. Don't twist to the side, don't let your buttocks or belly pop out, and don't bend your knees. Hold, then straighten up and bend to the right, leading with the heel of your right hand. Hold. When you do this correctly, you feel a stretch on both sides of your body, no matter which direction you bend. Stretches the sides of your trunk.

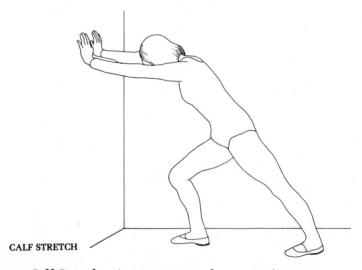

CALF STRETCH

19. Calf Stretches (same as universal warm-ups)

Stand about eighteen inches from a wall, facing it. Place both hands on the wall, about shoulder height and width. Stretch one leg out behind you, keeping the knee straight and the heel firmly on the floor. Center your body over the forward leg, bend that knee slightly, and plant the heel firmly in the floor. Slowly lean into the wall, sliding your hips forward and bending your arms until you feel a real pull. Hold. Repeat with the other leg. Stretches the calf muscles, lower hamstrings, and the shin muscles extending to your feet.

SUPER STRETCHING

If you want to be extremely limber, and you've already been working on progressive static stretches for several months, proprioceptive neuromuscular facilitation may give you the most stretch for the least pain, according to an article in *Medicine and Science in Sports and Exercise*. Although it was described by Margaret Knott in 1956, PNF spent more than twenty years in obscurity before it was rediscovered by athletes convinced that a little extra flexibility gives them a competitive edge. Now, more and more gymnasts, figure skaters, ballet dancers, and swimmers use pairs of PNF-based exercises to develop the extraordinarily loose joints required for their sports.

For the simplest forms of PNF, you stretch as far as you can, hold, then release. Then perform an isometric strength exercise to contract or tighten the same muscles you've been lengthening and stretching, hold it, then repeat the original stretching exercise. To choose which stretch goes with which isometric, select an isometric that tries to move your muscles in the opposite direction of the stretch. For example, to stretch your hamstrings using PNF, do a gravity toe touch for a count of twenty. Release carefully, then immediately do an isometric hamstring strengthener. My favorite involves standing with my back to a very heavy coffee table. I hook my heel under the table and then try to lift it up by bending my knee as if I could bring my heel up to touch my butt. (This is really a fifth-level hamster done against an immovable object.) Hold the isometric contraction for a ten to twenty count, slowly release, and immediately perform another gravity toe touch. During this second touch, you can reach much farther than the first. The toe touches elongate your hamstrings by straightening them; the isometric curls shorten them by bending the joint they move (the knee) against a resistance. To stretch your groin muscles, spread them with wall splits, then bring them together against a resistance by doing groin squeezes with a ball or unsqueezable object. If you have time, you can repeat the stretch-isometric-stretch sequence two or three times.

When you try to stretch a muscle beyond its usual range, it tightens up, hurts, and actually becomes shorter than before. PNF short-circuits this reflex but, in the process, removes your innate protection against muscle tears. The tightening reflex resembles a fuse in a fuse box. When the circuit becomes overloaded, the fuse blows, cuts off power, and prevents an electrical fire. PNF, used carelessly, is the penny some people place behind a fuse to keep it from blowing: The penny eliminates the temporary inconvenience of blowing a fuse, but it also eliminates the protection from fire the fuse is supposed to afford. Thus, PNF is dangerous unless you are already quite experienced in stretching and are very sensitive to the slightest signal that you might be overdoing it.

20. Achilles Stretches

Same as calf stretches, but bend your back knee very slightly. Keep both heels on the floor. Stretches the calf and the Achilles tendon.

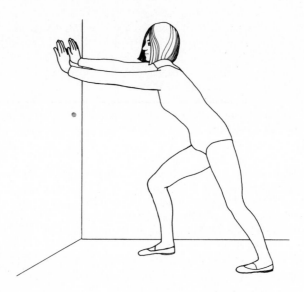

ACHILLES STRETCH

7 / Sports A to W

The sports in this directory will provide you with a lifetime of fitness and good health. To be included, each sport must provide at least two out of the three ingredients of good physical conditioning: aerobics, strength, and flexibility. If a sport doesn't have a training effect, you won't find it here, no matter how popular it is. Take bowling, for example. More than 4.2 million U.S. women compete regularly in 168,000 sanctioned Women's International Bowling Congress leagues throughout the country, so imagine how many bowl occasionally just for the fun of it. But bowling does nothing for your heart and lungs, muscle strength, or flexibility. If you rolled that heavy ball down the alley nonstop for thirty minutes, you'd probably develop strength and endurance in your arms and shoulders and even improve your wind. But bowling is a stop-start game, with more pit stops than playing time. Result: no training effect.

Golf is out too. The only exercise you get from golf is walking—if you do walk and leave the cart at the clubhouse—but that walking only lasts about three minutes at a stretch. To develop cardiovascular conditioning, you must walk briskly for at least thirty minutes without stopping. Furthermore, because of its intermittent nature, you don't loosen or strengthen your muscles, even if you carry your golf bag over your shoulder.

Also missing are table tennis, land and sea motor sports, flying and soaring sports, skydiving, shooting, archery, tai chi, croquet, sailing, pitching horseshoes, riding horses, throwing flying disks (Frisbee and its kin), and sledding of all sorts (although some forms do strengthen parts of your legs if you practice them several hours each day several months of the year). These sports, and their cousins, may have their occasional brief moments of strenuous bursts, but overall they stress coordination, a good eye, a steady hand, and, for many, a big dose of courage.

STERNOCLEIDOMASTOID
(turns, flexes, and extends head)

TRAPEZIUS

DELTOID
(lowers, raises and rotates arm out)

PECTORALS
(lower, raise, and rotate arm in)

BICEPS
(bends elbow)

RECTUS ABDOMINIS
(compresses abdominal cavity, bends
and rotates torso)

**FOREARM ROTATORS AND
FLEXORS**
(twist and bend wrist and hand)

TENSOR FASCIAE LATAE

*Thigh and
Hip Adductors*

PECTINEUS
ADDUCTOR LONGUS
ADDUCTOR MAGNUS
GRACILIS

ILIOTIBIAL BAND

PERONEUS LONGUS
(picks up outside of foot while
bending ankle inward, extends foot)

ANTERIOR TIBIALIS
(raises inner edge of foot while
bending ankle outward; flexes foot)

**LOWER LEG, ANKLE, AND FOOT
EXTENSORS,
FLEXORS AND ROTATORS**

CLAVICLE
(collarbone)

SERRATUS ANTERIOR
(pulls forward, upward; rotates,
abducts, and stabilizes shoulder
blade)

EXTERNAL OBLIQUE
(with internal oblique underneath,
compresses abdominal cavity, bends
and rotates torso)

ANTERIOR SUPERIOR ILIAC SPINE
(part of hip bone)

ILIOPSOAS
(hip flexor)

SARTORIUS
(knee flexor, outward thigh rotator;
weak hip flexor)

RECTUS FEMORIS
(hip flexor)
VASTUS MEDIALIS
(knee extensor)
VASTUS LATERALIS
(knee extensor)

*Three of the four muscles
of the quadriceps; the fourth,
the vastus intermedialis, lies
underneath the rectus femoris*

PATELLA (kneecap)

TIBIA

GASTROCNEMIUS

SOLEUS

ACHILLES TENDON

**SELECTED BODY MUSCLES, BONES,
AND TENDONS: FRONT VIEW**

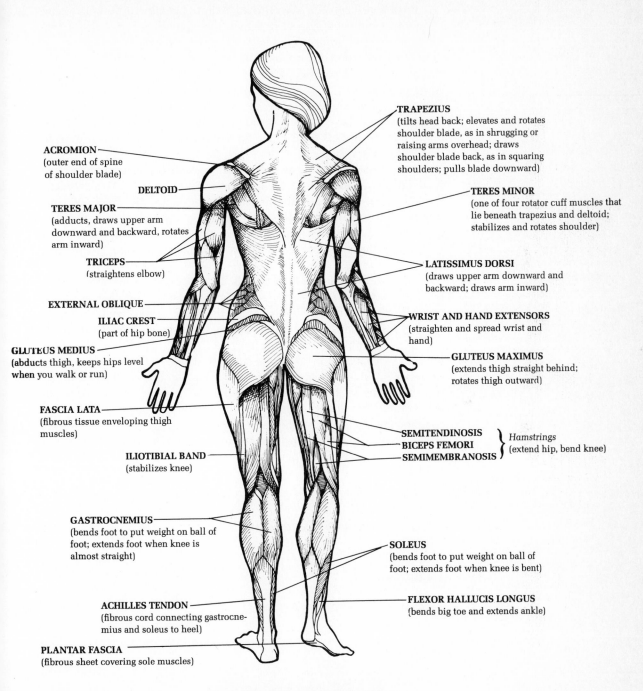

TRAPEZIUS
(tilts head back; elevates and rotates shoulder blade, as in shrugging or raising arms overhead; draws shoulder blade back, as in squaring shoulders; pulls blade downward)

ACROMION
(outer end of spine of shoulder blade)

DELTOID

TERES MAJOR
(adducts, draws upper arm downward and backward, rotates arm inward)

TRICEPS
(straightens elbow)

EXTERNAL OBLIQUE

ILIAC CREST
(part of hip bone)

GLUTEUS MEDIUS
(abducts thigh, keeps hips level when you walk or run)

FASCIA LATA
(fibrous tissue enveloping thigh muscles)

ILIOTIBIAL BAND
(stabilizes knee)

GASTROCNEMIUS
(bends foot to put weight on ball of foot; extends foot when knee is almost straight)

ACHILLES TENDON
(fibrous cord connecting gastrocnemius and soleus to heel)

PLANTAR FASCIA
(fibrous sheet covering sole muscles)

TERES MINOR
(one of four rotator cuff muscles that lie beneath trapezius and deltoid; stabilizes and rotates shoulder)

LATISSIMUS DORSI
(draws upper arm downward and backward; draws arm inward)

WRIST AND HAND EXTENSORS
(straighten and spread wrist and hand)

GLUTEUS MAXIMUS
(extends thigh straight behind; rotates thigh outward)

SEMITENDINOSIS
BICEPS FEMORI
SEMIMEMBRANOSIS
} *Hamstrings*
(extend hip, bend knee)

SOLEUS
(bends foot to put weight on ball of foot; extends foot when knee is bent)

FLEXOR HALLUCIS LONGUS
(bends big toe and extends ankle)

SELECTED BODY MUSCLES, BONES, AND TENDONS: REAR VIEW

Boxing also gets the downturned thumb, but for a different reason. I cannot recommend a sport in which the chances are so high for disfigurement, fatal brain hemorrhages, fractured hands, ruptured organs (because most women don't have as highly developed abdominal muscles as men), and painful, although rarely permanent, breast injuries. After all, the goal of a boxer is to hurt her opponent. If as great a fighter as Muhammad Ali may be suffering throat and brain damage, as some reports have suggested, no boxer is safe. Just because men are dumb enough to beat each other up doesn't mean that women have to make the same mistake.

Every sport makes its own demands on your body. Running a hundred miles a week doesn't mean you can hop on a bike and breeze through a ten-mile ride. Running has strengthened the backs of your legs but left the fronts weak. Bicycling, like downhill skiing, uses the quadriceps, the muscles running along the front of your thighs. You may finish the ride, but your knees will ache and your thighs will throb.

Because the principles of specificity and overload are as immutable as the First Law of Thermodynamics, you must train anew for each sport. Use the Index of Exercises at the back of the book to locate specific instructions. Some sports make surprisingly good bedfellows, however. Downhill skiing, bicycling, and speed skating use the same muscles of your legs in the same strength ratios (as the bicycle-racing successes of Olympic speed skaters Beth Heiden and Sarah Docter attest); bicycling in the summer will make you a better skier or skater in the winter. This doesn't mean that you should only play sports which complement each other—the more sports you play, the more muscles and joints you use, the fitter you become and the less likely you are to injure yourself—but complementary activities are included for each sport listed.

SPORTS DIRECTORY

Acrobatics

See GYMNASTICS AND ACROBATICS

Aikido

See JUDO AND AIKIDO

Alpine Skiing

The word "ski" is Norwegian, and the practice of gliding over snow and ice on wooden runners is recorded in a 2000 B.C. rock carving at Rödöy, in northern Norway. Although skiing is one of our oldest forms of travel, it wasn't adopted for use in the military until 1542 (in Sweden) and didn't become a sport until 1843 (at Tromsö, Norway). Alpine skiing was introduced into the Alps in 1883; the earliest formal downhill race was staged in Montana, Switzerland, in 1911.

Evaluation.   Skiing, says Elissa Slanger, founder and director of Woman's Way Ski Seminars, usually is an anaerobic activity because you ski in "short bursts"; however, "it can be aerobic if you work hard enough to raise your pulse rate to a training level and keep it there for a sufficient period (fifteen minutes or more). For example, when you ski down a mountain or a long run, or take a long powder run, you are skiing aerobically." Skiing strengthens your quads and your buttocks. It also builds your rectus and oblique abdominal muscles (during deep turns when you reach the advanced level), and your biceps and triceps (when you try to stand up after falling). It diminishes your flexibility, especially your hamstrings and Achilles tendons.

Training.   To strengthen your quads and buttocks, do dumbbell lunges and squats. In addition, do split shifts to strengthen your groin muscles and prevent accidents, killer sit-ups and twisting sit-ups to work your abdominals, and push-ups for upper body strength. Slanger also recommends ankle inversion and eversion strengthening exercises.

Effects of Alpine Skiing

Anaerobic
Strength: quadriceps, gluteals, abdominals

ANKLE INVERSION AND EVERSION

Ankle inversion: Sit on a chair with your feet flat on the floor. While pressing your feet down against the floor, rotate your ankles inward so that the outer edge of each sole comes off the floor. Repeat fifteen or twenty times. When this becomes too easy, place a soft ball or firm pillow between your ankles and then roll them inward, compressing the ball.

   Ankle eversion: Sit on a chair with your feet flat on the floor, as above. While pressing your feet down against the floor, rotate your ankles outward so that the inner edges of your feet lift up. Repeat fifteen or twenty times. When this becomes too easy, add resistance by tying your ankles together loosely with a scarf or loop of surgical tubing and then rotating your ankles outward as you push against the scarf.

"Skiing is virtually the only sport," Slanger says, "that uses the muscles rotating your foot. The weakest woman in a ski school has stronger ankle muscles than anyone on a football team." Before and after your strengthening exercises, do towel stretches for your hamstrings and Achilles tendons. Because skiing tightens your muscles, conscientiously perform universal warm-ups before you go up to the slopes.

Complementary sports.   Many snow-hungry skiers switch to grass skis during the summer. On a smooth grassy slope, these two- to three-foot miniature tank treads feel like snow skis and can attain speeds in excess of 55 miles per hour.

Bicycling and speed ice skating use the same muscles as Alpine skiing in the same ratios. They strengthen the quads only slightly more than the hamstrings. For this reason, people who cycle in summer can ski in winter with only the merest of pre-skiing conditioning. Running, on the other hand, strengthens the quads more than twice as much as the hamstrings and is much less suitable for a skier. If you do run, add uphill intervals to stress your quads. "I've taken up board sailing in the summer," says Slanger, "and it seems to go quite well with skiing. The balance is similar, and the position of bracing yourself with the sail against the wind builds your arms."

Injuries.   Overuse injuries are rare. Skiers who don't stretch their Achilles tendons may develop tendinitis, and those who ski every day throughout the season may develop knee problems, but the average weekend skier is unlikely to suffer these injuries. Traumatic ski injuries have declined in the last ten years as the result of better lifts and tows, better-groomed hills, better ski instruction, better release bindings, higher boots, and shorter skis. When an ankle sprain, torn Achilles tendon, or tibial fracture does strike, it is likely to be during the first hundred feet of the first run of the day, while your muscles are still cold and stiff. Pre-skiing strengthening exercises and thorough warm-ups will prevent most of these problems. "The high boots," says Slanger, "are also a tremendous advantage. Women tend to have weak ankles. The high boots give support and leverage to the leg and put more torque and leverage on the safety bindings, so women can twist out of them more easily. I broke both ankles before the modern boots came in, and I wouldn't be able to ski today without an operation if I didn't have high boots." Women get colder than men, says Slanger and Dinah Witchel, authors of *Ski Woman's Way*, because women can't get as much warming blood from the core of their body to their skin and extremities. So dress carefully, in layers, to adjust to fatigue, wind, and changes in temperature. When you ski downhill, you create your own wind, which must be added to the prevailing wind when you calculate your wind-chill factor (see Table XIV in chapter 10). Eat a carbohydrate-laden breakfast, to provide easily available calories for quick energy and warmth. Avoid heavy lunches if you plan to ski during a cold afternoon, because your fatigue combined with the reduced blood circulation during digestion will make you colder.

Skiers who ascend particularly high mountains may suffer from altitude sickness (see chapter 10).

Badminton

There are two kinds of badminton: "dink" badminton, in which people lazily bat a plastic bird over a volleyball net while they sip beer on a late summer's afternoon, and power badminton, a dizzyingly fast game of speed, power, and position played on an indoor court (to eliminate wind interference) with a five-foot-high net, a goose-feather leather-covered cork shuttlecock (the plastic ones are too fast for this already lightning-fast game), and 4- to 5-ounce rackets (a little lighter than squash rackets). The Chinese, Japanese, Indonesians, Malaysians, Singaporeans, and Thais dominate the world ranks of this primarily amateur sport, and for good reason. In Asia, badminton is *the* national sport, as soccer is in Europe and baseball is in the United States.

Effects of Badminton

Anaerobic
Strength: quadriceps, back, deltoid,
    triceps

Badminton is at least as fast as racquetball and squash. In a top-level game, a shuttlecock spends about 0.95 second in flight. A squash ball spends 1.3 seconds, and racquetball and tennis balls spend 1.5 seconds. The full swing of a power shot may last only one tenth of a second and send the bird across the net at a speed greater than 200 miles per hour. No wonder a long volley of twenty-five or thirty shots may last only twenty seconds. Badminton requires fast reflexes because the bird is not allowed to bounce.

Evaluation: "Badminton is not an aerobic sport because of its stop-start nature," says Christine L. Wells, a professor at Arizona State University in Tempe and a former competitive badminton player. "Although it is not a strength activity, it does minimally strengthen your triceps, deltoids, back, and the quadriceps in your thighs. It doesn't contribute much to your flexibility."

Training: Because the game requires high speed and stamina, players must augment their badminton training with some kind of aerobic exercise. Top players usually run, jump rope, and do intervals and calisthenics or circuit training. Squats, pull-ups, sit-ups, push-ups, dumbbell pullovers, and arm sprints strengthen large muscles in your legs, trunk, and arms. For power and snap in your wrists and arms, perform very fast reps of wrist curls with light weights. For flexibility in your back and your racket arm, shoulder, and wrist, perform wasp waisters, king of Siam kowtows, posture clasps, birds, and pigeon crawls. Bridges and door hangs are also very useful if you can do them comfortably.

Complementary sports: None, although volleyball uses similar back arching and spiking movements, and basketball, racquetball, and squash require similar sprinting and agility.

Injuries: Rare. Occasionally, a player develops bursitis in her racket shoulder; muscle strains in her trapezius, rhomboids, and deltoids of the shoulder, in the abdominal rectus, or in the gastrocnemius, soleus, or hamstrings of the leg; sprains of the forearm extensors, inside or outside of the ankle, or inside or outside of the knee. A low backache after several games indicates weak abdominals and inflexible back muscles. When played outdoors during hot weather or indoors in non-air-conditioned gyms, heat exhaustion is a danger.

Baseball

See SOFTBALL AND BASEBALL

Basketball

Effects of Basketball
Aerobic
Anaerobic
Strength: calf, quadriceps, hamstrings,
  hip and gluteals

Modern basketball was invented in 1891 in Springfield, Massachusetts, by a Canadian doctor, James A. Naismith. It was an exceedingly active game and for a few years was played as avidly by schoolgirls and college women as it was by boys and men. However, in 1895, Clara Baer of Newcomb College in New Orleans published a set of women's rules which scaled the game down to women's supposedly more modest abilities. There were to be six players on a side, and they played in fixed areas of the court. Only three of the six players were allowed to shoot the ball. The women's game became slow, complicated—and boring. In the last few years, however, women have been playing essentially the same game as men. They drive all over the court, feint, dribble, guard, pivot, and lay up shots the way every basketball player should. The women's game has become exciting again.

The result is revived interest. "Amateur and professional women's basketball is at the level now that women's tennis was in 1973 or 1974," says Don Meucci, public relations director of the San Francisco Pioneers in the former Women's Basketball League. "In Carol Blazejowski, Nancy Lieberman, and Molly Bolin, it has the role models it needs, people who can talk off the court about the excitement of women's basketball and the needs of the players, and can back up their talk by playing well on the court. Women's basketball stresses the fundamentals of the game better than men's. Women can't dunk or jump as high as men, but their style is more precise. Nancy Lieberman says, 'Come out and see us just once and you'll come back for more,' and she's right. Women's basketball is tremendously entertaining.''

Evaluation: Basketball played well is a highly aerobic sport, according to Marty Kennedy, basketball coach at the University of San Francisco. "It is one of the most aerobic sports there is," she says, "second only to running, field hockey, and soccer, because you're always moving up and down the floor," and it strengthens just about every part of your body except your back, abdominals, and arms. The jumping particularly develops your quads and gastrocs, while the running builds up your quads and hamstrings. It doesn't add to your flexibility, however.

Training: "Run about a mile and a half or two miles for LSD training," Kennedy says, "just to improve your general health, but on top of that, do sprints or interval training three times a week. In fact, if you just do distance running, you'll actually hurt your game because basketball is a game of sprints." Rope jumping and stair running develop your jumping ability while they build aerobic and anaerobic fitness.

To build strength for running and jumping in your quads, hamstrings and gastrocs, and ankles, do squats (straightening into a jump as you come up), run-'em-out-of-gym-class sprints, dumbbell lunges, heel and toes, and ankle inversion and eversion exercises. To prevent groin injuries, strengthen your hip abductors and adductors with split shifts. If you have a long trunk and long legs, you may have weak back and abdominal muscles, which will hamper your shooting and trunk stability. Do swimmer's kicks, killer sit-ups, and twisting sit-ups. To strengthen your arm and shoulder muscles so that you can stand farther away from the basket when you are shooting, do push-ups, dips, and chin-ups. To strengthen your wrists and fingers for shooting, do wrist curls and fingertip extensions.

FINGERTIP EXTENSIONS

Slowly straighten the fingers of one hand while applying resistance with the other hand.

In addition, practice volleyball jumping drills whenever possible and add high jumps.

HIGH JUMPS

Starting from a slight crouch, jump off both feet simultaneously while reaching up with your right hand as if you were going up for the ball. Repeat with the left hand for one rep. Do ten, twenty, or thirty reps per set.

To strengthen your shoulder for shooting and ball handling, hold onto a 1- to 3-pound dumbbell while repeatedly moving your arm and shoulder through its entire range of motion. Whenever you lift weights for basketball, use light weights and twenty or more reps. Low weights/ high reps build muscle endurance while they develop the moderate degree of strength you need for basketball.

Because basketball uses every part of your body, you must maintain a full-body flexibility with universal warm-ups. In addition, concentrate on stretching every part of your legs, especially your quads and gastrocs, with geisha kneels, extra calf stretches, and Achilles stretches. Add wasp waisters and king of Siam kowtows for your back, pigeon crawls for your hands and wrists, and finger pushes: One at a time, push and pull the fingers of one hand with the other. You need very flexible fingers and wrists in order to have a light shooting touch.

Complementary sports: Volleyball, for jumping.

Injuries: The injuries in basketball closely resemble those in volleyball, Kennedy says, but they are more serious in basketball because it is a contact sport. Serious ankle sprains are the scourge of basketball players, as are torn ligaments or cartilages in the knees. "Groin pulls are common," she says, "because people don't stretch enough before they go out and play this stop-start game. When they take off suddenly after an abrupt stop, they pull something." Basketball players often develop blisters from the constant irregular pounding and scraping on the bottoms of their feet. Charley horses in the thigh or upper arm can also occur.

Bicycling

See chapter 5

Board Sailing

Riding the waves on a little board with a sail attached is as venerable a sport in the South Seas as sliding down hills with barrel staves is in the snow belt. Nonetheless, board sailing didn't become a sport until 1967, when Southern California computer programmer Hoyle Schweitzer invented the free sail system. He fastened a mast to a surfboard with a universal joint and called his craft a Windsurfer, the trade name of America's most popular board. Today, more than 500,000 sailboards have been sold, a great proportion of them to Europeans; the world championships feature slaloms, freestyle, round-the-buoy course racing, and long-distance racing. Board sailing may become an event in the 1984 Olympic games.

"Women have an advantage over men in board sailing," says June Everett, veteran teacher of the sport. "The lighter a person is, the faster. Therefore, if a man and a woman have equal ability, the woman has a chance of beating the man."

Evaluation: Board sailing is not an aerobic sport. It has some anaerobic spurts, especially when struggling against high winds or rough waters, but you usually grapple with the sail and the winds for only three or four minutes, and then let the wind out of the sail in order to rest and catch your breath.

Board sailing strengthens your forearms, upper arms, and shoulder areas, as well as your pectorals, abdominals, gluteals, and quads, Everett says. It marginally increases the flexibility of your back, shoulders, and hips.

Training: Many board sailors run, bicycle, or swim to stay in shape. To win a short race of thirty minutes or the 15- to 30-mile long-distance races lasting two hours, you must have cardiovascular stamina and muscular endurance. However, you don't need endurance while you're on the board unless you race.

Many professional board sailors perform weight-lifting exercises such as wrist curls and dumbbell pullovers to strengthen their forearms and upper arms. En gardes strengthen your buttocks muscles, and kiddie kicks build up your quads. Killer sit-ups are essential for board control. However, Everett says, you don't have to be strong in order to begin board sailing. "If you start with a small sail in relatively calm weather," she says, "you can handle anything that comes along."

For flexibility, the universal warm-ups will stretch all the muscles you use in board sailing. Devote extra time to groin stretches and to toe flexers, ankle rolls, and foot twisters to prevent foot cramps.

Complementary sports: Alpine skiing, waterskiing, and cross-country skiing all provide endurance conditioning for board sailing and use similar muscles, Everett says. However, none of these precisely simulates your movements in board sailing.

Injuries: If you have weak forearms and must face particularly strong winds for four or five hours, you may develop very achy forearm muscles.

Effects of Board Sailing

Strength: quadriceps, gluteals, pectorals, abdominals, shoulder, upper arm, forearm

Flexibility: hip, back, neck, shoulder

Body Building

See WEIGHT LIFTING, POWER LIFTING, AND BODY BUILDING

Canoeing and Kayaking

Effects of Canoeing and Kayaking

Aerobic

Anaerobic

Strength: abdominals, shoulder, upper
    arm

In the early 1880s, canoes and kayaks graduated from efficient forms of transportation to sports, and the first canoeing and kayaking boom among white men was on. Specialized canoes and kayaks were developed for sailing, flat-water racing (an Olympic sport for women since 1948), marathon racing, wild-water racing, slalom racing, canoe poling, and cruising. The canoes of the 1880s were wooden, modeled after kayaks from Greenland. Every time a new, lighter material was invented, a new canoeing and kayaking boom hit the United States. In the twenties, it was wood and canvas; in the fifties came aluminum; then fiberglass; and now DuPont's Kevlar 49, lighter than fiberglass and five times as strong as steel. (Kevlar is also used in bullet-proof vests.)

Canoes and kayaks are immensely popular among hunters, fishermen, picnickers, and overnight campers—about 125,000 canoes were sold in the United States in 1979. Canoe and kayak sport racing is also growing in popularity. The United States won its first women's world championships in 1979, and in 1980 the women's and men's Olympic trials were broadcast on nationwide television.

Evaluation.   Canoes and kayaks are almost as efficient modes of transportation as bicycles; it is possible to paddle lazily across an entire bay without ever raising your heartbeat. Thus any discussion of training effect must refer to hard paddling—races or white-water runs. This type of paddling is highly aerobic, according to Eunice E. Way, Ph.D., professor and assistant dean of the School of Health, Physical Education, and Recreation at Central Michigan University in Mount Pleasant. Olympic-length kayaking races last up to thirty minutes, while marathon canoe and kayak races last as long as thirty-six hours.

Both sports strengthen your arms, shoulders, and upper trunk muscles. The shoulder is especially developed because the power of the trunk is transmitted through the shoulder to the paddle. In the trunk, the lats, obliques, rectus abdominis, and erector spinii muscles get particular workouts, Way says. Canoeists develop their biceps and triceps during their bent-arm stroke, while kayakers develop shoulder strength during their straight-arm stroke. Because you paddle on both sides of a kayak, your strength is developed more evenly than it is in a canoe. Elite canoeists paddle four or five strokes on one side of the boat and then four or five strokes on the other side, but they still favor their dominant side. They simply compensate for any strength imbalance by stroking harder once in a while or taking an occasional extra stroke.

Both sports are power events and do not increase an athlete's flexibility.

Training.   Way feels that you should run distances in order to develop the endurance capacity necessary to pull you through a thirty-minute or thirty-hour race. She prefers running to other aerobic sports because, she says, it demands the most work from your body during each workout. However, rope jumping or any other highly strenuous aerobic sport will also work. In addition, she recommends a generalized strength training program for the abdominals and upper body. Do killer sit-ups, twisting sit-ups, locusts, pull-ups, chin-ups, arm sprints, and dumbbell pullovers. Kayakers should do extra sets of arm sprints to develop endurance strength in their shoulders. Canoers should add isometric leg exercises for their gluteals and quads. "Although your legs are not involved in the actual act of paddling," Way says, "they are braced against the inside of the canoe to hold your position. For this, you need static strength." She suggests wall sits.

WALL SITS

Stand with your back against a wall, and bend your knees and hips until you look like you're sitting in a chair. Hold for ten, twenty, even sixty seconds, then stand up, for one rep. Do several reps throughout the day.

She also suggests doing pinches whenever you can.

PINCHES

Stand with your feet parallel and comfortably apart. Without actually moving your feet or legs, tighten and pinch in your buttocks muscles, the inside of your thighs, and your abdominal muscles. Pretend that you can bring your feet together, and hold for ten to sixty seconds, for one rep.

If you are interested in competing, Way says you must do canoe or kayak sport-specific exercises. One of the best involves tying one end of your boat to a tire and the other end to a tree. Get into your boat and paddle against the resistance of the anchor.

For flexibility, do universal warm-ups before and after each workout, adding birds, door leans, and posture clasps for your shoulders.

Complementary sports.   None. In fact, kayaking and canoeing don't even complement each other because they use different amounts of biceps, triceps, and shoulder and leg muscles.

Injuries.   Overuse injuries are concentrated in the shoulder, especially up toward the collarbone, for this area takes the brunt of the force of each stroke. An adequate stretching and strengthening program prevents many of these injuries. A kayaker may dislocate the front of her shoulder if her paddle is dragged outward at the end of the backstroke by a high wave. Prevent this injury by turning your trunk toward the end of each stroke so that your arm doesn't have to straighten out fully. "The greatest hazard in canoeing or kayaking," Way says, "is falling in the water. Most water is very cold. If you tip over, you can be a victim of hypothermia even if it's a nice summer day."

Climbing

See MOUNTAIN CLIMBING; ROCK CLIMBING

Cross-Country Skiing

Effects of Cross-Country Skiing

Aerobic

Strength: lower leg, upper leg, hip, gluteals, front of trunk, shoulder, upper arm

Cross-country skiing was introduced to the United States by Norwegian sailors jumping ship in San Francisco during the Gold Rush. Long skinny skis were first used as transportation over the meadows of the high Sierra but soon became one of the few forms of entertainment during the long mountain winters. The first recorded Nordic ski races in North America took place during this time in California.

In the last ten years, cross-country skiing has drawn 3 million participants, most of them new to the sport. Nordic skiing is easy to learn and inexpensive—$85 buys a full package of moderate-quality light touring skis, boots, poles, and bindings. Skiers follow the snow, kicking and gliding along machine-made tracks, hiking and biking trails, bridle paths, golf courses, abandoned roads and railway tracks, meadows, city parks, mountains, and backpacking areas. Citizens' races, so-called because the entrants are recreational skiers, have sprung up all over the country. Experts predict that, by 1985, cross-country skiers will outnumber Alpine skiers in this country.

Evaluation.   "Cross-country skiing is definitely aerobic," says Christine L. Wells of Arizona State University, "and is one of the best sports of all because it involves so many muscles. In fact, you have to start slowly, because it is so vigorous you get tired quickly." It strengthens the fronts and backs of your legs because you have to lift your skis as well as straighten your legs, and it strengthens your hips and abdomen as well or better than most other leg sports. It also builds strength in your arms and shoulders because you are constantly poling and pushing against the ground with your poles. It contributes only a small amount of flexibility to each of these areas. "It's great for weight loss," she says, "because it's such vigorous exercise. Even if you're just walking at cross-country skiing, you expend a great many calories. It's also beautiful, quiet, and serene."

Training.   The poling and scissoring glide-and-kick of cross-country skiing is peculiar to that sport, and few exercises duplicate these movements effectively. However, a woman who has good upper body strength has a definite head start in Nordic ski poling. Push-ups and pull-ups prepare your arms and your heart for the ski touring season. (Your heart beats faster during arm exercise than leg exercise.) To strengthen your arms specifically for ski poling, you must develop the muscle fibers at the beginning of each swing. The resistance is greatest then, just after the pole is planted in the snow in front of your body and you are pushing yourself forward. For this reason, most weight and pulley exercises don't help; their resistance is greatest at the end of each swing. Summer ski poling will condition your arm—and leg— muscles for the real thing come winter: Walk up a grassy hill leaning forward in the classic diagonal stride, stretching your legs out behind you, pushing off your toes, bending your forward knee, and pushing back and through with your pole. Thrust yourself up the hill with each pole push. Start with a gentle grade and progress up steep slopes. Serious cross-country skiers train during the summer on roller skis. These wheeled platforms, costing $150 and up, imitate the diagonal stride and double poling motions of real Nordic skiing but don't develop your hill or turning techniques.

For flexibility, do posture clasps, pigeon crawls, birds, Achilles stretches, calf stretches, geisha kneels, runner's starts, and wall splits.

Complementary sports.   No sport really imitates the motions of cross-country skiing. Cycling involves a resistance at the end of each leg swing (the upstroke), as does cross-country skiing (the lift after each push), and challenges the athlete with up-and-down hills. Running builds leg endurance but uses different muscle ratios. Nonetheless, many competitive cross-country skiers run up and down hills during the summer as well as a couple of times a week during the racing season to condition their bodies for the intense anaerobic bursts of an uphill climb and the restful recovery of a downhill sweep. Although swimming and rowing build strength in the arms, they do not use the muscles in patterns similar to those of Nordic skiing.

Injuries.   Overuse injuries in cross-country skiing are uncommon. It is much easier on the knees than Alpine skiing because your heels are free, and the smooth gliding stride does not stress that delicate joint as much as bicycling or running does. Prevent calf, hamstring, groin, and quadriceps muscle strains and tendinitis by stretching those areas with calf stretches, Achilles stretches, towel stretches, runner's starts, and storks. Prevent shoulder aches due to weak upper body musculature

with push-ups and pull-ups. Prevent backaches caused by double poling with locusts, swimmer's kicks, and killer sit-ups. Broken legs and
hips caused by falls and collisions while speeding downhill occur, but
rarely. Every skier should wear sport goggles to keep twigs from
scratching or piercing the eyes (see chapter 10). Gamekeeper's thumb
(see chapter 10) crops up occasionally when a ski pole applies leverage
to a thumb during a fall.

Guard against cold injury. Dress in layers so that you can peel off
outer clothing during vigorous skiing to minimize sweating. If you do
perspire heavily, the sweat may freeze against your skin, subjecting you
to frost nip, frostbite, or hypothermia. Replenish your fluids by drinking water or diluted fruit juices. If you feel cold, don't drink alcoholic
beverages because they cause your surface blood vessels to dilate and
give up precious body heat to the air.

If you have flat feet, you may be susceptible to plantar fasciitis
from strain during the kickoff. If none of the suggestions in chapter 10
help, see a podiatrist for an orthotic for your ski boots.

ORTHOTICS

An orthotic is a corrective device molded from a plaster cast of your
foot and inserted into your shoe to correct imbalances and abnormalities in your feet which can affect your stride, posture, and spinal con-
figuration. Usually prescribed by sports podiatrists, these arch supports, heel wedges, cradle-like full shoe inserts, and other prostheses
tilt your foot and lower leg back into a neutral position and correct
heel spurs, uneven leg lengths, pronated (inturned) ankles, and many
other problems, as well as cushion your feet while you run. These appliances aren't foolproof, however; the cure rate is only about 75 percent, and they themselves may cause blisters and aches during the
breaking-in period. If you don't have any foot or leg problems, orthotics won't improve your performance or prevent injury any more than a
pair of eyeglasses will improve the vision of someone with normal eyesight. However, if you do have some abnormal foot function, orthotics will prevent overuse injuries. A pair of orthotics from a podiatrist
cost about $300 when the examination, fitting, x-ray, and laboratory
fees are figured in.

If you have any kind of heart disease, consult your physician before you begin cross-country skiing. The cold, the altitude, the use of
your arms in poling, and the uphill grades all place great stress on your
heart.

Dance

Dancing is one of the most athletic endeavors you can undertake. At its highest levels, it requires a discipline, dedication, and total body conditioning far greater than the most demanding team or individual sport. Professional dancers adhere fanatically to a grueling regimen of class, rehearsal, and performance, six days a week, all year long. Because they have no off season, they are always in shape. No wonder that top ballerinas are fitter by far even than most professional women athletes and score higher on fitness tests than many top male athletes playing body contact sports. Ballet training may be the most demanding of all dance arts, but if you dance at your target heart rate continuously for at least thirty minutes three times a week, you get a training effect, be it modern dancing, folk dancing, square dancing, Appalachian clog dancing, belly dancing, tap dancing, jazz dancing, disco dancing, jitterbugging, or social dancing.

Dancing knows no age limit. You may begin serious dance lessons as young as two or three or as old as eighty or ninety. The average professional ballet dancer performs well into her thirties and forties. At fifty-five, Dame Margot Fonteyn danced *Romeo and Juliet* with Rudolf Nureyev and received more than forty curtain calls. In 1978, at the age of fifty-six, Alicia Alonso triumphed in the role of Giselle at the Kennedy Center in Washington.

Evaluation. During the actual thirty- or forty-minute dancing segment of any ballet or modern dance class, you get as good an aerobic workout as running or cross-country skiing, as long as you work at or above your target heart rate. If you tap dance in an active, athletic style, says Ellen Jacob, author of *Dancing: A Guide for the Dancer You Can Be,* you get an extremely good workout, because many of the intricate weight transfers involve hopping or jumping. If you folk dance without rest breaks between each dance, you work as hard as most runners or cyclists. If you jazz dance, on the other hand, you rarely work with the intensity and full body use necessary to develop good cardiovascular conditioning.

The first half of every ballet and modern dance class consists of a systematic warm-up to strengthen and stretch every part of your body. Ballet dancers perform most of this warm-up at the barre, while modern dancers work on the floor. Thus, ballet emphasizes the legs and feet, and modern dance emphasizes the torso. Although the actual act of dancing doesn't appreciably strengthen your muscles, the warm-ups do. Ballet exercises, Jacob says, "are over 350 years old and take you through your body bone by bone to strengthen and stretch you from head to toe." Tap dancing, which has very little pre-dance warm-up, primarily strengthens the thighs, calves, pelvis, and abdomen and, to a

Effects of Dance, Ballet

Aerobic
Anaerobic
Strength: all over, with emphasis on leg
   and foot
Flexibility: all over

Effects of Dance, Modern

Aerobic
Anaerobic
Strength: all over, with emphasis on
   trunk
Flexibility: all over

Effects of Dance, Folk

Aerobic
Anaerobic
Strength: lower leg

Effects of Dance, Tap

Aerobic
Anaerobic
Strength: calf, quadriceps, hip flexor,
   gluteals, abdominals, back

Effects of Dance, Jazz

lesser extent, the back. Jazz dancing works the back and trunk muscles, but not enough to condition the body. For this reason, jazz dancers who want all-around conditioning must add ballet or modern classes to their training.

The warm-ups also stretch your body and make it increasingly limber. However, the degree of strengthening or stretching you get during class depends on the orientation of the teacher. Some teachers concentrate on timing, others on strength, and still others on flexibility. Select a teacher who focuses on your particular needs.

Training.   The amount of cardiovascular conditioning you get from dancing depends on how hard you work and how continuously. At social dances or in beginning dance classes, you don't dance nonstop for twenty or thirty minutes. You take a break between each three- or five-minute dance, or you watch whenever the teacher corrects a movement, explains a step, or requests another run-through. Under these conditions, you get a moderate anaerobic workout but little aerobic conditioning, so you need some kind of cardiovascular exercise for good fitness and endurance. As you become more advanced, you dance more continuously, but even top-level dancers run, bicycle, or swim to develop enough endurance to last all the way through a demanding performance. "Swimming's wonderful," Jacob says. "It develops a useful kind of strength because it is tied to functional movement. Bicycling is also good because it's smooth, rhythmical movement, and extends your legs if your seat is the right height. Running is okay, but if you run, stretch afterward, because running makes you very tight." Jazz, square, and social dancers need supplementary aerobic training because their arts rarely condition the heart and lungs.

Dancers need strength to protect themselves from injury as well as control their movements. "Strong muscles support your body and give consistency and smoothness to your movements," Jacob says. Most ballet and modern dancers get enough strengthening exercises from their warm-ups, but those who need more have recently turned to circuit training with free weights or Nautilus machines. If you attend dance class only two or three times a week, add a full circuit training program (chapter 6) to your daily routine.

If you need more flexibility than you develop during your dance warm-ups, or if you only dance two or three times a week, perform a daily concentrated stretching lap (chapter 6). Jacob says that many dancers now practice Yoga outside of class because it uses static stretches the way dancing does and emphasizes controlled breathing. If your style of dancing doesn't include the codified warm-ups used in ballet and modern dance, add strength and flexibility circuit training at least four times a week.

Complementary sports.   Gymnastics and ice skating share many similarities with ballet and modern dance. The exercises are done against the resistance of your own body weight, a piece of equipment, or a heavy pair of skates, so the movements increase your range of motion and add variety to your training. Asian martial arts have heavily influenced modern dance choreography in the last ten years and provided dancers with a new attitude toward movement. Although they haven't yet been incorporated into training exercises, many of the highly controlled martial arts movements and warm-ups add flexibility, strength, and power to any dancer's repertoire without shortening or tightening the long muscles dancers need.

Injuries.   Most dancers don't get hurt as much as other athletes because they warm up thoroughly before they move across the floor. When they do get hurt, they usually suffer an overuse injury caused by poor technique, inexperience, or exhaustion. The foot, ankle, knee, and back are the most vulnerable to plantar fasciitis and arch strains, bunions, shin splints, Achilles tendinitis, stress fractures in the foot bones, sprained knees, and spinal disk problems. Muscle pulls occur throughout the body. Most of these can be prevented by good technique. If your teacher doesn't correct you when you pronate, sickle (put weight on the inner side of your knee, ankle, and big toe), point your knees forward in a demi-plié, or take off from a jump on the ball of your foot (you should press your heels into the floor instead), find another teacher. If you have pain under the big toe and the heel when you stand on half-toe, try a wider pair of shoes before you decide you have the arthritic growth of *hallux rigidus*. If your shoe is too narrow, it squeezes your toes together and the ridge of the ballet shoe sole presses into your foot.

Diving

In Olympic and World Competition, there are two diving events: one- and three-meter springboard, consisting of five required dives; and three-, five-, seven-and-a-half-, and ten-meter platform (or highboard), consisting of eight voluntary dives. Each dive is performed in any one of three positions: straight (body unbent at hips, knees, or ankles; feet together, toes pointed); piked (body bent at hips; legs straight, toes pointed); or tucked (whole body curled into a fetal position; knees together; hands on lower legs; toes pointed). Twists may be performed in any position. The body must always be straight and vertical or near-vertical when entering the water. The dive is finished only when the body is completely submerged.

Evaluation.   Diving provides neither aerobic nor anaerobic con-

Effects of Diving

Strength: quadriceps, hip flexor, gluteals, abdominals, back

Flexibility: thigh, hip, back, neck, trunk

ditioning. If you train hard enough, it strengthens and limbers your abdominals, hip flexors, back, buttocks, and thigh muscles. Otherwise, diving doesn't change your condition at all.

Training. Patricia McCormick, who earned double gold medals in high and springboard diving in the 1952 Helsinki and the 1956 Melbourne Olympic Games—an Olympic women's record for individual gold medals in water events—believes that you must be a good, fit athlete in order to be a good diver. Build a solid aerobic base by Long Steady Distance running or swimming or following some other aerobic program. You also need overall strength and flexibility. Strong back and trunk muscles hold your body straight and vertical, while strong abdominals and hip flexors bend your hips into the pike and tuck maneuvers and rotate your body in the difficult twist dives. Killer sit-ups, swimmer's kicks, locusts, hanging curls, mermaids or dumbbell pullovers, and run-'em-out-of-gym-class sprints help you reach and hold your diving positions better. Strong shoulder muscles and triceps, built up with dumbbell pullovers, pull-ups, chin-ups, and dips, withstand the impact of the water.

McCormick says that 90 percent of all diving is board work. "If you can't get off the board consistently," she says, "you can't dive." Strong gastrocs, Achilles tendons, quadriceps, hamstrings, and gluteus muscles provide strength and height in the hurdle and spring off the board or platform. She suggests jumping up stairs, using both feet, and then hopping up stairs using only the hurdle leg. When stairs become easy, advance to a bench. She also recommends practicing your hurdle away from the board whenever possible, with or without ankle weights. "Just take three or more steps and hurdle to what would be the end of the board," she says. "I used to walk down the street practicing my hurdle. People thought I was nuts." To add height to your spring, do jump squats.

JUMP SQUATS

Hold a dumbbell weighing one quarter of your body weight in each hand. Squat down until your knees are bent a little less than 90 degrees, then straighten up and spring into the air in one smooth movement, for one rep. Do not bend your knees more than 90 degrees or you may damage them. Work up to two or three sets of fifteen or twenty reps three times a week.

All dives require a high degree of flexibility, but the pike requires the most. In it, your forehead must touch your thighs and your toes must be pointed. To limber up your hamstrings, lower back extensors, and shin muscles, perform plows, runner's starts, towel stretches, king of Siam kowtows, and geisha kneels.

Complementary sports. Gymnastics and diving use the same fundamentals, according to McCormick. Trampoline gives you the spring off the springboard. However, it is a very dangerous sport, particularly for women with poor strength and flexibility. Figure skating and dancing use similar movements and muscles in similar ratios.

Injuries. Like gymnasts, many divers suffer low back problems from hyperextension (overarching). Strengthen your trunk muscles with killer sit-ups, twisting sit-ups, and dumbbell pullovers, and your lower back muscles with swimmer's kicks and locusts. Some of the modern dives dictate unusual entry positions which strain the shoulder muscles. These injuries may be prevented by strengthening the shoulder muscles. Prevent pulled biceps muscles with chin-ups, and pulled quadriceps muscles with squats or kiddie kicks. Shin splints and knee problems occur occasionally. The rare catastrophic accident occurs when a diver hits the board or the bottom of the pool.

Fencing

When gunpowder and bullets made warfare with swords obsolete, swordsmanship developed into elaborate rituals of dueling and defense of honor. It became a sport when dueling declined during the nineteenth century and was organized for competition in the United States in 1891. The United States entered men's Olympic competition at the St. Louis games in 1904. Women's Olympic competition began in 1924 in Paris. Although men fence in tournaments using all three legal weapons—the foil, the epée, and the saber—women are restricted to the foil, the lightest of the three. Women train, however, with all three weapons. International rules state that the fencer is allowed to thrust only with the foil (a flexible four-sided 500-gram-or-less rapier with a blunt tip) and the epée (a 770-gram-or-less rapier with a three-sided blade and a guard over the tip), but can thrust and cut with the saber (a 500-gram-or-less sword with two cutting edges and a blunt point). The beginner starts with the foil, because it requires less arm strength than the other two.

Like chess, fencing is not a spectator sport unless you know all the moves and stratagems. It develops hand-eye coordination, quick reflexes, gamesmanship, imagination, and subtlety. Moreover, it exercises just about every muscle in your body in one way or another. Because of the interplay of mind and body, women of any age can fence. "When I was fencing," says Christine Haycock, M.D., "we had fencers in their seventies, and they were as agile as they come."

Effects of Fencing

Aerobic
Anaerobic
Strength: lower leg, quadriceps, upper
  arm
Flexibility: all over

Evaluation.   "Fencing is an aerobic activity during practice," says Haycock, associate professor of surgery at New Jersey Medical School, "but not during competition. Fencing matches last only five minutes and are primarily anaerobic." In practice, however, you may do one hundred lunges against a wall, or spend thirty minutes or an hour alternating between advances, retreats, and lunges—definitely a cardiovascular workout. Fencing strengthens just about all of the muscles in your upper arms, lower legs, and thighs because you are lunging and running backwards and forwards, using the back arm for balance and the forward arm for parrying. You strengthen the thighs and legs because you spring off your legs and bend your knees. The abdominals may be the only muscles not directly strengthened. It increases the flexibility in every part of your body.

Training.   Although fencing practice does provide an aerobic workout, it is seldom enough to keep you totally fit. Supplement your fencing with an endurance sport. Jump rope to improve your hopping and jumping ability; run distances to increase your cardiovascular capacity; run intervals for anaerobic conditioning. Fencing movements and postures are not natural. At first, they seem awkward and tiring. Although diligent practice quickly strengthens the necessary muscles, you can hasten the process by doing split shifts, en gardes or dumbbell lunges, run-'em-out-of-gym-class sprints, and twirling jumps.

TWIRLING JUMPS

To perform twirling jumps, jump a quarter turn to the right, then a quarter turn to the left, a half turn to the right, a half turn to the left, a three-quarter turn to the left, and, finally, a three-quarter turn to the right.

Chin-ups and pull-ups increase the strength of your upper arms. Because fencing develops the dominant side of the body, do extra reps of each exercise on your nondominant side to balance your development.

Injuries.   Rare, except for the occasional painful but not dangerous blow to the breasts if you forget to wear chest pads.

Field Handball

See TEAM HANDBALL

Field Hockey

Field hockey became an Olympic sport for women at the 1980 games in Moscow. (Men's field hockey had been an Olympic event since 1908.) In the United States, field hockey is played mainly by girls, be it in elementary school, high school, or college. Many women, however, play it throughout their adult lives. It is as fast-paced and exciting a spectator sport as its more publicized cousin, ice hockey. Ireland's national sport, hurling, which is played with a lightweight ball resembling a softball, and Scotland's shinty, whose ball is smaller and even lighter, are also relatives of field hockey and require the same sort of training regimen.

Evaluation.   Field hockey is a demanding, exhausting game involving continuous running and sprinting in front-line and halfback positions. Fullbacks do not run as much, and goalies run even less. For the active positions, it is excellent aerobic exercise. The running strengthens the quadriceps, hamstrings, and buttocks, while the stickwork and shooting contribute some strength to the latissimus dorsi, deltoids, triceps, pectorals, and biceps. Because the sticks are relatively short, you run and shoot in a bent-over position, which is good for your back, according to Christine L. Wells, Ph.D. Field hockey does not make you more flexible.

Training.   Although field hockey gives you an ample aerobic and anaerobic workout, you seldom play it three or more times a week. Therefore, you must augment your playing time with workouts to guarantee enough stamina to get you through a game. Both Long Steady Distance running and some form of sprinting are necessary, since you will use both in every game. Fartlek, or speed-play, incorporating running, sprinting, and some sudden stops and starts, is ideal. Practice your stickwork during fartlek for added benefit. In addition, practice twirling jumps. To improve your grip and shooting strength in your wrists and hands, do wrist curls at high speed, and grip-strength exercises. To increase the endurance of the upper body muscles used for stickwork, do shoulder shrugs, chin-ups, dips, and pull-ups. To strengthen the musculature around your knee and prevent knee injuries caused by sudden stops or changes in direction, do hamsters. Because field hockey contributes nothing to your flexibility, pay special attention to your warm-ups—especially toe touches and Achilles stretches—and add posture clasps and birds to limber up your arm and shoulder muscles.

Complementary sports.   Ice hockey and lacrosse.

Injuries.   Bruises are common, stick injuries to the teeth, mouth,

Effects of Field Hockey

Aerobic

Anaerobic

Strength: quadriceps, hamstrings, gluteals, pectorals, latissimus dorsi, deltoid, upper arm and eyes occur frequently in field hockey, as do dislocated knees and shoulders and fractures caused by collisions with another player. Shin guards prevent painful bruises and fractures to the lower leg. Of the self-generated injuries, ankle sprains are the most common. Knee injuries also occur frequently, because great stress is placed on that joint during the stopping, starting, and twirling movements of a typical game.

Figure Skating

Effects of Ice Skating, Figure
Aerobic
Strength: lower leg, quadriceps, gluteals, abdominals, back, neck, shoulder
Flexibility: all over

According to the *Guiness Book of Women's Sports Records*, figure skating went from relaxing recreation to art with E. W. Bushnell's invention of the steel skate blade in 1850. Fourteen years later, while in Vienna, American ballet master Jackson Haines transferred the movements and choreography of classical dance to the ice. The first skating organization in the world, the Amateur Skating Association of Canada, was founded in 1878 by Louis Rubinstein, one of Haines's pupils, followed in 1879 by the National Skating Association of Great Britain, in 1887 by the Skating Club of the United States, and in 1892 by the Internationale Eislauf-Vereinigung (International Skating Union) in the Netherlands. The International Skating Union governs international competition, world championships, and Olympic figure skating events to this day.

After years of languishing in dark, chilly rinks, figure skating has become a premier spectator sport. The world championships now play to standing-room-only crowds, nationwide tours of internationally acclaimed skaters fill the largest, most elaborate of indoor skating facilities, and ice shows, competitions, and exhibitions are broadcast regularly on network television. The United States Figure Skating Association's 1981 contract with ABC Television nets the USFSA some $200,000 each year, and the world championships have become a million-dollar property.

Figure skaters, like dancers, have proven that an athlete's physical peak is much later than we believe. "I don't think that nineteen is a biological peak," says figure skating and ice hockey trainer Laura Stamm. "I think it's much closer to thirty. An American athlete peaks at nineteen not because her body is at its best, but because she has reached her peak in determination and psychology. After nineteen, she has other responsibilities and can't train as singlemindedly. Russian athletes stay in their sports much longer than ours because they're supported. They don't have to go out and get a job to support their families. The Protopopovs [two-time Olympic champions Ludmila Belousova and her husband, Oleg Protopopov] are in their late forties and they're still skating. They're probably the best figure skaters that ever lived. It's just a matter of being able to stay with it and not take a day off. As you get older, your rate of recovery is slower and much more difficult."

Evaluation.   Figure skating is a highly demanding aerobic sport during daily practice sessions. "Skating is extremely hard work," Stamm says. "It's much more work than running the same distance. And you're not just circling the rink slowly. Your legs must generate enormous amounts of speed and make it look easy. In addition, you are doing very difficult moves out there, and the legs are working extremely hard."

Figure skating strengthens all the leg muscles, especially the feet, ankles, quadriceps, and buttocks, Stamm says. "You can always tell a skater because she has big thighs and a big butt. She uses the big muscles in her thighs and buttocks to push, and she pinches in her gluteus muscles to control her spins and rotations." Skating strengthens your abdominal and back muscles because you begin your push from your trunk, and it develops your shoulder and neck muscles because you control and hold your position with your upper body. In pairs skating, the lifts and other maneuvers strengthen your arm and chest muscles almost as much as they strengthen your partner's. Figure skating also markedly increases your flexibility, for its movements require as much limberness as those of ballet or gymnastics.

Training.   A figure skater requires endurance in order to get through a four-minute program consisting of one difficult move after another, interlarded with purely anaerobic bursts for triple toe loops and other jumps and twists. Until a few years ago, figure skaters trained by practicing their school figures and freestyle maneuvers over and over again. However, many now do a half hour of moderate interval training each day to build up their aerobic capacity. "Speed is not essential in figure skating," Stamm says. Figure skaters aren't racers, after all, so sprinting around a rink doesn't make you a better figure skater. Stamm puts her students through two-stride laps to develop wind and leg endurance. Each student skates around the rink, taking the two straightaways in only two strides apiece. "A rink is two hundred feet long," she says, "which means the straightaways are two hundred feet long. If you can take only two strides to get down the straightaway, you are making eighty to one hundred feet on each glide. You've got to have tremendous power in your legs to do that." Stamm also suggests that you do ten minutes of circles (she calls them crossovers) for wind and leg endurance and that you practice leg movements and exercises at different speeds. The only way you can learn to skate at slow, medium, and fast speeds is to skate slowly, moderately, and quickly every day.

Beginning skaters often complain of weak ankles. Stamm feels that most wobbly ankles are the result of poorly fitted, loose skates rather than inherent muscle weakness. Skates should fit snugly without curling or bunching up your toes. Many skaters wear skate boots two or three full sizes smaller than their street shoes, not because they want their boots to fit like plaster casts but because they want their boots to fit like gloves. If you do suffer from weak ankles, however, strengthen them with ankle inversion and eversion exercises and by walking on your heels and toes. Tilting on a balance board strengthens peroneal muscles on the outside of your ankle while developing your balance. Center a three-foot board on a perfectly round log or four-by-four post. It should look like a seesaw. Place one foot at each end of the board and tilt back and forth, first slowly, then quickly.

Strengthen your shoulders and arms with door hangs, chin-ups, pull-ups, and dumbbell pullovers. Strengthen your arms and chest with push-ups. Strengthen your abdominals with killer sit-ups and twisting sit-ups, and your back muscles with swimmer's kicks, and locusts.

Skaters must work for extremes in flexibility. You must be able to do splits and bridges (back bends) and have the total body flexibility of a ballet dancer or gymnast. Stretch your groin with wall splits, then

---

BRIDGE OR BACK BEND

Lie down on your back with your knees bent, your feet on the floor, and your hands flat on the floor above your shoulders. Arch your back and lift yourself onto your hands and feet, positioning your feet so that you can straighten your knees. Straight legs force you to arch your back to reduce the strain on your knees. Your arms should be straight and shoulders should be directly over your hands. Hold for ten to twenty seconds and return to your starting position. Take it easy with this exercise. It is extremely taxing when you first attempt it.

---

slowly advance to floor splits with your foot flexed, not pointed. Work your way up to well-arched straight-legged bridges. To prevent injuries, stretch your calves and Achilles tendons with calf stretches and Achilles stretches and your hamstrings with towel stretches and runner's starts.

Complementary sports. Most serious figure skaters study ballet for flexibility, grace, agility, and strength as well as choreographic style, says Stamm, who is herself a former ballet dancer. Gymnastics also provides the same types of strength, flexibility, and balance. To develop your quadriceps and your aerobic capacity, bicycle for at least thirty minutes four or five times a week. Cycling builds up your leg muscles the same way skating does. Alpine skiing, waterskiing, and board sailing use your quads similarly. Although ice hockey is complementary to figure skating, it exposes you to groin injuries with its sudden stops and turns. Scandinavian-style skate touring on specialized long blades over frozen streams or lakes builds up your aerobic capacity while exercising your skating muscles.

Injuries.   Figure skaters are close runners-up to ballet dancers in the ugly feet contest. Their feet are usually bruised, swollen, calloused, and full of corns and bunions. In addition, knee problems of various sorts and pulled muscles in the thigh are also common. Groin injuries are rare, but they can occur during some unusual stretching movement. Freestyle skaters frequently suffer back injuries caused by the impact shock of landing on one foot after a powerful twisting or high jump.

Most broken bones, serious bruises, muscle and tendon injuries, dislocations, and damage to internal organs, however, are due to falls. "Considering how often a skater falls," Stamm says, "it's amazing there are so few injuries." Learn to fall in a relaxed, controlled roll instead of a panicked flailing. Do not fall on a straight outstretched arm or try to break your fall by grabbing a friend or the side of the rink.

Football

Football has always been a preserve of male violence and brute strength. Men occasionally allowed women to play in pick-up touch football games, and even smiled as women formed touch football teams sponsored by local bars and competed in their own national championships. But tackle games on the old gridiron . . . well, any woman who donned shoulder and kidney pads, helmet and mouth guard to go out and hit other women was certainly a freak. No one wants to provide corporate backing for the $10,000 to $30,000 it takes to buy equipment and insurance each year, rent a stadium, and pay travel expenses. As a result, after more than ten years of ups and downs, the Women's Professional Football League is reduced to five official teams, four of them in Ohio. There are also professional teams in Oklahoma, California, and Texas, but their affiliation with the league is so loose that the league management can't predict at the beginning of the year how many teams will actually play during the coming season.

Women play as aggressive a game as men and like hitting as much as men do. However, most adult women are afraid of being hit because they didn't grow up playing the game and learning how to avoid injury during body contact. Girls who play the game as children and teenagers are as savvy about hitting and falling as boys and build up the

Effects of Football
Anaerobic
Strength: lower leg, upper leg

football-specific muscular strength and flexibility to make them exciting, effective football players.

Evaluation.   Football is not an aerobic sport. Even the longest
runs extend only a hundred yards or so. If you play or practice it three
days a week or more, however, you develop anaerobic sprinting capacity. The practice sessions strengthen every part of your leg, says Peggy
L. Lau, athletic director at the Naval Education and Training Center
in Newport, Rhode Island, and former athletic trainer of the Detroit
Demons women's professional football team. "Running on grass or turf,
with its stopping, turning, and pivoting, makes you lift your leg high,
and that strengthens your muscles," she says. "The act of playing football increases the flexibility in your ankles, lower legs, waist, and
hands, but only to a very limited extent."

Training.   A good football player needs endurance to last an entire game, Lau says, and should be able to run three to five miles on
each of three or more days a week without becoming exhausted. To
develop your sprinting ability, run goal-to-goal intervals during practice. Starting at one goal line, sprint as fast as you can to the ten-yard
line and back, then immediately turn and sprint to the twenty-yard
line and back, then to the thirty-yard line and back, and so on, until
you run from goal line to goal line. These ten nonstop sprints comprise
one set and are grueling in the extreme. Well-conditioned football
players run two or three sets nonstop during each workout. If you can't
do your speed work on the playing field, run either intervals or sprint
jogs. For sprint jogs, the whole team runs single file at an easy pace.
After a few minutes, the last person in line breaks away and sprints to
the front of the line. Then, as the line continues to run, the person who
becomes last in line sprints to the front, and so on until every person
has sprinted several times during a three- to five-mile run.

A football player must be very strong and flexible to withstand
injury and tackle effectively. Lau recommends Nautilus machines "because they give you a total body workout through your complete range
of motion." Other trainers still prefer free weights, concentrating on
strengthening all the leg muscles, the lower back, and the upper body.
For overall strength, run through the strength circuit at least three days
a week. Perform your squats with a jump at the end of each rise, and
include swimmer's kicks, shoulder shrugs, chin-ups, and pull-ups. To
protect your neck from injury, do neck-strengthening exercises four
times a week.

Flexibility in the neck, back, lateral abdominal muscles, hips, hamstrings, and ankles helps you absorb the stress of rapid accelerations,
sudden stops, and changes of direction, as well as the impact of getting
hit from all sides. Instead of the universal warm-ups before a game or

NECK STRENGTHENING EXERCISES

You need a partner to act as the resistance. She applies enough force to make the exercise difficult, but not enough to make it impossible. You should be able to do twelve reps per set with only mild fatigue. For additional protection, increase the resistance so you can do only six reps per set, but expect your neck to thicken.

Neck extension: Sit on a chair. Your partner stands behind you and places her hands on the back of your head. Roll your chin onto your chest, then arch your head back against her resistance, taking four seconds to get all the way back. Return to starting position for one rep.

Lateral neck flexion: Sit on a chair. Your partner kneels alongside and places her hands on the side of your head. As she pushes against your head, incline your head and try to touch your ear to your shoulder. (Your ear won't actually touch your shoulder.) Do not slump, and do not lift your shoulders. Return to starting position for one rep. When you complete the set on one side, repeat with the other side.

Neck flexion: Sit on a chair. Your partner kneels in front of you and places the heels of her hands on your cheekbones. Her fingers rest on your forehead so that there is no pressure on your eye socket. As she resists, push down against her hands until your chin touches your chest. Then resist your partner's hands as she pushes your head up until you look at the ceiling for one rep.

Rotary neck: Sit on a chair with your posture erect. Your partner kneels beside you and places her hands on the side of your face. Swivel your head as if it were possible to see behind you like an owl, while your partner resists your movement. Do not move your shoulders or torso. Resist your partner as she pushes you back to the starting position for one rep. When you complete the set, repeat with the other side.

training session, limber up with the concentrated stretching circuit, adding head twisters, plows with straight and bent knees, and towel stretches. For your ankles, Lau suggests walking very slowly and carefully on the outsides of your feet, trying to get your ankles to touch the ground. Do not do this exercise if you have weak ankles or knees.

Complementary sports.   Lau stresses alternate team sports during the off season. Soccer, field hockey, lacrosse, and rugby improve your football skills because they force you to work with teammates and develop your hand-eye coordination and your passing and running skills.

Injuries.   Bent, sprained, and broken fingers are the most common injuries afflicting women football players, Lau says, followed by sprained or fractured ankles and pulled muscles around the ankle.

"When people are falling on you," she says, "it's difficult to keep your body in a position that won't twist your ankle." Twisted knees are endemic to football, as are muscle strains and disk problems in the lower back. "Women haven't been taught to use leverage when they hit," Lau explains. "They lean over and use their weaker back muscles instead of using the stronger muscles in their legs." Prevent most of these injuries by strengthening all the involved muscles. The new soft, moldable mouth guards prevent most split lips, broken teeth, fractured and dislocated jaws, and cut gums and reduce the incidence of concussions and neck injuries.

HOW TO FIT A FOOTBALL HELMET

Whether you buy a suspension, padded air, or fluid liner helmet, try it on with your hair the length and arrangement you will wear it during practices and games. A properly fitted helmet should fit so tightly that you can barely turn it on your head. When you press down on the top of the helmet, you should feel the pressure on the rubber crown and not on your forehead. If you do feel pressure on your forehead, the helmet is too low. The crown should sit about one finger's width above your eyebrows. The neckband should be snug without rolling up, to prevent the helmet from slipping too far over your forehead. The jaw pad should also fit snugly and the chin strap should fasten tightly, with even tension on both sides. These prevent lateral movement of the helmet and keep your mouth closed. The chin strap should have a quick-release feature so that you or someone else can easily remove your helmet if you are injured.

Effects of Gymnastics

Anaerobic
Strength: all over
Flexibility: all over

Gymnastics and Acrobatics

Although the United States Sports Acrobatics Association and the United States Gymnastics Federation make hair-splitting distinctions between the two sports, acrobatics and gymnastics have so many aspects in common that they are here lumped together under one rubric to include tumbling (with its emphasis on flight and horizontal movement), acrobatics (with its emphasis on static poses or discontinuous single feats of tumbling—a triple somersault over a six-foot man, for example), trampoline, uneven and parallel bars, balance beam, vaulting, pommel horse, horizontal high bar, and other apparatus exercises. Rhythmic gymnastics, a women-only sport consisting of five disciplines—ribbons, clubs, balls, rope, and hoop—is taught to schoolchildren throughout Eastern Europe but is virtually unknown in the United States. In 1980, there were only about 500 competitive rhythmic gymnasts in this country, but more and more adults are attracted to it each year because it has been accepted as an Olympic event and because it demands less tumbling and physical strength than artistic gymnastics and stresses agility, hand-eye coordination, and grace.

Gymnastics is a girls' and woman's sport. A ten- or fifteen-year-old girl has long legs in proportion to her torso, the greatest ratio of strength to body weight she will ever have, and a high center of gravity. Once she matures, her proportions shift; she puts on fat and lowers her center of gravity. These changes may give her less muscle in proportion to her weight and make it harder for her to do explosive, powerful acrobatic and tumbling skills, but Dick Mulvihill, director of the National Academy of Artistic Gymnastics in Eugene, Oregon, is not so sure. "It's appealing to watch daring young girls—the Korbuts, Comanecis, and Talaveras—whittle their way through [difficult routines]. I call this the Shirley Temple syndrome. But in some cases, the actual beauty and aesthetic aspects are omitted." Mulvihill, who is Tracee Talavera's coach, believes a gymnast reaches her physical peak between twenty-four and twenty-nine and points out that at the 1964 Olympics in Tokyo, the Russians fielded gymnasts aged forty-one, thirty-eight, and thirty-six; the Americans had twenty-six- and twenty-five-year-old competitors; the Japanese had a twenty-eight-year-old champion; and the Czechs won three medals with twenty-two-year-old Vera Caslavska-Odlozil. Four years later, at the Mexico City Olympics, twenty-six-year-old Caslavska-Odlozil won four more medals. Most American gymnasts don't last this long, he says, because they can't afford to remain in training. Unlike athletes in many other sports, gymnasts receive no financial assistance or salaries. "After a while, they go toward other, less intense professions where they're going to be paid."

Many women over thirty do continue to perform and compete in gymnastics by moving into the master's level. Moreover, a woman can begin to learn gymnastics at any age, says Carol Elsner, gymnastics and exercise instructor at the YWCA in New York City. "I've seen a thirty-year-old with no previous experience learn back handsprings and do floor skills and a child acrobat now in her sixties who can still do the splits." Anyone at any age can learn gymnastics-related exercises from a competent teacher or even a gymnast daughter.

If you have an exercise mat or carpet with heavy underpadding, you can work out at home on the most basic of gymnastic exercises. It is better to find an adults' gymnastics class, though, because this is one sport in which form is extremely important. For example, on as elementary skill as a bridge (or back bend), you must curve your entire back. If you bend only your knees, you will strain your lower back. Or if you hang from a bar and do leg lifts in a pike (straight-legged) position instead of a tuck (bent knee) before your abdominals are strong, you will again injure your back. A competent coach knows this and fastidiously corrects your technique. She also spots (holds and catches) while you learn cartwheels, handsprings, and other exercises. To find a trustworthy coach, look for someone with a solid ballet background, because she is more likely to be versed in the technical aspects of correct body position. (Not all gymnastics coaches are qualified. There is no national certification program for gymnastics coaches, and many instructors have neither a ballet background nor a degree in physical education.)

Evaluation.   Gymnastics is not an aerobic sport, according to Jackie Walker, coach of the women's gymnastics team at Stanford University. "Each skill, whether it's a walkover, a handstand, or a cartwheel, takes only a few seconds, and then you rest for fifteen seconds or more. Even if you learn a complete gymnastics routine, it still takes only one and a half minutes, so it's more similar to running sprints—it's anaerobic. Gymnastics improves your overall flexibility and coordination first, and then, as you get good at it, you develop strength and power throughout your body. Gymnastics is a much more interesting activity than, say, jogging, because it involves so much variety. And you can't believe how good you feel when you can do a cartwheel and land on your feet!"

Training.   Although gymnastics doesn't condition your heart and lungs, you need good endurance in order to practice and perform well. For this reason, Coach Walker requires fifteen-minute running workouts each day. Aerobic types of dance classes would probably work as well for noncompetitive gymnasts, she says.

If you are taking gymnastics classes three or more times a week, the warm-ups, cool-downs, and gymnastics skills you learn there give you all the stretching you need. However, all gymnasts need additional weight training to prevent injuries, and if you practice gymnastics-related skills at home, or take only one class a week, you also need extra stretching. After universal warm-ups, jog or jump rope for three to five minutes to raise your heart and respiration rates. Then stretch again by progressing through one lap of the concentrated stretching circuit, emphasizing groin flexibility with wall splits and back flexibility with plows. Add bridges (back bends) when you feel strong and flexible enough. When single bridges become easy, lift one leg to a vertical position, hold for a few seconds, return it to the floor, and lift the other leg. After your workout, stretch again, then run through one lap of the strength circuit, including pull-ups, chin-ups, and hanging curls and working up to fifty killer push-ups and fifty killer sit-ups. (Gymnastics requires more strength than almost any other sport.) Finally, jog slowly for five minutes to cool down.

Complementary sports.   Ballet dancing not only provides the grace and style for floor exercises but lays down a technical basis for moving your body. Figure skating, calisthenics, and even diving use gymnastics-style skills.

Injuries.   At beginning and intermediate levels, injuries are relatively infrequent, as long as you work out on mats 1½ inch thick or more and have a competent coach who provides thorough spotting and is a stickler for technique. When you advance to the bars, you may develop hip pointers unless you wear pads underneath your leotard.

Trampolines are dangerous for everyone. Even the strongest, most flexible, and most adept gymnast can accidentally land on an edge of the tramp or on the floor and sustain crippling or permanently paralyzing head or neck injuries.

The child gymnast who works out with a rigor surpassing many adult athletes is stressing her body during her most active growth period. Many gymnastics coaches demand fifty or one hundred repetitions of difficult airborne stunts, applying tremendous torque and strain to the still-developing body of an eight- to fourteen-year-old. As a result, young girls in increasing numbers are sustaining such overuse injuries as damage to their growth plates, Osgood-Schlatter disease, chondromalacia patella, stress fractures, and vertebral disk problems (see chapter 10). Before the gymnastics boom, disk problems were rare in children. Mothers of gymnasts should question their children after each gymnastics class and listen for symptoms of serious injury. For example, a little girl who complains of low back pain and, later, pain down the buttocks into the leg may have tight hamstrings. If she does, the extreme hypertension (back arching) of many gymnastics poses may have forced one vertebra to dislocate forward of the vertebra below it, a condition called spondylolisthesis. Consult your doctor.

Handball

Court handball and the very similar British game called rugby fives are played by two players (singles) or two pairs (doubles) in a walled court. The object of the game is to hit a small hard ball (rubber in handball, cork-covered leather in rugby fives) with a gloved hand in a way that is impossible for the opponent to return. Rugby fives must be played on a four-walled court; handball may be played against one, three, or four walls, but the four-walled version is the most popular. (The completely unrelated game of team handball is discussed separately.)

Evaluation.   Handball is an anaerobic or short-burst sport. A game of twenty-one points lasts about fifteen minutes at championship level, but play isn't nonstop. Play stops for a few seconds whenever a

Effects of Handball
Anaerobic
Strength: lower leg, upper leg, shoulder, upper arm, lower arm
Flexibility: lower leg, upper leg, back, neck, trunk, shoulder, upper arm

point is scored, while the server takes her position in the server's box and the opponent sets her position toward the back of the court. In addition, there are three thirty- to sixty-second time-out periods for rest. As a result, play is intense for perhaps forty-five seconds or a minute, and then the players recover slightly as they resume position.

Handball strengthens your arms, shoulders, and legs, according to Rosemary Bellini, 1980 national women's handball champion. Although your dominant arm is favored during the game, you develop the muscles of both arms because you use them both. There is no racket in handball, so there is no backhand; you must use your nondominant arm for shots to your nondominant side. Handball makes you more flexible, Bellini says, "because you have to stretch up for high shots, bend down low for low shots. You limber up your whole body because you don't have the added reach that racket sports give you. You really have to stretch out to reach some difficult shots."

Training. Most handball players—even the champions—are in bad shape because they do nothing to build their strength or stamina; some of them don't even warm up before a game. However, "Anything that builds up your aerobic conditioning will help your handball game," Bellini says. "Swimming is the best because it uses the whole body just as handball does." In addition, running ten to twenty short sprints (20 to 30 yards) two or three times a week will give you the anaerobic stamina to maintain a rally. For handball, you need overall upper body strength as well as endurance strength in your legs and arms. To develop general upper body strength, do slow-motion push-ups, killer sit-ups, pull-ups, and chin-ups. To build endurance strength in your legs, ankles, back, and shoulders, do fast reps of squats, ankle inversion and eversion exercises, run-'em-out-of-gym-class sprints, split shifts, swimmer's kicks, shoulder shrugs, and arm sprints. Several times a day, practice quick, snappy wrist curls with as heavy a weight as you can tolerate for twenty or thirty reps per set. "The speed you get on the ball," says Bellini, "comes from snapping your wrist." Work for extremes of flexibility in your Achilles tendons, hamstrings, groin, back, and shoulders by doing Achilles stretches, calf stretches, towel stretches, runner's starts, hunkers, plows, wasp waisters, door leans, posture clasps, and birds. In addition, if you have strong knees, abdominal muscles, and back muscles, try some straight-legged bridges (back bends).

Complementary sports. "Softball or any other sport which increases hand-eye coordination will help you," Bellini says. However, although racquetball and handball make similar demands on the body, she doesn't wholeheartedly recommend racquetball for handball players. "I feel that handball is good for my racquetball game, but racquetball is terrible for my handball. In racquetball, you have a racquet for extra reach so you get a little lazy. After playing racquetball, I don't hustle as much to set myself up for shots in handball, because I think I still have that racquet in my hand."

Injuries.   Very few injuries afflict handball players, Bellini says. Bone bruises on palms of hands and fingers occur when the player strikes the hard men's ball with the flat of her hand or has uncalloused or inadequately warmed-up hands, but they rarely happen when the player uses the soft "family" ball. (Women in tournaments are required to use the softer family ball, but many women, including Rosemary Bellini, prefer playing their daily games with the hard ball because it is heavier, more responsive, and easier to control.)

Hard-plastic impact-resistant goggles are essential for protection against the variety of eye injuries a speeding handball can inflict. They are mandatory in juniors tournaments, and in the last year or two many adults have begun to wear them too. "It takes several times to get used to playing with them," Bellini says, "and I used to worry that I was giving away four to five points a game because they were bothering me, but I decided I would rather give up four or five points in a few games than lose an eye."

Hockey

See FIELD HOCKEY; ICE HOCKEY

Ice Hockey

Girls and women's ice hockey is quietly growing in the United States. In the last ten years, approximately 300 women's club teams have sprung up in various parts of the country. (A club team is an amateur group not affiliated with a school or university.) In addition, colleges and universities in eastern and northern states now boast highly competitive collegiate teams. The Amateur Hockey Association also has a program of girls' hockey teams similar to the Little League program in baseball.

Effects of Ice Hockey
Anaerobic
Strength: calf, foot, quadriceps, hip abductor, hip adductor, gluteals, abdominals, back, lower arm

Evaluation.   Ice hockey is an anaerobic rather than an aerobic game, according to Laura Stamm. Stamm has trained men's professional teams in skating technique as well as such individual National Hockey League players as Bobby Nystrom of the New York Islanders, Greg Fox of the Chicago Black Hawks, Mel Bridgeman of the Philadelphia

Flyers, and Bobby Lalonde of the Boston Bruins. During a game, you skate intensely for about one and a half minutes, racing down the ice, stick handling or shooting the puck or checking. Then play stops and you rest. It strengthens your back, abdominals, quadriceps, gluteals, thigh adductor and abductor muscles, calves, feet, and toes. Stick handling, shooting, and checking also strengthen your arms and wrists, but most hockey players must lift weights in order to play well. Hockey does not limber you up. Until hockey players discovered stretching a few years ago, they were among the stiffest athletes in American sports. This stiffness accounted for most of their overuse injuries.

Training. A good hockey player needs a good aerobic base in order to last through a whole game and play effectively, says Stamm, author of *Power Skating the Hockey Way.* Cycling is especially good for skaters because it uses the same ratios of quadriceps and hamstring muscles as skating does. Many professional hockey players, in fact, train on stationary bicycles. Others run. Whichever you prefer, do both Long Steady Distance and speed intervals. For cardiovascular staying power and anaerobic sprinting capacity, alternate between cycling or running at moderate speed and sprinting as fast as you can for ten seconds. Do this for twenty minutes, the time of one hockey period.

Strengthen your groin, thighs, and ankles with split shifts or side leg lifts, dumbbell lunges, squats, ankle inversion and eversion exercises, and heel and toes. Upper body strength is very important for power skating. Strengthen your back with swimmer's kicks and your abdominal muscles with killer sit-ups and twisting sit-ups. For general upper body strength, do chin-ups, pull-ups, and push-ups. Tie ankle or wrist weights just above the blade of your stick and use that weighted stick to practice your slap shots and strengthen your arm muscles. Wrist shots require strength in your hands and lower and upper arms. Practice this shot over and over again with a weighted stick, and do grip-strength exercises several times every day to build up your hand muscles. To prevent injuries from hitting the boards, body checking, and other body contact, do neck strengthening exercises.

Do your universal warm-ups conscientiously before and after every game and practice session because the cold stiffens your muscles. Power turns, shots on goal, and scrambles for the puck overdevelop your groin and thigh muscles, making them short and tight. Stretch them before and after every game and practice session with runner's starts, storks, and geisha kneels; stretch your hamstrings with towel stretches, your calf muscles with calf stretches and Achilles stretches, and your lower back with wasp waisters and king of Siam kowtows. To prevent injuries when you hit the boards or fall on the ice, stretch your shoulder muscles with birds.

Complementary sports. Bicycling builds aerobic endurance while developing your quads in the same ratios that skating does. Board sailing uses the same leg muscles and teaches you balance. Figure skating helps you perfect your skating technique and control, while soccer makes the same aerobic and anaerobic demands as ice hockey does. In fact, many European hockey players play soccer during their off season in order to stay in shape.

Injuries. The most common overuse hockey injuries affect the groin and knee. Both parts of the body are stretched or stressed during sudden stops or sharp changes of direction. Muscle pulls in the thighs also occur frequently. Prevent many of these injuries by maintaining flexibility in these two areas. Shoulder, neck, and back problems stem from shooting before you are warmed up or from weak back and abdominal muscles. Because you skate bent over, your back is constantly under stress. Strengthening your abdominal muscles, as well as your back muscles, relieves some of the pressure on your back. Shoulder separations and knee damage are often caused by falls, as are broken ankles, wrists, and arms. Now that junior and women hockey players wear helmets with cages or face masks, most of the facial injuries have disappeared. The only time they occur is when a player wears a cage with a large space between the bars. The bars should be spaced narrowly enough to screen out the blade of the stick. The chin strap of the helmet should protect your chin, not just hold your helmet in place. Stamm also advises wearing the clear plastic mouthpiece football players wear. Buy it in sporting goods stores and mold it to your own shape by softening it in hot water and then inserting it into your mouth.

There is a myth that flat-footed people can't skate or play ice hockey. This isn't true. If you have flat feet, buy your boots and blades separately; then position the blade on the boot to counteract any pronation or posture defects. If this isn't enough, ask your sports podiatrist for orthotics.

Ice Skating (Speed)

Women were competing in organized speed ice skating races in the Netherlands by 1805. The first world championships for women were held in 1936, and in 1960 women's speed skating became an Olympic event at the Squaw Valley Olympic Games. In 1975, Tatiana Averina of the USSR skated the 1,500-meter race in world record time of 2:09.91, a pace which would have won the 1973 men's world speed skating championships. American speed skater and cyclist Sheila Young has been clocked on skates at over twenty-seven miles per hour.

Evaluation. Speed skating is an excellent aerobic sport, accord-

Effects of Ice Skating, Speed

Aerobic
Anaerobic
Strength: quadriceps, gluteals, hip flexor, hip extensor, lower back
Flexibility: upper leg, hips

ing to Dianne Holum, coach of the 1976 and 1980 American Olympic speed skating teams, but the training, not the racing, conditions your body. In competition, women skate 500-meter, 1,000-meter, 1,500-meter, and 3,000-meter races. The longest race lasts only about four and a half minutes at world championship levels. The shortest events, the 500- and 1,000-meter races, last less than fifty seconds and one and a half minutes respectively. However, training involves an hour or more of nonstop distance skating. Because speed skaters do not specialize in one distance, the way runners do, but must skate all four distances in world competition, skaters develop their anaerobic as well as their aerobic capacity.

Speed skating strengthens your quads, gluteals, hip extensors and flexors, and lower back, says Holum, who won a silver and a bronze medal in the 1968 Olympics and a gold and a silver in the 1972 Games. It increases the flexibility of your hips and thighs, but "speed skaters *never* count on skating itself to increase flexibility. They do specific flexibility training."

Training. "Although a top international skater trains eleven months a year," Holum says, "she spends only about thirty to forty percent of her time on the ice. The rest of the time, she does dry-land training. She does a lot of cycling and running and an awful lot of simulation exercises to imitate her movements on the ice." Bicycling is best because it uses the same muscles in the same ratios as skating does. Bicycle long distances and sprints or intervals to develop both aerobic and anaerobic capacity. If you want to improve your performance in sprint events, an hour of distance cycling three days a week is probably enough. The other four days, ride hills and intervals. For the 3,000-meter race, concentrate on distance and do intervals two or three days a week for tempo. A standard cycling regimen is ideal for speed skating. Elite skaters also run and sprint ten or twenty yards because it not only gives them a cardiovascular workout but simulates their start. "The start in speed skating," Holum explains, "is similar to running uphill, because you bend your knees. To simulate your turn, run sideways up a gradually sloping hill doing crossover steps and leaning into the hill the way you lean into a turn." Holum also suggests simulating the gliding stride by bending into your skating position and pushing or jumping to the side on grass as if you were gliding on ice. If you watched the 1980 winter Olympics coverage on television, you probably saw Beth and Eric Heiden sliding sideways across a room on a slide board. This is the ultimate aerobic simulator. Holum, who coached the Heidens, first in Madison, Wisconsin, and then on the Olympic team, sells a manual that includes directions for building and using your own slide board. (See Selected Readings for address.)

Speed skaters need overall strength and specific muscular strength. Elite speed skaters run circuits several days a week and then strengthen their quads, hip abductors, hip adductors, gluteals, lower back, and abdominals with low weight/high rep weight training. Light weights and twenty or more reps develop muscular endurance while increasing your strength moderately. Combine your circuits and muscle endurance training by running through the full circuit program three times and then adding extra sets of squats or jump squats. Do one set while holding the dumbbells against the front of your shoulders, to strengthen your quads just above your knee. Also perform kiddie kicks, hamsters, swimmer's kicks, side leg lifts, and killer sit-ups. In addition, elite skaters do high resistance exercises to develop explosive strength and sprinting power in their legs, particularly their thighs. Two or three times a week, do dumbbell lunges, squats, *and* jump squats while holding so much weight that you can only do six or seven reps before you are exhausted.

As a speed skater, you must stretch your calves (gastrocs), hamstrings, hip flexors, and groin very carefully. Spend fifteen or twenty minutes every day working your way through the universal warm-ups and the concentrated stretching circuit. Emphasize the groin stretch, gravity toe touch, stork, towel stretch, runner's start, calf and Achilles stretches, and hunkers.

Complementary sports.   Bicycling and running, as described. In addition, Holum suggests rowing because it uses the quads and gluteals as well as the upper body muscles.

Injuries.   "The only really common injuries," Holum says, "are spiking injuries, when a skater cuts herself with her own skate blade. Otherwise, there are very few injuries in speed skating."

Judo and Aikido

Judo and aikido evolved out of jujitsu systems of Japanese martial arts in the middle of the eighteenth century. Both use throwing and pinning techniques: The judo player grapples, using the knee, ankle, or hip as a fulcrum; the aikidoist relies on momentum throws and uses swords, four-foot sticks, and knives as well as empty hands. Judo developed in Japan as a competitive sport rather than a martial art. The first women's world championships were held in New York in November 1980. Aikido, on the other hand, is a lifelong martial art, a soft, flowing style of self-defense which uses the opponent's own force to throw her off balance and therefore provides very little muscular endurance or respiratory training effects. Its injuries resemble those of judo.

Effects of Judo and Aikido

Aerobic
Anaerobic
Strength: all over
Flexibility: all over

Evaluation.   Intense two-hour judo practice sessions are aerobic, says Rusty Kanokogi, former coach of the U.S. women's judo team and tournament director of the first women's judo championship. An actual five-minute match, however, is anaerobic. Judo develops strength all over your body, she says, but it is primarily isometric body building because two bodies trying to manipulate each other or turn each other over are effectively immovable objects during most of each maneuver. Judo players emphasize lower body strength as much as upper; thus you develop and use the large strong muscles below your waist. The sport develops and requires overall flexibility, for you must be able to get into and out of all sorts of positions.

Training.   According to Kanokogi, a judo practice session is a total aerobic, strength, and flexibility workout. You don't need anything else. To illustrate, she challenges you to do judo push-ups. "They're probably the best exercise in the world," she says. "If I could do just one exercise, this would be it. Swimmers and basketball and baseball players use it in their training. Try it—but don't send me your doctor bills!"

JUDO PUSH-UPS

Crouch in a crab position, with your weight on your hands and the balls of your feet. Spread your arms and legs as wide as possible for balance, bend your knees, and stick your rear end up. Leading with your head, slowly swoop down and forward and rub your chest, abdomen, and thighs on the mat. Tuck your buttocks in tight during this shoveling thrust. Return slowly to the starting position, for one rep. Do ten reps slowly and ten reps quickly. Builds strength in the lats, triceps, pectorals, abdominals, quads, and even the shins.

Also included in Kanokogi's judo workout: half squats done slowly and then quickly, killer sit-ups, jogging slowly and quickly in place, plows with both feet angled first over your right shoulder, then over your head, and finally out over your left shoulder; and judo shoulder shrugs.

Complementary sports.   "Every single sport helps a judo player," Kanokogi says, "and judo helps with your coordination, strength, and movement in every other sport. Volleyball, for example, gives you the spring you need for judo. Spring is bending your knees and lifting with your hips. Your judo spring helps in handball and racquetball, and learning the eight natural directions of the body we use in judo will

JUDO SHOULDER SHRUGS

Stand with your arms extended out to the sides and your fingers pointed. Exaggeratedly shrug your shoulders forward ten times, then backward ten times. Next, extend your arms straight above your head and touch the backs of your hands together. Shrug forward ten times, then rearward ten times.

help you when you're playing squash. If you were using running to train for squash, you'd only learn to move in one direction. Judo teaches you how to keep your balance and recover in basketball. A kid who plays judo learns greater pain tolerance and the fighting spirit.''

Injuries.   Aikidoists and judo players frequently catch and break their toes on practice mats. Miscellaneous bruises, sprains, and strains are also common as the result of bad falls, poor throwing techniques, worn-out mats, and aborted throws. Dislocations and fractures of the clavicle or other structures in the shoulder occur more often in judo than in aikido, as do knee injuries, because the knee is used as a fulcrum during a throw. Aikido has relatively few injuries overall, because it is noncompetitive.

Karate, Kung Fu, and Tae Kwon Do

These three martial arts form a continuum. Karate is the Japanese form of empty-handed punching, kicking, striking, and blocking combat. At least 50 percent of its techniques are sharp, straight-line, ballistic punching and striking movements. Except in actual warfare, it is a non-contact martial art, in which students are trained to stop before they touch their partners. There are about one hundred different styles of karate. China's kung fu, also known as gung fu or wu shu or shaolin chuan ta, also uses hand and foot blows but favors circular, clawing, stabbing, striking motions with the hands. There are more than four hundred different kung fu styles. Tae kwon do is Korea's contribution to empty-handed martial arts. Like karate, it favors straight-line ballistic movements, but about 70 percent of its techniques involve hip rotating, high kicks, and smashing movements with the feet. It is an attacking, contact offensive martial art; tae kwon do players are trained to make contact even during their training. (Players wear body armor during training and matches.) Hapkido, moo duk kwon, and tang soo do are a few of its substyles. At many schools, elements of karate, kung fu, and tae kwon do are taught as the teacher's own conglomerate system.

Effects of Karate, Kung Fu, and Tai Kwon Do

Aerobic
Anaerobic
Strength: all over
Flexibility: all over

In these martial arts, you continue to improve as long as you practice regularly. People in their sixties become more efficient and learn to use less motion to gain the advantage over younger, more physical opponents. And yet, all forms of karate are good skills for beginners, according to Marcia Hall, the first American (male or female) to win a gold medal in the international tae kwon do competition. "Unlike football or basketball," she says, "you don't have to be skilled in order to get into it. It teaches you whatever you need to know; takes in weak people and makes them strong." She feels that tae kwon do, with its emphasis on kicking, is best suited to women because women have more strength in their legs than in their arms. They are usually limber enough to find the kicks relatively easy to do, and their well-padded hips add weight, and therefore force, to the hip rotation used in most kicks. Tae kwon do women's competitions are the best organized of all the Asian martial arts in the United States. Karate competitions for women exist at the regional level and, weakly, at the national level, but only in forms (choreographed matches). Tae kwon do competition is fully organized in forms and free fighting at the regional, national, and international levels, and is divided into eight ten-pound weight divisions. Finally, Hall says, because tae kwon do is a contact sport, it makes women feel less vulnerable and more confident.

It it difficult for a beginner to find a reputable, reliable school. "The martial arts community has a lot of shysters," Hall says, "and a lot of people teaching things they shouldn't be teaching to beginners." Not even a certificate from a school or federation in Japan or Korea is a guarantee of competence, for some of these organizations don't test or evaluate their pupils. What's more, says Hall, "there are a lot of good instructors who don't have certificates and are just as good as people from Asia." Before enrolling in any school, observe several classes. "Be suspicious of any studio that won't let you watch a class," Hall says. Look for control, discipline, decorum, and cleanliness. Chaos or rough-housing indicates a frivolous approach to the art. If possible, choose a school which incorporates meditation into each class, because this indicates that the instructor treats karate as a serious philosophy rather than a fun-filled way of imitating Bruce Lee. Talk to the students, especially the women. Ask them whether their physical condition has improved as much as their karate skills since starting to study at the school, and whether they have ever been injured. (At a reliable school, injuries are extremely rare.) Choose a school which has several other women students because this indicates that the teacher understands their special physical attributes.

Evaluation.   All forms of karate develop aerobic capacity during the repetitious training patterns, according to Susan Borger Budge, owner of the Omine Karate Dojo in San Bruno, California. Each of these form drills, called *kata* in Japanese, emphasizes explosive power in specific parts of the body, and a whole series of repetitions lasts more than fifteen minutes. In addition, during warm-ups and sparring, there are many bursts of anaerobic effort. Because tae kwon do relies on kicking—a more strenuous movement than punching—it gives you better aerobic and anaerobic training effects than karate, but neither one conditions you to the extent that running and jumping rope do.

All forms of karate systematically develop strength in all parts of your body during the warm-ups and *katas*. However, karate focuses on your upper body strength while tae kwon do's kicking preferentially builds up your quads.

The warm-ups and *katas* of all styles of karate are designed to develop flexibility in every joint in your body, and tae kwon do's head-high kicks add an extraordinary degree of limberness to the hamstrings, groin, and hips.

Training.   Marcia Hall, who was tae kwon do world champion in her weight division for three consecutive years (1978–80), advises running five or six miles a day, three or more days a week, in order to develop a high level of cardiovascular fitness and to build aerobic and anaerobic endurance for competition. She also suggests intervals or other speed work. In karate competition, she says, you spar intensely for a few seconds or a couple of minutes until a point is scored and then rest until your next match, so you need good anaerobic capacity. In tae kwon do competition, you play three consecutive three-minute rounds, interrupted only by one-minute intermissions, so you need a combination of anaerobic and aerobic endurance.

Karate movements are sharp, forceful, explosive outward blows. There is very little pulling involved. Thus, any strength training should replicate these kinds of movements throughout your body, but particularly in your lats, triceps, forearms, quads, groin, and calves. In addition, if you play tae kwon do, strengthen your hamstrings to balance your overdeveloped quads and prevent injuries. Most schools have some form of makiwara, slightly flexible padded striking posts for punching and kicking against a resistance. Instead of or in addition to practice against the makiwara, do arm sprints; push-ups, first with your hands flat on the floor and then on your knuckles with your hand clenched into a fist to strengthen your wrists as well as your chest, shoulders, and arms; wrist curls; squats; split shifts; and run-'em-out-of-gym-class sprints. Finally, build up your abdominal muscles with killer sit-ups and twisting sit-ups. These muscles are used to support and control every movement in your body.

Both Budge and Hall feel that the warm-up exercises built into each karate system make you very limber without any supplementary programs. If you play tae kwon do, give extra attention to groin, quad, and hip stretches and practice wall splints, hunkers, geisha kneels, and wasp waisters at home as many times a day as you can.

Injuries.   Karate has surprisingly few injuries, because thorough warm-ups and proper technique are stressed at every reputable school. Most of the injuries are sprains or strains to the hamstring, groin, thumb, or toe caused by kicking or striking incorrectly or with cold muscles. Occasionally, karate players fracture their little fingers or their first, second, or little toes, but even these injuries are rare.

Kayaking

See CANOEING AND KAYAKING

Korfball

See SOCCER

Lacrosse

Effects of Lacrosse
Aerobic
Strength: upper leg

Lacrosse is derived from a North American Indian game in which teams of hundreds of players moved a wooden or deerskin ball from one end of a field to the other. The fields had no boundaries or side-lines and were sometimes several miles long. The participants carried and passed the ball in loops attached to one end of a three- or four-foot stick. Today, lacrosse is played with wooden or plastic sticks with a basket attached to one end. The rubber ball is slightly larger than a softball. (A similar non-contact stickball game, marketed either as STX-ball or McWhippet, is played with a soft, spongy ball and a flexible stick with a bigger basket than the usual lacrosse pocket. It has become increasingly popular with children and older women.)

Lacrosse is an eastern sport, immensely popular in high schools and colleges in Baltimore and Philadelphia, for example, but virtually unknown in California. Women's lacrosse remains closer to the original Indian game than the men's game. The men play on a field with established boundaries, use plastic sticks, and wear protective helmets and equipment. The women play on a field limited only by natural boundaries, use wooden sticks, and with the exception of the goalie, wear little or no protection gear. (Some women wear shin guards and gauntlets or padded gloves.)

Evaluation.   Lacrosse is an aerobic sport, according to Maggie

Faulkner, lacrosse coach at Towson State University in Maryland. "Lacrosse is more demanding than soccer, field hockey, or basketball," she says, "because the field (also called a pitch) has no boundaries. It's 100 yards from goal line to goal line, but the field can go from 120 to 140 yards in length and 60 to 90 yards in width. There are no sidelines as such." Although play stops every three or four minutes when a foul is committed, the rest periods are thirty seconds or less—not enough to classify lacrosse as a short-burst sprint-and-stop sport. Lacrosse strengthens only the leg muscles involved in running and contributes nothing to your flexibility.

Training.   A good lacrosse player should have the aerobic capacity to run two miles in fourteen minutes, says Faulkner. She suggests running three to five miles a day at an LSD pace and running intervals two or three times a week. The women on her teams run "quarters": six quarter-mile intervals, or a total of a mile and a half, in one minute and forty seconds or less, allowing themselves about two minutes of rest between each quarter. "I prefer they run each quarter in 1:20," she says, "but I'll take 1:40."

Upper body strength is important for stick handling and checking in lacrosse. Build overall strength with push-ups, chin-ups, and pull-ups and add shoulder shrugs for your trapezius muscles, dumbbell pullovers for your pectorals and triceps, and squats for your legs. Faulkner recommends grip-strength exercises to give you an advantage in stick handling.

You need flexibility, Faulkner says, to prevent injury. Before each game perform the universal warm-ups for twenty minutes instead of the usual ten.

Faulkner stresses that a good lacrosse player is able to hold her stick with either hand uppermost. (The hand closer to the basket dominates the swing.) When you handle a stick ambidextrously, you always swing with the power of a forehand, no matter which side the ball comes toward you. "This is much the same as dribbling a basketball with your left hand," Faulkner says, "instead of bringing the basketball across your body to dribble on your right side." Drill yourself by running and stick handling alone or with a friend, giving as much time to your nondominant hand as your dominant one.

Complementary sports.   Field hockey resembles lacrosse, although hockey's downward stick handling differs from the upright stick handling of lacrosse.

Injuries.   Pulled quads and hamstring muscles occur frequently in lacrosse and can be prevented by adequate stretching programs. Sprained ankles caused by twisting falls are epidemic. Although lacrosse is a contact sport, the contact is usually body-to-body rather than stick-to-body, so injuries more serious than bruises are rare. However, "Occasionally you get bumps on the head from a stick," Faulkner says. "The way you get the ball from an attacking player is by checking. That means you try to hit your stick on her stick. Occasionally, you miss her stick and hit her head." A helmet-and-face mask with a vertical bar reinforcing the horizontal bars prevents most of these injuries.

Mountain Climbing

Effects of Mountain Climbing

Aerobic

Anaerobic

Strength: lower leg, upper leg, hip, gluteals, shoulder, upper arm

The sport of mountain climbing was born on July 24, 1760, when Swiss naturalist Horace-Benedict de Saussure offered about $60 to the first man who could climb Mont Blanc, the highest mountain in Western Europe. Two Frenchmen collected the prize twenty-six years later, beginning a tradition of all-male mountain climbing that was to last until 1970, when an all-woman expedition reached the summit of Mount McKinley. In 1978, a group of women climbers proved that "A Woman's Place Is on Top" (the motto of their fund-raising T-shirts) in an expedition to 26,504-foot Annapurna I, the tenth-highest mountain in the world and one of the Himalayas' most elusive and difficult peaks. "We're not superwomen, or super athletes," expedition organizer Arlene Blum has said in several interviews. "We just showed that women can do hard things and succeed."

Evaluation.   Mountain climbing is aerobic at the lower levels, according to Barbara Drinkwater, Ph.D., associate research physiologist at the Institute of Environmental Stress, University of California at Santa Barbara. "When you get up to high altitudes of about 20,000 feet," says Drinkwater, who accompanied the Indian-American women's group ascent of 22,218-foot Bhrigupanth Peak in India, "you are doing an aerobic work because the demands exceed maximum aerobic capacity. You're taking one step and then breathing seven times." The sport builds upper and lower body strength, particularly the fronts and backs of the thighs and lower legs during climbing and the upper arms and shoulders when you work the ropes or use ice picks. It develops a moderate amount of flexibility when you make awkward or reaching movements.

Training.   A high level of aerobic capacity is very important, says Drinkwater. Many climbers run with or without a loaded backpack to build their endurance capacity, but bicycling works almost as well and develops your quads. Running up and down stadium stairs is another favorite conditioning exercise because you pull yourself up with your thigh muscles as you do in climbing. When stadiums become tolerable—they never feel easy—run them while wearing an increasingly heavy backpack. Killer sit-ups, push-ups, and pull-ups develop your abdominals and upper body. "The best type of training," Drinkwater says, "is to find an easy hill-and-mountain trail, put on a heavy pack, and just go up. Then go down, for it's every bit as difficult going down as coming up, and the descent uses different combinations of muscles."

Injuries. "Avalanches and falling in crevasses are all too common in the Himalayas," says Drinkwater, and that statement applies to most of the highest climbs. Strained hamstrings and other overuse injuries occur frequently to climbers in poor condition. Heat is as much a danger in high altitudes as cold, and sunburn afflicts most climbers. The sun's rays, less filtered and more intense in the thin air, attack a climber directly from above and indirectly from below when they reflect off the white snow. A sunscreen is required equipment on any expedition. And altitude sickness threatens susceptible climbers with anything from headaches and nausea to pulmonary edema.

Consult your doctor before embarking on a moderate- or high-altitude mountain-climbing outing if you have: high blood pressure, asthma, cardiopulmonary problems, breathing or exertion problems, detached retina, supersensitivity to the sun, diabetes, anxiety (nervous people have less tolerance to altitudes), or emphysema, angina, chronic pulmonary obstructive disease, or any other problem involving lowered oxygen tension.

Power Lifting

See WEIGHT LIFTING, POWER LIFTING, AND BODY BUILDING

Race Walking

Anyone who has ever watched race walking knows that it is very different from normal walking. Race walkers must have one foot on the ground at all times. They are not allowed to spring from one to the other while spending a split second with both feet in the air the way runners do. If they do spring off the ground—it's called "lifting" in race walkers' parlance—they are disqualified. Race walkers must also fully straighten each leg and lock the knee once during each stride. If they don't, they are "creeping" and, again, disqualified. These two rules force a style in which the race walker lands on her heel, rolls to the outside of her foot, and then onto the ball of her foot. Instead of pushing off with the back leg as a runner does, she pulls the ground under her with her forward leg as if walking on a treadmill, according to world-class race walker Lori Maynard. In the course of each stride, she must rotate her hips in order to straighten her leg and pull with the front of her foot. The thrusting hips and concomitant arm pumping make her look like an angry duck.

Effects of Race Walking
Aerobic
Strength: shin, ankle, foot, hamstrings, back, triceps
Flexibility: hip, shoulder

"Race walking has many advantages over other aerobic sports," says Maynard, who ranks number one in the master's division (over forty years of age) and among the top ten nationally in the open division (nineteen years and older). "It uses more of the muscular system than running, so you get a whole-body workout instead of just a lower-body effect. It is less jarring to the skeleton because there is less impact than in running or jumping rope. People can continue to race-walk relatively injury-free much later in life than they can run. It can be used as a recreational activity, a competitive activity, or both. And the sport has a special camaraderie. Maybe because our numbers are so small compared to many other sports, all walkers welcome new walkers as if they are long-lost friends. All walkers give tips willingly. You don't have to prove yourself in order to be accepted."

Evaluation. Race walking gives you an excellent aerobic training effect—about 90 percent of the effect you get from running. Maynard says some race walkers, in fact, have maximal oxygen uptakes comparable to distance runners. The gait strengthens your hamstrings, shins, and the muscles along the front and outside of the foot and ankle, and the churning arm motion strengthens your triceps and back. The rotation in your hips improves the flexibility of your pelvic region, and the pumping motion loosens up your shoulders.

Training. Race walkers need no other aerobic conditioning. Because strong arms add miles to your endurance, strengthen your upper body by holding 1-, 3-, or 5-pound dumbbell in each hand and pumping your arms race walker–style until they are exhausted. Low-weight/high-rep lifting builds muscle endurance while moderately increasing your strength. In addition, strengthen your abdominals with killer sit-ups to add endurance to your trunk muscles.

Flexibility is extremely important for a race walker, Maynard says. In addition to universal warm-ups, she suggests conscientiously stretching your back, shoulders, hamstrings, calves, Achilles tendons, and the tops and fronts of the feet and ankles. Do extra gravity toe touches, calf stretches, Achilles stretches, towel stretches, geisha kneels, wasp waisters, king of Siam kowtows, and shoulder circles.

Complementary sports. "Cross-country skiing is an excellent sport for race walkers," Maynard says. "It is prime aerobic exercise and uses a forward motion like race walking and an arm swing. Although it's not precisely complementary, bicycling would help race walking because it's a fine conditioning exercise."

Injuries. Race walking has far fewer injuries than any of the running sports. It is usually safe exercise for people with knee problems because the knee is straight rather than flexed when the foot touches

---

SHOULDER CIRCLES

Stand up and hang your arms down at your sides. Move your shoulders forward and back and in circles without moving any other part of your body.

---

the ground. This permits the whole leg to absorb the impact of the foot strike. (In running, the bent knee absorbs much of the impact.) However, medial knee pain does occur if you over-pronate and turn the shinbone inward. Most back problems are eased by race walking, but swaybacks may be made worse. Hip-joint strain, hamstring pulls caused by straightening the leg while extending the heel at contact, anterior shin splints, and tendinitis of the large cord running just above the ankle also occur occasionally. Most may be prevented with adequate stretching.

Racquetball

Between 1976 and 1979, racquetball became the fastest-growing participatory sport in the United States, according to an A. C. Nielson Company survey. The sport increased by 283 percent during those years. Today, although the growth rate has slowed, at least 11 million people play this young brash cousin of squash.

In both squash and racquetball, you hit a small rubber ball with a racquet inside a boxlike, enclosed, four-walled court. However, you need more power to play racquetball because the short-handled racquetball racquet prevents you from using torque to make the ball go faster. You must put more arm and shoulder muscle into each stroke. Use of the ceiling and the entire front wall makes racquetball an easier game to learn and muscle your way through than squash. Outdoor racquetball, a sociable summertime sport played in several states, has a three-walled court and features waist and chest-high shots, in contrast to indoor racquetball's low bending shots.

Racquetball is a "mental" game—players must predict each other's moves as accurately as they read the angles and creases of the four walls. "Experience is a tremendous factor," says Heather McKay, top-ranked women's professional racquetball player now and formerly women's world champion in squash for many years. "But fitness is important. I'm peaking now at thirty-nine, and I think I can play winning racquetball for another two to three years at least. My shots and skills may improve, but my fitness won't. In professional racquetball, you're on the downhill grade at forty or forty-one."

Effects of Racquetball

Anaerobic
Strength: calf, quadriceps, lower back, forearm

McKay's standards, it should be noted, are higher than most. She owned women's squash for twenty years, losing only two matches (early in her career). She was also regional junior and senior women's tennis champion for three years in her teens and twice played on the All-Australia field hockey team. "Heather is a true athlete," says Lynn Adams, number-two-ranked women's player on the professional racquetball circuit, "not just a good racquetball player." At the amateur level, Adams points out, you can play good racquetball throughout your life.

Evaluation. Racquetball is rarely an aerobic sport, according to Adams; it is an anaerobic game of sprinting rallies and short rest periods. "At the lower levels," she says, "you don't really put the ball away a lot, so rallies go on for a long, long time—about thirty seconds—and you are constantly moving. Then you rest for fifteen or twenty seconds while you are setting up again. The higher you go, the shorter the rallies tend to be and you work in very short spurts."

The running and bending of indoor racquetball strengthens your quads, your calves, and your lower back. Hitting the ball strengthens your forearm muscles. In outdoor racquetball, your lower back isn't strengthened because you don't bend. Your upper arms are strengthened slightly, however, because you hit more balls at chest level.

Many professional racquetball players are very stiff because they don't have to stretch as far as squash players. The game of racquetball, by itself, does not increase your flexibility.

Training. "To improve your game," Adams says, "you should run. You rely on lung capacity, even though racquetball isn't an aerobic sport, and you need anaerobic training to last through the rallies and allow you to come out faster." Adams recommends running two or three miles a day, at least three days a week, and then running intervals, hills, or court sprints the other three days. When she runs court sprints, she works with a partner, "and we try to see who's meaner. I start in the middle of the court and my partner stands by the door of the court. I run as fast as I can to wherever she points, using racquetball footwork, across the court, backward, forward, sideward. She keeps me going until I can't move my legs anymore and then I do it to her. We alternate fifteen or twenty court sprints in a workout." In addition, Adams recommends "stadiums" (running stadium stairs) to strengthen your thighs and calves for the slightly bent position you use in racquetball, and jumping rope to strengthen your calves stand for standing on your toes. "In any type of racket sport," she explains, "you've got to stay on your toes. You can't play flatfooted."

If you are very serious about your racquetball performance, improve the strength and muscle endurance in your forearms and the front and backs of your legs with wrist curls, grip-strength exercises, run-'em-out-of-gym-class sprints, dumbbell lunges, and squats. "Your leg is where you get most of your power," Adams emphasizes. Strengthen your lower back and abdominals with swimmer's kicks and killer sit-ups, and build up your shoulders and upper arms in order to put more power into your stroke with chin-ups and pull-ups. Because you use only a small amount of your upper arms in a racquetball stroke, these last two exercises are optional. In addition, practice typical racquetball strokes while holding a 1- to 3-pound dumbbell in your hand or a weighted racquet. (To make a weighted racquet, tie a weight or piece of brick to the top of an old racquet.)

Racquetball doesn't require the flexibility, reaching, and stretching that squash and many other sports do. However, you should perform your universal warm-ups conscientiously in order to prevent injuries. Pay special attention to the gravity toe touches, storks, groin stretches, Achilles stretches, and calf stretches.

Complementary sports.   Bicycling not only develops your cardiovascular capacity but strengthens the front of your thighs in ways similar to racquetball. Other racket sports improve hand-eye coordination and use similar muscles. However, only badminton and squash use the flexible, flicking wrist motion required in racquetball.

Injuries.   There are relatively few overuse injuries in racquetball. Occasionally a player sprains her ankle or tears her calf muscle, but strengthening and stretching exercises prevent most of these sorts of injuries. Wearing basketball, volleyball, or racquetball shoes instead of running shoes also helps. Tennis elbow, caused by too many wrist flicks, should also be called racquetball elbow. Swimmer's shoulder, caused by making too many ceiling shots, can be prevented by learning an underhanded technique. Swollen and sore racquetball wrist, caused by turning over your wrist during a follow-through with an overly heavy racquet, may be prevented by using a lighter racquet.

Among the injuries caused by getting hit with the ball or your opponent's racquet, eye injuries are the most serious; they can lead to permanent blindness. Eye guards should be required equipment on every racquetball court. In addition, never turn around to see what your opponent is doing, or you risk getting a racquet or ball smack in the face. Stay away from players who swing their racquets wildly.

Racquetball players sometimes intentionally subject themselves to quite memorable ball marks—vivid five-color circular bruises—because blocking the ball in a way that looks like an accident results in playing the point over.

Rock Climbing

Effects of Rock Climbing

Anaerobic

Strength: all over

Flexibility: all over

Rock climbing used to be an extremely dangerous sport, but the introduction of climbing shoes with high-friction sticky rubber soles, Perlon braided filament ropes (which manage to be strong and stretchy at the same time), chrome-molybdenum-alloy carabiners, and other advanced equipment have made the sport one of the fastest growing in America. However, you still need expert instruction before you step out onto your first narrow rock ledge.

Many people lump rock and mountain climbing together, as if the two form a continuum, with rock climbing just done at lower altitudes. Although the history and traditions are similar, these two sports place very different demands on the body.

Evaluation.   Rock climbing, according to Barbara Drinkwater, is only minimally an aerobic sport. Primarily, rock climbers rely on anaerobic muscular capacity. Rock climbing builds strength in every part of the body, but especially in the hands, forearms, and shoulders used to pull yourself up. Its contortions develop amazing flexibility throughout your body by forcing you into contortions.

Training.   Although general cardiovascular fitness gives you the stamina to endure anything, specific aerobic training isn't as important here as it is in many other sports. Any kind of aerobic exercise will help—running, stair climbing with or without a pack, bicycling, or swimming. On the other hand, you must develop both specific and overall body strength. Women rock climbers tend to emphasize balance, technique, and leg strength to compensate for their weak arms and shoulders, but building upper body strength gives you a tremendous advantage. Do chin-ups, push-ups, shoulder shrugs, arm sprints, wrist curls, and grip-strength exercises, as well as run-'em-out-of-gym-class sprints, split shifts, squats, dumbbell lunges, and heel and toes for your lower body. For flexibility, do as many of these exercises in the concentrated stretching circuit as you can, paying special attention to the groin (wall splits), shoulder (posture clasps, door leans, and birds), and hamstrings (towel stretches, runner's starts, and gravity toe touches).

Injuries.   A trained and experienced rock climber rarely suffers injuries from misuse or overuse. Most injuries are traumatic, and occur when something unexpected happens. Scrapes and bruises are so common that climbers don't consider them worthy of mention. Dislocations, fractures, cuts, and other damage come from falls or being hit by falling rocks.

Roller Skating (Artistic)

Artistic skating, roller skating's equivalent of figure skating, is an international sport with annual world championships held in a different country each year. It is an event in the National Sports Festival, sponsored by the U.S. Olympic Committee, and in the Pan-American Games. Artistic skaters do the same compulsory figures as figure skaters do, have similar freestyle events, and are judged by a system very similar to that of ice skating.

Evaluation.   Artistic roller skating is an aerobic sport, according to Kathleen O'Brien Di Felice, 1980 U.S. Senior Ladies Singles Champion and silver medalist at the 1980 World's Competition. A skater trains two hours a day, four days a week, and skates continuously for fifteen or twenty minutes before she takes a five-minute rest break. (Elite skaters practice three to six hours a day, six or seven days a week throughout the year.) It strengthens your quads, buttocks muscles, calf muscles, and shoulders. "You use your shoulders," Di Felice says, "to keep your arms out to the sides and when you do jumps and spins. You also use your lower back, although to a lesser degree, to keep your body erect." It increases the flexibility of your legs, particularly the hamstrings, and your lower back.

Training.   In addition to artistic skating, Di Felice suggests that you bicycle to build up your aerobic condition and the muscular endurance of your quads. She also stresses ballet classes. "Ballet is a very important part of artistic skating," she says, "for aerobic capacity, style, and flexibility." Running doesn't exercise your skating muscles, she says, but she runs because it helps her control her weight. She also feels a skater must develop some anaerobic ability because the international competitions feature a two-minute freestyle program which is a kind of sprinting exercise. (The national competitions require a four-minute program.) "The way to develop stamina for the two-minute program," Di Felice says, "is to skate through your two-minute program five or ten times back to back, without stopping."

Di Felice believes skaters should do resistance training in order to strengthen their legs for skating. She works on isokinetic machines, but you can approximate her workout with squats, run-'em-out-of-gym-class sprints, split shifts, front leg lifts, side leg lifts, and swimmer's kicks. When you begin doing the last three exercises, wear your skates instead of ankle weights. When this becomes tolerable, add ankle weights. In addition, do knee rises. When you are away from the rink, practice jump squats while wearing your skates. For your shoulders, hold a light dumbbell (1 to 3 pounds) in each hand and straighten your arms out to the side. Without moving your arms, move your shoulders

Effects of Roller Skating, Artistic

Aerobic

Strength: calf, quadriceps, gluteals, back, shoulder

Flexibility: lower leg, upper leg, lower back

Knee Rises

While wearing your skates, hold one leg straight out in front of you and squat down on the other leg as if you were going to do a sit spin. Straighten out of the seated position for one rep. Do ten to twenty reps on one leg, and then repeat with the other leg.

forward, back, and up. Press them down (without changing the position of your arms) to lower your shoulders back to their starting position, for one rep. Do as many reps as you can, several times a day.

To increase your flexibility, take ballet classes every day. In addition, do bridges (back bends), toe touches, and forward-and-back splits. For the splits, start gradually, going down only as far as is comfortable and holding that position for twenty to sixty seconds. If you are naturally flexible, you will be able to lower yourself all the way to the ground within a year. To limber up your back and sides, add wasp waisters to your universal warm-ups. If you have stiff ankles, do foot circles, baby foot flexers, and football ankle walks.

Complementary sports.   Bicycling is the best non-skating exercise a skater can do because it uses the same leg muscles in the same ratios as skating. Ice figure skating is also complementary, although you will have to strengthen your ankle muscles for ice skating. "In roller skating," Di Felice explains, "you have a wider bottom on your skate, so you must bend and press with your ankle in order to press edges. In ice skating, you keep your ankle stiff and press your edges with the whole foot and lower leg."

Injuries.   Sprained ankles and back problems are the most common types of injury in competitive artistic skaters, Di Felice says, with various knee problems coming in a close third. However, among recreational skaters, sprained or fractured wrists head the injury list because these skaters fall more often and put their hands out to catch themselves. Falls also contribute to a plethora of facial cuts, bruises, and even fractures.

Roller Skating (Speed)

Effects of Roller Skating, Speed
Aerobic
Anaerobic
Strength: quadriceps, gluteals, hip
   extensor, back

Speed skating on roller skates is virtually identical to speed skating on ice skates. Women race the same distances—500 meters, 1,000 meters, 1,500 meters, and 3,000 meters—and the times are only a few seconds slower. For example, Sue Dooley set the 500-meter record at the 1980 national championships with 56.6 seconds and the 3,000-meter record with 6 minutes and 9 seconds. For comparison, in 1976, the world's ice-skating record in the 500 meter was 40.68 seconds (Sheila Young) and in the 3,000 meter was 4 minutes and 31 seconds (Galina Stepanskaya). Roller and ice speed skaters use the same bent-over posture, running start, and crossover turns and must be able to skate several distances rather than specializing in just one or two. However, roller skaters have the added difficulty of skating on two or three surfaces. They qualify for tournaments by skating on an indoor rink, but they skate the world championships outdoors on concrete or asphalt. For this reason, roller speed skaters must practice indoors and out throughout the year.

Evaluation.   Although the races themselves are so short that they use anaerobic or a combination of anaerobic and aerobic metabolism, a speed skater must train by skating long distances. Sue Dooley, for example, skates ten miles nonstop outdoors every day. Thus, speed skating, when pursued seriously, is an excellent aerobic sport. If you practice short races as well as long ones, it also gives you good anaerobic conditioning.

Speed skating strengthens your quads and, to a lesser extent, the rest of your legs, as well as your gluteals, hip extensors, and lower back, Dooley says. It does not increase your flexibility to any appreciable degree.

Training.   Dooley believes that speed skaters must add other aerobic training to their program. "I've been bicycle riding ever since I became a top speed skater," she says, "and it's always helped me." She recommends both distance and speed training. Ride for an hour a day, choosing a twenty-mile route with a few hills to develop your anaerobic power and sprinting abilities and "to adjust your legs to recuperating quickly." Or ride the same four-mile route five times over. If there are no hills in your area, practice interval training by sprinting as fast as you can as long as you can, then pedaling easily until you *almost* catch your breath, and then sprinting again. Between the regional and national championships, when Dooley is training her hardest, she bicycles fifty miles every day and a hundred miles at least once a week. Running, she feels, does skaters more harm than good because it is too jarring and it trains them to pick their feet up too high.

"I'm a firm believer that your whole body must be in good physical condition in order to take the low times with the high times," Dooley says. She believes a good skater must follow an overall strength training program such as the circuit training program, with added emphasis on the gluteals, quads, groin, hip extensors, and lower back: run-'em-out-of-gym-class sprints, side leg lifts, and swimmer's kicks. (For other suggestions, see ICE SKATING.)

As a speed skater, you must stretch your calves, hamstrings, hip flexors, and groin very carefully. Work your way very slowly through the universal warm-ups and the concentrated stretching circuit, focusing on the groin stretch, gravity toe touch, stork, towel stretch, runner's start, calf and Achilles stretches, and hunkers.

Complementary sports. Bicycling. Ice speed skating also works most of the same muscles in similar ratios.

Injuries. Except for floor burns from falling and an occasional groin pull caused by running your start on cold muscles, injuries in roller speed skating are rare, Dooley says. The unusual broken bones, she says, are caused by freak accidents, such as bumping into someone who has stopped to tie her shoelace in the middle of the track.

Rope Jumping

See Chapter 5

Rowing

Effects of Rowing

Aerobic

Anaerobic

Strength: calf, quadriceps, pectorals, abdominals, shoulder, biceps

Rowing has two categories: sweeps and sculls. In sweeps, each rower pulls a single twelve-foot oar; in sculls, she pulls two nine-and-a-half-foot oars. Women's Olympic events include: coxed fours (four oars-women pulling one oar apiece plus one coxswain over a 1,000-meter course); double sculls (two oarswomen pulling two oars apiece over a 1,000-meter course); coxswainless pairs (two oarswomen pulling one oar apiece over a 1,000-meter course); single sculls (one oarswoman pulling two oars apiece, plus one coxswain, over 1,000 meters); and eights (eight oarswomen pulling one oar apiece, plus one coxswain, over a 1,000-meter course).

Traditionally, sculling races have been sexually segregated. Women rowed these shorter races, and men rowed longer races such as the 2,000-meter Olympic races; the five-mile Doggett's Coat and Badge, first rowed from London Bridge to Chelsea on August 1, 1716; and the Oxford–Cambridge University race along the River Thames, first rowed in 1829. However, in 1981, British women's Olympic coxswain Susan Brown moved to the front of the bus when she coxed the otherwise male Oxford crew to victory in the annual Oxford-Cambridge duel.

In addition, there is recreational rowing. If pursued vigorously enough, rowing across a quiet bay or down a river gives the same training effect as a row in a match, as any mile-a-day rower will attest. Because rowing uses natural, logical, non-jarring, easy-to-learn movements, your half mile soon stretches to five or ten as you scull alone on a foggy lagoon, free of traffic, smog, and muggers.

Evaluation.   Rowing training is one of the best all-around exercises and is "tremendously aerobic," according to Penn State's Dorothy Harris. In a three- or three-and-a-half-minute 1,000-meter race, however, you start off anaerobically, go into an aerobic phase for a short time, and then finish anaerobically again. It builds strength in the upper legs, especially the quads, because you push with your legs as the seat slides, and it builds strength in your calves, shoulder girdle, biceps, chest, and abdomen when you stroke with your arms. Because it puts very little stress or flexion on your back muscles, rowing is good exercise for people with low back pain. In fact, using a rowing machine is often prescribed by sports physicians for people with low back and disk problems.

ROWING MACHINES

Rowing machines provide excellent cardiovascular conditioning and strengthen your arms, upper back, and upper legs. A good rowing machine has a smoothly sliding seat, comfortable foot straps, separate, easily calibrated tension adjusters for each oar, cushioned hand grips, sturdy construction, and a price tag of a few hundred dollars or more. Machines used to train competitive rowers also have featherable oars. (Electrified machines that do the rowing for you while you just hang on for dear life give you zero exercise.)

Because you use your upper body when you row, your pulse shoots up faster than it does in leg sports. If you are in poor or fair condition, start out slowly. Row at low tension and a fifteen- to twenty-stroke-per-minute pace for one minute, rest for one minute, and then row again, for a total of fifteen minutes. Aim for a target heart rate of 60 to 80 percent. Coordinate your arm strokes and leg pushes; your legs should be straight when your hands reach their highest point (close to your chest); your legs should be fully bent when your arms are straight and your oars reach their lowest point. This way, your legs pull the oars as much as your arms do. Increase the rowing intervals and decrease the rest periods as this pace becomes easy. When you can row for fifteen minutes nonstop, increase the tension on the oars.

Wear socks and shoes to keep the straps from cutting your skin, and expect blisters on your hands from the oars.

Rowing doesn't increase your flexibility, says Pat Sweeney, head women's crew coach at the University of California at Berkeley. However, Sweeney says, "You must have good flexibility in your lower back and ankles in order to reach full compression, in which the chest is right up against the thighs and the shins are vertical. You reach from the shoulders, so you need good flexibility there too."

Training.   Sweeney recommends running for endurance, with some sprint intervals for anaerobic capacity; plus running stadium stairs to build explosive power in your legs. If you can't run, cycling will build endurance. Do chin-ups, push-ups, jump squats, and squats for strength. For flexibility, add geisha kneels or hunkers, plows or king of Siam kowtows, posture clasps, and birds.

Complementary sports.   In addition to running, Sweeney suggests swimming, because it develops upper body strength and flexibility, and cross-country skiing, because it is even more demanding than running and forces you to develop your arms as well as your legs.

Injuries.   "Most injuries occur outside the boat doing dry-land training," says Sweeney. "There are very few injuries inside the boat. The main one is sore hands and blisters early in the season, but after three weeks your hands harden up. You always know a rower because when you shake hands with her, it's like shaking hands with a piece of sandpaper."

Rugby

Effects of Rugby

Anaerobic

Strength: all over

A rugger's definition of her game: "A hooligan's game played by gentlemen. And ladies. Sometimes together."

Women's rugby is growing steadily in the United States. In 1975, there were no women's rugby clubs in this country. Now, there are about 150, each with fifteen to twenty-five members. These clubs belong to statewide unions which administer both men's and women's clubs. The statewide unions belong to one of four territorial unions, which in turn belong to the United States of America Rugby Football Union, a nonvoting member of the Rugby Football Union of Great Britain. In most parts of the country, you can find an active women's side (team) to play with, but if not, you may be able to talk your way onto a men's side.

Rugby is the ultimate contact sport, and yet women can play against men. "It all depends on the position you play," says Paula A. Cabot, director of the information and resource center of the Women's Sports Foundation. On a men's team a woman rarely plays a forward position, reserved for the largest players on the team. A forward must be able to win possession of the ball from set scrums, rucks, mauls, and lineouts. Weight, strength, power, height, and the ability to jump high are prerequisites for good forwards. Women play backs in a men's game because backs run with the ball, pass, or kick it with the sole intent of scoring. They must be able to handle and kick a ball, and speed is the main prerequisite, to outrun and outmaneuver the opponents. Cabot played standoff, "a quarterback-type position," for four years on the men's rugby side at the University of Massachusetts at Amherst.

Evaluation. "Rugby is a very demanding sport," says Cabot, "probably suitable only for the most ardent of amateurs, but strictly speaking it is not aerobic because you rarely see people running up and down the field for fifteen minutes without stopping. Play only stops when there is an infringement of the rules (or when the ball goes into touch—out of bounds, that is—or a try, or a goal, is scored), but you rarely go for fifteen minutes without some infringement on the rules." Rugby is an anaerobic or sprinting sport, although every rugby player must be in top cardiovascular aerobic condition in order to play. It develops strength all over your body but doesn't do much for your flexibility. You must already be flexible in order to play without injury.

Training.   "You need aerobic conditioning in order to play well," says Cabot, who coached the Smith College Rugby Football Club and was New England Rugby Football Select Side (all-star). "Running is better than cycling. If you're a forward, run distances of four to six miles four days a week. If you are a back, run shorter distances of three to four miles, four days a week, but run faster. The other two days, do speed work—a lot of sprinting, some 220s, a couple of 110s, especially if you are a back." Intervals or fartlek are also effective.

You need strength in your legs, upper body, and shoulder girdle because rugby is a tackling sport. "If you are a back," Cabot says, "build explosive power in your legs in order to drive through a tackle. If you are a forward, you want explosive pushing power in your legs during a scrum. Squats are the best exercise for overall strength building." Also do chin-ups, pull-ups, push-ups, run-'em-out-of-gym-class sprints, arm sprints, and killer sit-ups.

Flexibility is particularly important in your hip joints, backs, arms, and shoulders. Supplement the universal warm-ups with wasp waisters, runner's starts, king of Siam kowtows, posture clasps, and birds.

Complementary sports.   The physical demands of soccer are very similar to those of rugby. However, few ruggers supplement their rugby games with soccer because the two sports have the same season.

Injuries.   Bruises, scrapes, and cuts are so common in rugby that,

Cabot says, "bruises aren't really injuries." Jammed fingers occur in almost every game, and sprained ankles beset people with weak leg muscles. Do ankle inversions and eversions for preventive strengthening. "A lot of pitches (fields)," says Cabot, "are full of bumps and crevices. If your legs are strong, there's less chance they'll give out. During the first two years a woman's club or team is established, you have a lot of injuries because the women aren't in good enough shape. You get a lot of broken collarbones because their upper bodies are weak, and you get a lot of broken noses. Once they're in good shape, they're less likely to hurt themselves."

Running

See chapter 5.

Skating

See FIGURE SKATING; ICE SKATING; ROLLER SKATING

Skiing

See ALPINE SKIING; CROSS-COUNTRY SKIING; WATERSKIING

Skin and Scuba Diving

Effects of Skin and Scuba Diving

Aerobic
Strength: lower leg, upper leg, hip flexor, abdominals

Skin and scuba diving are the culmination of our primordial desire to walk and breathe under the sea. Once you master the techniques of diving with and without tanks, you are free to roam through brilliant worlds more fantastic than Jules Verne ever imagined—to wander among schools of multicolored fish, hunt for abalone or rock scallops, photograph undersea life, or search for artifacts on sunken ships. This is one sport, however, you must not learn from a book or on your own, for one stupid move endangers your life and the life of anyone diving with you. A safe diver must know basic skin and scuba diving skills, basic physics and the principles of gases, safety and rescue skills, how to use the equipment and the dive tables, how to swim on the surface and underwater, and much more. Courses leading to certification in basic diver training usually last at least thirty hours and are available through dive shops, some colleges, and many Ys. Make sure your instructor has been trained and certified by the National Association of Underwater Instructors (NAUI), the Professional Association of Diving Instructors (PADI), the YMCA, or the Los Angeles County Department of Parks and Recreation. These four organizations have the oldest and most rigorous training programs in the country.

Evaluation. Whether or not diving gives you an aerobic workout depends on how you do it, says Kenneth W. Kizer, M.D., former president of the Hawaii Undersea Medical Association and the North Pacific Chapter of the Undersea Medical Society. "If you dive in the Caribbean or other calm water, and you make a straight slow descent from a boat, stopping very often to take pictures, you are not getting any cardiovascular conditioning. Conversely, if you are diving off the California coast to collect rock scallops or search for artifacts in choppy water, and you come up against a current, you are swimming for thirty to fifty minutes, moving your muscles isotonically against the resistance of the waters, working the whole time, and getting a good training effect." However, few people live in an area that permits diving three or more days a week, every week of the year, and so must augment their diving with some other sport. Diving also gives you a small amount of anaerobic conditioning if you swim through the surf or against a current to reach the site of your dive, or if you climb a long ladder to get back into the boat at the end of a dive, but this effect is minimal.

If you dive at least three days a week, skin and scuba diving will strengthen your rectus and oblique abdominal muscles, your hip flexors (iliopsoas), and the fronts and backs of your upper and lower legs. Because you propel yourself through the water entirely by kicking, the actual dive does very little for your upper arms. However, lifting tanks, taking off tanks, and carrying your other gear strengthens your upper body muscles to a small degree. Diving does nothing for your flexibility.

Training. If you dive at least three days a week for at least thirty minutes a session, every week throughout the year, you do not need supplementary aerobic training. However, if you can't dive all year round, supplement your diving by kicking laps to build aerobic endurance as well as to train your muscles specifically for diving. Wearing fins, snorkel, and mask, swim laps in a local pool, working up to a minimum of a half mile each workout. To develop the small amount of anaerobic capacity you need at the end of each dive, kick your last two to six laps at a sprinting pace.

Strength training is unnecessary for diving, Kizer says. Out of the water, handling a 200-pound diving rig is merely a matter of technique, not brute strength, he says, and once you are in the water everything becomes lighter. Strong and weak people becomes equals. If you want to develop good overall physical conditioning, however, play an upper-body sport or do circuit training.

Because a diver needs to stretch only to prevent injury, the universal warm-ups are all you need. Flexibility is neutralized once you are in the water—the water provides so much resistance that you can't make the quick, reaching movements you do on land.

Complementary sports.   Swimming provides the ideal aerobic conditioning, even though its movements are not specific to diving. Water polo and underwater hockey, on the other hand, teach you to maneuver against the resistance of the water. Many scuba teachers use these games during scuba classes.

Injuries.   Despite myths to the contrary, women do not have a greater propensity for accidents and injury in diving than men do. Kizer says there is a small theoretical chance that women are more prone to decompression sickness than men, but it has never been proven to exist in real life. The most common injuries come from coral scrapes and cuts; mild envenomations or rashes from Portuguese men-of-war, some irritating seaweeds, and other sea life; rashes from oil, gasoline, and other pollutants in the water; and bruised fingers smashed under fallen tanks. The next most common injuries are barotraumas, those pressure-change injuries called the squeezes. If your muscles are weak or stiff, you may develop cramps in your calves or hip flexors.

Before taking up scuba diving, consult your doctor if you have chronic ear or sinus conditions, vertigo, heart or circulatory problems, asthma or chronic lung disease, epilepsy, or previous head injury, or if you are taking medications that impair your vision or slow down your reaction time.

Soccer

Effects of Soccer

Aerobic
Anaerobic
Strength: quadriceps, hamstrings, hip
   abductor, hip adductor, gluteals, lower
   back, neck

Soccer, called association football in Great Britain and just plain football elsewhere, is played in more than 150 countries and is probably the most popular team sport in the world. It is easy to learn and requires no special physical attributes, esoteric skills, or expensive equipment. Bring a few people together with a ball on an empty lot, a schoolyard, or a grassy meadow, and you have a soccer game. Unlike American football, with its set plays and position specialists, soccer gives everyone a chance to move the ball and set up plays.

Women's amateur soccer leagues have sprung up throughout the country in the last five years, with teams concentrated in Texas, Florida, the Northeast, and California. Most leagues have two divisions, the under-thirty and the over-thirty, and conduct local, state, and regional championships before sending the top four teams to national championship playoffs. If played right, soccer is a thinking game, rewarding control over speed. Seattle coach Mike Ryan's Blue Angels, most of whom are in their forties, regularly beat younger teams, and he expects his under-thirty Ramlösa (named after their Swedish mineral-water sponsor) to continue to dazzle their opponents at age fifty.

Speedball and korfball make similar demands on the heart, lungs, and muscles as soccer. Speedball strongly resembles soccer, but players may use their hands as well as their feet. Goals are scored by kicking or American football-style touchdowns. Korfball, very popular in Holland, is another hands-on soccer game, but here the goals are scored by shooting the ball into a wicker basket 11½ feet off the ground. Each korfball team must include six men and six women.

Evaluation.   Although soccer looks like a stop-start short-burst an-aerobic activity, it makes strong aerobic demands on your body, ac-cording to Sue Torok, women's coordinator for the Metropolitan D.C./ Virginia Soccer Association. An aggressive player moves constantly during each forty-five-minute half, running, sprinting, walking, ball handling, fighting for the ball, and jumping. Often the rests between activity during a game are not long enough to allow even partial recov-ery, and the exercise is even more continuous in practice sessions. Thus, top-level soccer develops aerobic and anaerobic capacity for all players except the goalie. The referee, if she is officiating alone or with only one other referee, gets an especially good workout. She must run con-tinually, following the ball all over the field.

Soccer strengthens your quads when you run; your hip abductors and adductors, gluteals, and lower back when you dribble, kick, and trap the ball; your hamstrings when you kick and leap; and your neck muscles when you head the ball. It increases your lower body flexibility to a small degree, according to Torok, but not enough to prevent injury or make you limber.

Training.   If you play aggressive soccer at least three times a week, it provides an adequate amount of cardiovascular conditioning. However, if you want a higher level of fitness or want to be a better soccer player, run about three miles a day at least three days a week and add some intervals, sprints, or other speed work during or at the end of each workout. Speed work is essential, especially if you play forward. If you play halfback or fullback, run more and sprint less but include some anaerobic training.

Soccer players do not need upper body strength, although you may want to develop strength in your back, shoulders, and arms for overall physical fitness. If you are a recreational soccer player, you may not need any strengthening exercises at all. If you are a serious soccer player, strengthen your neck muscles with neck-strengthening exercises, your ankles (to prevent ankle sprains) with heel and toes and ankle inversion and eversion exercises, your lower back with locusts and swimmer's kicks, and your quads, gluteals, groin, calves, and shins with squats and dumbbell lunges. In addition, practice kiddie kicks if you have weak knees—soccer is especially hard on the knees.

Flexibility in your ankles, knees, hips, back, and running muscles is extremely important to a soccer player because it prevents injury as well as improves performance. Universal warm-ups are excellent if they are augmented by baby foot flexers, hunkers, runner's starts, king of Siam kowtows, birds, and towel stretches. If you have reasonable flexibility in your hamstrings, groin, and hips, add alternate kicks to your stretching regimen. Torok's teammates, who won the eastern regional over-thirty championship in 1981, do tai chi exercises to systematically stretch every part of the body in a controlled way.

ALTERNATE KICKS

Stand up with both hands extended in front of you at chest level. Kick up and try to touch your right hand with your left foot, while swinging your left arm behind you for balance. Return to the starting position, then kick your left hand with your right shoe, swinging your right arm behind you. Return to starting position for one rep. Do ten or twenty reps each day.

Complementary sports.   Now that soccer is played indoors as well as outdoors, it has become a year-round sport. Many avid soccer players play nothing else. Torok, however, feels that the twisting stop-start movements of tennis are similar to those of soccer, and that each game improves her performance in the other.

Injuries.   Soccer is a fast-moving contact sport, and if you play it you are going to get bruised. Other players collide with you or kick you by accident; the ball hits you with full force; you fall or crash into some obstacle. In addition, suddenly accelerating from a standstill and stopping, twisting, and turning to change direction or to reach, kick, and trap the ball frequently tear the muscles or ligaments in the ankle, knee, hamstring, and groin. Daily strengthening and flexibility exercises for these areas prevent many of these injuries. Ankle sprains are also common, as are, to a lesser extent, knee cartilage injuries. Black toe occurs when someone steps on your foot or when you kick the ball with your toe instead of the top of your instep. Broken noses, legs, arms, and wrists happen occasionally, but they are due to freak accidents and are relatively rare. Once in a while, a player develops migraine headaches from heading the ball. After all, a 14- to 16-ounce ball kicked about ten yards strikes your head with a force of about 400 pounds. Overall, however, although there is a high incidence of bruises, bumps, and minor sprains in every soccer game, most soccer injuries are mild. This is especially true of youth soccer, which is one of the least dangerous of all organized youth team sports.

Softball and Baseball

At the most sociable level, just about anyone of any age can play fast- or slow-pitch softball, baseball (hardball), rounders (in Great Britain), and even cricket. Its slow, meditative, undemanding pace makes it the perfect game for family outings. But there is about as much training effect in a casual baseball game as there is in the beer bust afterward. Softball provides neither aerobic nor anaerobic conditioning for any player. The only players who exercise at all during any kind of baseball game, even during a hard-fought game between two top-level teams, are the pitcher and catcher, because they work consistently throughout their "ups." The pitcher strengthens her deltoids, trapezius, latissimus dorsi, forearm extensor and flexor muscles, and, to a lesser extent, her biceps. Christine Haycock, M.D., associate professor of surgery at New Jersey Medical School, says that the circumference of her right arm was much larger than her left during the thirty years she was pitching and catching softball. The catcher strengthens her quadriceps, hamstrings, gluteus, and calf muscles each time she moves in and out of her squat. No position in softball increases your flexibility.

Training.   For overall fitness as well as stamina for batting and base running, follow any all-around aerobic program of cycling, running, or swimming. To strengthen your hips, shoulders, triceps, wrists, and hands for batting and your lattisimus dorsi for throwing, perform run-'em-out-of-gym-class sprints, en gardes, pull-ups, wrist curls, and grip-strength exercises. If you are a catcher, do split shifts and groin stretches. For flexibility, the universal warm-ups meet your basic needs, but augment them with towel stretches or plows and birds to avoid pulled muscles and other injuries.

Injuries.   Most softball injuries occur when a player is in poor condition. She tries to steal second base, or twists as she hits for right field, and suddenly she's pulled a muscle or strained her back. Blisters on the fingers of a pitcher's throwing hand can force her out of the game. To prevent blisters, apply moleskin or Spenco Second Skin before the game begins. Mallet finger, caused by the ball's hitting the tip of an extended finger, is common in catchers. Pitcher's elbow may afflict people who play three or more times a week.

Effects of Softball, pitcher
Strength: deltoid, trapezius, latissimus dorsi, lower arm

Effects of Softball, other positions
none

Speedball

See SOCCER

Squash or Squash Rackets

Effects of Squash

Aerobic

Anaerobic

Strength: quadriceps, hamstrings,
    gluteals, shoulder, forearm

Flexibility: groin, upper leg, hip flexor,
    hip extensor, shoulder, upper arm

Squash and racquetball are intimately related. Both are played inside a boxlike room, using rackets to rebound a small hollow rubber ball against all four walls and the floor in a duel of angles and strategy. However, squash, which boasts about 100,000 enthusiasts in the United States, uses a longer-handled racket, a smaller, slower ball, and a smaller court and prohibits ceiling shots. The result is a game of finesse, with longer rallies, shrewder defensive strategies, and less power than the much more popular racquetball.

Evaluation. "Squash is a combination of aerobic and anaerobic exercise," says Barbara Maltby, 1980 and 1981 U.S. national women's open champion. "The rallies consist of short sprints, but a match might take one or one and a half hours with very little rest between rallies." If you are a typical squash player, you run and hit for half to three quarters of the time you are on the court, and your rallies last from five to ten seconds. These rallies give you some anaerobic conditioning, but they also improve your cardiovascular system because your intervening rest periods are so brief.

Squash strengthens your quads, hamstrings, and buttocks muscles, Maltby says, as well as the forearm and shoulder of your stroking arm. It does not strengthen your upper arm significantly because you snap your wrist rather than stroking with your whole arm as you do in tennis.

Reaching for the ball in squash increases the flexibility throughout your legs, but particularly in your groin, quads, hamstrings, hip flexors, and hip extensors. It also stretches your shoulder and arm joints.

Training. Leg aerobic exercises increase your endurance during a match, Maltby says. She suggests running one to three miles a day or riding a bicycle about five miles a day at least four times a week. In addition, she stresses the importance of interval training for anaerobic capacity. Intervals, she says, resemble the stop-start nature of squash rallies.

For bicycle intervals, either ride up and down hills or pedal a stationary bicycle with alternate high and low resistance. For running

---

STAR DRILLS

As fast as you can, run back and forth between the six points on a squash court: the two front corners, the two back corners, and the two points where the short line meets the court walls. Run to each point two or three times for one set. Rest only enough to *almost* catch your breath. Run as many sets as you can.

intervals, try star drills on the squash court. If you don't have access to a squash court, run standard intervals on a track.

Develop your arm and shoulder strength in order to hit the ball harder. Do chin-ups, pull-ups, push-ups, and dips for your shoulders, triceps, and biceps, and do wrist curls to strengthen your forearm muscles for wrist flicks. In addition, practice typical squash racket strokes with a 1- to 3-pound dumbbell or a weighted squash racket (an old racket with a weight or piece of brick tied to the top).

To be a good squash player, you must be able to reach for balls with your shoulders and arms and stretch for them with your legs. Limber up your legs with universal warm-ups, stressing toe touches, groin stretches, calf and Achilles stretches, and storks. In addition, do towel stretches, runner's starts, and even wall splits if you are flexible enough. For your upper body, do extra reach-for-the-skys and add wasp waisters, if you notice stiffness in your sides, or birds, if your shoulders are tight.

Complementary sports.   "All racket sports—tennis, racquetball, squash, and badminton—are good for one another," Maltby says, "because they use the same basic movements and muscles even though the timing, swings, and techniques are different."

Injuries.   Sprained ankles, pulled hamstrings, or groin or quadriceps muscles, and occasional twisted knees are the commonest squash injuries. Because the racket and balls are light, tendinitis and other shoulder overuse injuries are rare. Maltby recommends wearing eye guards to protect your eyes from flying squash balls. The squash ball is small enough to fit inside the bony cage (or orbit) around the eye and can permanently blind you if it makes a direct hit.

Surfing

Riding the crest of a wave is one of the few sports native to the United States. Hawaiians surfed on their long wooden olo and shorter omo boards long before the New World was discovered by the Europeans. Although it has been popular for centuries throughout the tropical Pacific, it wasn't until the flexible wet suit was perfected in the early seventies that surfing became a year-round sport in California, Oregon, Texas, North Carolina, South Carolina, and Florida. In New Jersey, New York, Massachusetts, Maine, and even in Michigan (on Lake Michigan), the wet suit, replete with hood, booties, and gloves, permits surfers to catch a wave in all but the coldest weather.

Evaluation.   For the recreational surfer, surfing is a sport of short-burst exertions. It provides no aerobic conditioning but does offer

Effects of Surfing

Anaerobic

Strength: ankle, calf, quadriceps, back, neck, latissimus dorsi, trapezius, triceps

Flexibility: ankle, knee, back, shoulder

some anaerobic benefit. The recreational surfer expends a great deal of effort paddling out beyond the surf, then waits and rests three or four minutes before choosing the best wave to ride back to shore. The ride itself, also strenuous, lasts anywhere from one to five minutes. However, if you surf the way Margo Oberg does, you get a good twenty-minute aerobic workout. Oberg, amateur world champion surfer in 1968, 1969, and 1970, top professional surfer in 1975, 1976, and 1977, and world champion in 1980, never stops moving during each intense surfing workout. She paddles out beyond the breakers, an activity akin to swimming without using your legs, immediately turns around, catches a wave, and surfs in, now relying on her legs for control and strength. As soon as she pulls out of that wave, she turns around and paddles right back out, so she has no rest periods between exertions.

Surfing strengthens many of the muscles in your upper and lower body, Oberg says. "When you're paddling, you strengthen your triceps, the muscles in the back of your shoulder, and, most of all, your lats. If you look at surfers, they have nice narrow waists and then they wing out at the chest. You also develop your back and neck muscles from paddling with your back and neck arched to keep your face from getting splashed. The bulk of my muscle is in my back." Riding big waves back to shore strengthens your quads and calf muscles because you surf in a squatting position, and strengthens your ankles and the muscles immediately around your knees in the turns. "Surfers' legs are strong," Oberg says, "but they're not bulky. Their muscles are long, like dancers' muscles."

Surfing forces you to bend and stretch and so limbers up your shoulders, knees, ankles, and, to a lesser degree, your back. However, it is not an overall stretching exercise, and surfers usually practice some form of careful stretching to stay in condition.

Training. "Anyone who is serious about surfing," Oberg says, "should build up her heart and lungs." Most surfers run or swim. Swimming is best because it builds your upper body strength for paddling as it develops your aerobic capacity. Running is not a complementary sport, but it is popular among surfers in California and Hawaii. Bicycling is an excellent conditioner for surfing because it develops the quads, although not in a way analogous to riding the waves. During surfing season, which is year-round in some areas, build your aerobic capacity by paddling long distances on your board. Just hop on your board, paddle out beyond the breakers, then turn and paddle parallel to the shore for about half an hour.

Most serious surfers work out with free weights or Nautilus equipment. Recreational surfers aren't required to build strength in order to surf, but even a few exercises of low weight/high reps will give you an edge in muscular endurance and strength. Do not use heavy weights because you want long muscles. Perform squats for your quads and gluteals; dumbbell pullovers for your triceps, pectorals, and middle back; a few chin-ups for your biceps and lats; dumbbell lunges for your hamstrings; and locusts for your back.

Surfing requires flexibility in your back and hamstrings. Universal warm-ups, supplemented by towel stretches, plows, and even bridges (back bends), if you are limber enough, provide the minimum daily requirement of stretching exercises, but you should also stretch the paddling muscles in your shoulders with door leans, birds, and posture clasps. (Any stretching exercises suitable for swimmers work for surfers too.) Most professional surfers, Oberg says, dance, do Yoga or an Asian martial art in order to keep their bodies limber and agile.

Complementary sports. Swimming, running, bicycling, and martial arts.

Injuries. Since time immemorial, surfboards have slammed into surfers' knees, leading to bruising, swelling, and occasional housemaid's knee. But knee overuse injuries have been relatively infrequent. Now, however, with the introduction of the new superlight boards, knee cartilage injuries are increasing rapidly. The new boards respond much faster and permit sharper, more radical twists and turns. The result is a sudden, shearing force on the knee and torn cartilage.

When you fall off your board, you risk getting hit by your own or somebody else's board. Learn to fall by shooting your board away from you. Do not use springy elastic or surgical-tubing leashes. Instead, fasten your board to your ankle with a urethane leash that is at least one or two feet longer than your board. Urethane stretches out but doesn't spring back the way elastic does. After you haul the board back, the urethane returns to its original length. If you are surfing near someone who can't control her board, bail out and dive under the water rather than risk a collision and a head injury.

Lacerations are common in surfing but rarely serious. They occur when you fall in shallow water and scrape or cut yourself on a rocky bottom or coral reef. Surfers' ear, a benign bony growth inside the ear, develops only after surfing in cold water for many years. With the advent of wet suits, hypothermia from surfing in cold water is rare, but does occasionally occur.

Swimming

See Chapter 5

Tae Kwon Do

See KARATE, KUNG FU, AND TAE KWON DO

Team Handball

Effects of Team Handball

Aerobic

Anaerobic

Strength: quadriceps, hamstrings, gluteals, pectorals, abdominals, back, deltoid, latissimus dorsi, triceps

When team handball, also known as field handball, came to the United States in 1959, someone should have changed its name. In this country, it conjures up visions of two gangs of players crashing into each other on the tiny four-wall handball court. It is, however, an entirely different game, a combination of soccer with the hands and water polo without the water. Invented in Europe in the late 1920s, and now almost as popular as soccer in Western and Eastern Europe, team handball is played indoors on a court about a third again as long as a basketball court. Each team has seven players, six court players and one goalie. Players may throw, pass, dribble, or run three steps with the ball, which looks like a small one-colored soccer ball and is 21 inches in circumference (23 inches for men) and weighs 13 ounces (16 ounces for men). Players are not allowed to kick the ball or otherwise control it with their feet. To score a goal, a player throws the ball into a miniature soccer-goal net. The front of the goal is protected by the semicircular goal area. No one but the goalie may step inside the goal area—with one exception: If a player jumps from outside the goal area and throws the ball before she lands, she may come down inside the goal area. This adds an exciting vertical basketball-like dimension to an otherwise horizontal game. It is officially a contact sport because players are allowed to use their bodies the way basketball players do to block or obstruct their opponents. There are no time-outs during each thirty-minute half unless a player is seriously injured or the ball gets stuck in the ceiling.

Team handball is now played in sixty-five countries on six continents. Some 3 million *registered* players belong to the International Handball Federation, and countless million unregistered children and adults play casual pick-up games on lazy Sunday afternoons. Of those 3 million players throughout the world, four hundred are in the United States.

Although the game has been an Olympic sport for men since 1972 and for women since 1976, the United States has never been able to qualify a team for the Olympics—until now. Because the United States is the host team for the 1984 Olympic games in Los Angeles, they are given the honor of fielding a team handball team whether or not it can survive the elimination matches. This, says Mary Phyl Dwight, captain of the 1980 women's national team, gives American athletes a rare opportunity. The sport is so new in this country that it has only a few players. An athlete who begins early enough may have a chance to work her way onto the Olympic team.

Evaluation. Team handball is an extremely aerobic sport, Dwight says, even more so than basketball. "In basketball, you have time-outs for free throws and conferences," she says. "In team handball, you don't have any time-outs except for a major penalty, and they only happen four or five times in an entire game. The official never handles the ball. If there's a foul or an out-of-bounds or a goal, the official points to the spot where the ball should be put into play, and the team picks up the ball and runs with it. So you're running up and down the court nonstop for thirty minutes, and everyone except the goalie is getting an aerobic workout." In addition, wings frequently go out for fast breaks and so have several anaerobic sprinting bouts per half.

Team handball strengthens your quads, hamstrings, gluteals, and quads—your running and jumping muscles—as well as your latissimus, deltoid, pectoral, and triceps muscles in your arms, shoulders, and chest—your throwing muscles—and your back and abdomen—used for throwing and maintaining your position. "When you shoot the ball," Dwight says, "you try to get your total body into the ball in order to get more power." It does very little to increase your flexibility, although you need flexibility in order to dive into the circle or reach up to block a pass.

Training. Team handball requires both aerobic and anaerobic capacity. To have the endurance and stamina to play an entire game of team handball, supplement your games with three days of distance running and two days of speed or interval work each week.

A generalized weight-training program strengthens your muscles and provides muscular endurance as long as you work with medium weights and ten to twelve reps per set. A basketball weight-training program satisfies most of your needs. Build up your quads, hamstrings, gluteals, gastrocs, and ankles for running and jumping by doing jump squats, dumbbell lunges, run-'em-out-of-gym-class sprints, heel and toes, and ankle inversion and eversion exercises. Develop your abdominals with killer sit-ups and twisting sit-ups and your back muscles with swimmer's kicks. For generalized arm strength, do wrist curls, push-ups, dips, and chin-ups. In addition, practice your throwing motion while holding a 1- to 3-pound dumbbell or a small weighted ball. The throwing motion in team handball is fast and flexible. Do not push or force the ball through its arc. Instead, think of your arm as a whip, and snap the ball into the goal. To improve your jumping, practice the high jump and volleyball jumping drills.

In order to stretch and reach in team handball, you must be moderately flexible in your hamstrings, shoulders, back, quads, calves, and Achilles tendons. In addition to the universal warm-ups do door leans, birds, geisha kneels, wasp waisters, and king of Siam kowtows.

Complementary sports.   Although soccer and basketball share some elements with team handball, they are not similar enough to keep you in condition for team handball.

Injuries.   Sprained ankles plague team handball players, as do finger and hand injuries caused by impact with the ball. Knee injuries from quick movements or jumping are not as common but are far more serious. The myriad bruises from falls, dives, or other body contact are rarely serious.

Tennis

Effects of Tennis

Aerobic

Anaerobic

Strength: lower leg, upper leg, hip, gluteals, shoulder, upper arm

Flexibility: knee, hamstrings, hip, shoulder

Women have figured heavily in the history of tennis. A woman, Mary Ewing Outerbridge of Staten Island, New York, introduced tennis to the United States in 1874. She had played the game, then called "lawn rackets," "pelota," or "lawn tennis," in Bermuda and brought the balls, rackets, and nets back home with her. The first American court was set up that same year at the Staten Island Cricket and Baseball Club. One of the directors of that club was Ms. Outerbridge's brother. The British Championships at Wimbledon, England, were established in 1877 for men only. Women's singles were added in 1884. The first non-British winner at Wimbledon was an American woman, May Sutton, who won the singles title in 1905.

Today, tennis is one of the most popular and fastest-growing sports in the country. In 1978, 14 million people said they played tennis regularly (more than twice a week) and 35 million said they played once in a while. In the next two years, the figure for occasional players doubled, so that by 1980, 84 million people played tennis.

Platform tennis, a doubles game played with a short-handled wooden paddle and a sponge ball on a screened-in court about one third the area of a standard tennis court, follows most of the rules of tennis. Players must hit the ball over the net, as in tennis, but they may play the ball after it rebounds off the fence, as in racquetball. It is easier to learn than either sport and requires less stamina and strength.

Evaluation.   If your tennis rallies are long and you hit the ball hard and far, tennis gives you aerobic conditioning, according to Ann Valentine, tennis coach at Brigham Young University. If you alternate short-burst rallies with long rests between points, you are getting a small amount of anaerobic training but no aerobic conditioning. And if you rarely return a serve, and spend more time bending over to pick up balls than running and hitting, you probably get no training effect at all from your tennis game. For the purposes of this discussion, we will assume you play tight nonstop tennis matches.

Playing and practicing tennis regularly strengthens your legs, hips, biceps, triceps, and shoulders. Your tennis serve increases flexibility in your shoulders; running in the bent-kneed position as well as bending and reaching for balls limbers your knees, hips, and sometimes the backs of your legs.

Training.   Valentine recommends jumping rope to improve your coordination, leg strength, and cardiovascular endurance. In addition, she suggests non-partner and partner drills. When you don't have a partner to play with, run the court to develop agility: Run forward and touch the net, then run backward to the baseline, then sidestep to the center service line; run forward and touch the net again, back pedal to the service line, slide over to the single service line; run forward to touch the net again, back pedal to the baseline, slide across to the center of the baseline; and so on. Steadily increase the distance of your court runs or decrease the time it takes you to run a set distance to build your endurance. When you have a partner for practice drills, she should hit the balls to all parts of the court. If she makes you run for the balls, you develop cardiovascular endurance while you learn how to return the ball. In addition, Valentine says that serious tennis players should do Long Steady Distance running (about three miles a day) and intervals. LSD gives you the stamina to last throughout an entire match, and intervals give you the anaerobic energy required for fast rallies. Because tennis is mainly a sprinting game, intervals are even more important than LSD running.

Strengthen your hands with grip-strength exercises and your forearms with wrist curls. In order to be a good tennis player, Valentine says, you must have strong abdominals. Killer sit-ups and twisting sit-ups give you the torso strength to hit balls while you are stretched awkwardly or bent over. Chin-ups, push-ups, and pull-ups give you the upper body strength tennis players need to stroke the ball forcefully. Strengthen your quads and hamstrings with squats or hamsters or dumbbell lunges. To develop sport-specific strength, leave the racket cover on while you hit balls against the backboard. (Or fasten a 1-pound weight or part of a brick to the top of an old racket and pretend to hit balls with it.)

Tennis players need flexibility in their shoulders in order to serve and do overheads well, Valentine says. Do posture clasps and birds and arm circles. Hanging from a chinning bar both stretches and strengthens your rotator cuff, a common area for injuries in tennis. Stretch your back with bridges if you use twisting serves. For other shots, Valentine

---

ARM CIRCLES

Stand with your arms out to your sides. Swing your arms slowly in large circles in one direction for a count of twenty, and then in the opposite direction for another twenty count.

---

says, use less back stretching and more knees. "There's a lot of lunging and stretching in tennis," she says, "and you have to be able to hit the low balls with your knees bent so that you get rotation through the hips. If you keep your knees stiff and bend your back, you just 'shoulder' or 'muscle' the ball, and your shot isn't nearly as effective." Stretch your lower legs, hamstrings, and quads with calf stretches, Achilles stretches, towel stretches, runner's starts, and geisha kneels.

Complementary sports.   Bicycling develops your legs and hips and gives you the free movement through the knees and hips you need for tennis, Valentine says. Racquetball develops your hand-eye coordination and your running and hitting skills, although it gives you too much flexibility in your wrist.

Injuries.   Tennis elbow, tennis shoulder, and rotary cuff tears are the most common injuries in serious tennis players. Calluses are usually the athlete's friend, but if you play on a variety of surfaces in a variety of temperatures, heat and moisture are trapped inside your shoe, the calluses lift up, and liquid accumulates between the layers of skin. If this is a recurring problem for you, powder your shoes and socks thoroughly, change socks part-way through each workout, or experiment with another pair of tennis shoes or a variety of foam shoe inserts. Occasionally cysts or calcium deposits accumulate inside the wrist. Heat injury is always a threat during moderate or hot weather.

Volleyball

Effects of Volleyball

Aerobic

Anaerobic

Strength: calf, quadriceps, hamstrings, rotator cuff, upper arm, lower arm

Volleyball was invented in 1895 by the Holyoke, Massachusetts, YMCA's physical director, William G. Morgan. The game he called Mintonette was supposed to be the middle-aged businessman's answer to the highly strenuous, newfangled game called basketball (invented in 1891), but it was soon adopted by a younger crowd and became cutthroat and extremely demanding. By the early 1900s, Canadians, Central and South Americans, and Filipinos were competing in volleyball, and by the beginning of World War I, Europeans and Britishers had caught the bug. Ironically, although the game was invented here, the United States didn't become a world volleyball power until recently. For years, Japanese and Soviet women dominated the sport, but recently Cuba and the United States have challenged their supremacy. American women always made better showings in international volleyball competition than men because volleyball has been a highly organized high school and college women's sport for more than forty years. Even today, most schools don't have men's teams.

Evaluation. Volleyball, like many other games, may be played as a simple afternoon's idyll or as a highly competitive, aggressive, demanding sport. If you play a casual game with as many picnickers on each side as you can cram onto the lawn, you will get no training effect from it at all. However, if you play classic beach or power (competitive) volleyball, you get both an aerobic and an anaerobic workout. At the highest levels of play, beach volleyball is a doubles game played on outdoor sand or grass and is more physically taxing than power volleyball, according to Marty Kennedy, head volleyball coach and assistant basketball coach at the University of San Francisco. Power volleyball, with its six players per side and its indoor hardwood floors, permits more strategy, more offensive plays and defensive shifts, so fewer demands are made of each player. However, few beach volleyball players practice their game for several hours each day, four or five days a week, the way power volleyball players do, so competitive volleyball players usually derive a far greater conditioning effect from their sport. At moderate levels, both power and beach volleyball are stop-start anaerobic sports.

Jumping in volleyball strengthens your quads, gastrocs, and most of the other muscles in your legs. Hitting the ball strengthens your rotator cuff, upper arms, and forearms. Volleyball doesn't increase your flexibility.

Training. In addition to playing volleyball intensely enough to maintain your target heart rate for at least fifteen minutes, Kennedy suggests that you run two or three miles of Long Steady Distance each day "for your general health." However, LSD, she says, is not as important for volleyball training as running intervals three times a week, because every volleyball game has many episodes of sprinting and anaerobic rallies. Deborah Gellermann, a world-class volleyball player, suggests that you also run stairs, for anaerobic and aerobic training, and

---

JUMPING DRILLS

Jump straight up in the air; then jump up and pull your knees in; then jump back and forth over a low bench or other obstacle. Do each of these jumps ten, twenty, or thirty times before moving on to the next.

do jumping drills. Jumping rope also builds your jumping muscles as well as your heart and lungs.

Strengthen your leg muscles with jump squats. For your hamstrings, do hamsters or run-'em-out-of-gym-class sprints. Strengthen your back with swimmer's kicks, your abdominals with killer sit-ups and twisting sit-ups. "You really need your abdominals to spike and attack," Gellermann says. Build up your upper body with dumbbell pullovers, push-ups, dips, arm sprints, hang-ups, and wrist curls.

Most volleyball players complain that they are too stiff. In addition to your universal warm-ups, stretch your gastrocs with extra calf stretches and Achilles stretches. Stretch your back with king of Siam kowtows and wasp waisters. Add runner's starts for your hamstrings and groin and posture clasps and birds for your shoulders. Do every stretching exercise twice as long on your dominant arm.

Complementary sports.   Both Kennedy and Gellermann recommend basketball because "there is a lot of overlap in the movements," says Kennedy. Gellermann also bicycles: "I think it helps my quickness and strength in volleyball to pedal up hills fast." Although other net sports such as badminton and tennis use entirely different kinds of techniques, they, like volleyball, are games of angles and help you sharpen your net-playing strategy.

Injuries.   Jammed, sprained fingers are the most common injury by far, and their treatment differs from most other injuries, Kennedy says. If you jam your finger, wrap it in an ice pack but continue to move it during and after the ice therapy. "If you don't move it constantly," she says, "the joint will swell, stiffen up, and hurt for days." Ankle sprains plague volleyball players, as do shoulder tendinitises on the hitting side. Less frequent but more serious are the ligament and other knee injuries common to all jumping and lunging sports.

Walking

See chapter 5; see also RACE WALKING

Water Polo

Effects of Water Polo

Aerobic
Anaerobic
Strength: all over
Flexibility: all over

Water football, the ancestor of water polo, was played more than a century ago in England as a vicious form of ritualized gang warfare: Two teams of bathers slugged, bit, kicked, and punched a soccer ball past their opponents and plunked it into a rowboat to score a goal. Refinements and codified rules led to the first organized leagues in London and Manchester in the 1890s, and the sport quickly spread throughout Europe. In Yugoslavia and Hungary, water polo is the second most popular sport (soccer is the first), and these two countries, with Italy, have dominated the world standings for the last twenty-five years. Recently, the Russians, East Germans, and Cubans have also become water polo powers, The United States still trails far behind, but the sport is growing now as a result of well-developed high school, college, and masters programs, particularly in California.

Water polo is an aggressive, active, exciting game for players and spectators alike. It takes years to develop the swimming, strength, and ball-handling skills required of a good player. As a result, water poloists peak in their late twenties to middle thirties. Water polo is one of the few sports in which top high school women players can compete against men at their level of proficiency. Their smaller hands make it harder to handle and shoot the ball, and they have trouble because they can't palm it or pick it up, but their strong swimming and exceptional finger dexterity more than compensate.

Evaluation. "Water polo is one of the most strenuous sports there is," says Pete Snyder, University of California at Santa Barbara head coach of the women's water polo team, one of the top teams in the country. "It combines aerobic and anaerobic exercise, although there are more explosive and sprinting movements than aerobic ones." You must be a fast and strong swimmer in both the crawl and the backstroke, able to swim constantly through all four of the five-minute playing periods. It strengthens every part of your body, developing your shoulders and arms as you swim and throw the ball, your abdominals and hip flexors as you maintain a vertical body position, and your legs as you hold your head and upper body high above the water to shoot or intercept the ball. Water polo increases your flexibility more than swimming does, although it does not limber you up as much as gymnastics, wrestling, or dancing does.

Training. For specific aerobic conditioning, Snyder suggests swimming laps in freestyle, breaststroke, and backstroke while holding your head above the water. He also recommends practicing laps of the eggbeater or frog kick (a vertical breaststroke kick) while keeping as much of your head and trunk out of the water as possible. High body position is the key to good water polo and requires very strong legs, abdominals, and back muscles. Bench squats, kiddie kicks, dumbbell lunges, pull-ups, chin-ups, dumbbell pullovers, shoulder shrugs, and killer sit-ups develop strength in most of your prime movers.

Complementary sports. Swimming LSD and interval laps develop your aerobic and anaerobic capacity, while playing basketball builds your ball-handling skills. Running and cycling use your legs in ways similar to the vertical eggbeater kick and give them stamina and strength.

Injuries.   The cushioning effect of the water prevents broken bones, leaving cuts, nicks, and abrasions from elbows as the most common impact injuries. The shoulder suffers the most overuse in water polo. Shoulder bursitises, muscle pulls, and tendinitises are frequent, for the shoulder is used for swimming, maintaining body position, and passing and shooting the ball. Prevent these injuries with shoulder strengthening exercises and by stretching the area with posture clasps, door leans, and birds. Water polo players don't wear goggles and so are susceptible to swimmer's eye. Ear guards prevent most ruptured eardrums. Without ear guards, an elbow to the ear can force water in your ear canal through your eardrum.

Waterskiing

Effects of Waterskiing

Aerobic
Anaerobic
Strength: all over
Flexibility: lower leg, upper leg, back, neck, shoulder, upper arm

Waterskiing began centuries ago as plank gliding or aquaplaning but entered its present form in the early 1920s. Waterskiing was developed either by Ralph W. Samuelson on Lake Pepin, Minnesota, in 1922, or by an unnamed Frenchman on Lake Annecy in France in 1920, depending on whose claim you believe. World championships were established in jumping, slalom, and trick events in 1949 and later, in a separate tournament, in women's speed skiing.

Fifteen to eighteen million Americans water-ski, ranging in age from eighteen months to eighty years. (Eighteen-month-old babies ride on two skis attached together to form a sled and are pulled behind a boat moving at idling speed.) More than many other sports, waterskiing is a family activity. Whole families spend the day on the water taking turns driving the boat and skiing, and many families spend their entire vacations together at waterskiing camps or schools in Florida and California. (Contact the American Water Skiing Association for a list.)

Evaluation.   Waterskiing is both aerobic and anaerobic, according to Liz Allan Shetter, who was master's overall cup champion nine times. Once you are past the very beginning stages, you ski each set nonstop for fifteen to eighteen minutes at a strong aerobic pace. During each set, you make eight to ten passes, and these twenty-second passes are extremely strenuous short bursts—the equivalent of sprints in running. Most skiers ski five sets a day, allowing intervening rests of about forty-five minutes.

Waterskiing strengthens just about every muscle in your body, says Shetter, who is one of the most titled women in the sport. "I can't think of one muscle that doesn't get a workout. It improves the flexibility of your back, shoulders, arms, and legs when you ski the slalom and trick events. In jumping, however, you restrict motion to stay in control and stay rather tight and balled up."

Training.   Shetter emphasizes that recreational water-skiers don't need any special training at all. However, if you are a serious skier and live in a warm climate, you should ski almost every day. If you ski throughout the year, you don't need any other aerobic training. If you live in a winter climate, stay in shape by running or cycling distances for endurance. Intervals and other speed training are unnecessary because they don't give you the proper sort of explosive anaerobic strength you use in waterskiing.

Because waterskiing uses very specific movements not duplicated by dry-land activities, it is difficult to design a weight-training program to incorporate the pulling your arms do when you hold onto the handle and the lifting your legs do as you rise from the water. Generally, strength is important, however, especially in your lower back, abdominals, forearms, shoulders, quads, and buttocks. Perform a program of swimmer's kicks, locusts, killer sit-ups, wrist curls, grip-strength exercises, and dumbbell lunges. If you ski trick events, add twisting sit-ups and rope drills.

ROPE DRILLS

Attach one end of a rope to a doorknob and the other end to a water-skiing handle. Keep the tension on the line taut, and practice switching the rope back and forth, turning backward, doing 360s and other maneuvers with your hands and feet in order to improve your coordination.

Fifteen minutes of universal warm-ups before skiing your first set limbers up your muscles and prevents injuries. Focus on the stork, gravity toe touches, knee-nose touches, and reach-for-the-skys.

Complementary sports.   If you can't water-ski year-round, Shetter recommends cycling, running, Alpine and cross-country skiing, and weight training for your upper body. Not even cross-country skiing, she feels, strengthens your arms sufficiently for waterskiing. "A lot of water-skiers, especially in Europe, snow-ski in the winter," she says, "because the agility they develop from waterskiing makes snow skiing easier. It's not as easy to go from snow skiing to waterskiing, though."

Injuries.   The average recreational water-skier has very few injuries unless she skis for several hours when tired, weak, or out of condition. The serious ski jumper, however, is subject to torn knee cartilages and ligaments. This overuse injury rarely afflicts slalom skiers, although it does occasionally strike trick skiers. If you are skiing at high speeds when you fall, the water feels as hard as concrete and can break or separate ribs or cause fatal head injuries. "In jumping," Shetter says, "the boat is going 30 miles an hour, but you generate speeds of almost 65 miles per hour. To date, the longest jump by a woman was 129 feet, made by Deena Brush in 1979. In slalom, the boat is going 34 miles per hour, and you cut back and forth across the wake. The slowest part is the turns, about 20 miles per hour, but when you cut and accelerate, your speed goes up to about 60 miles per hour." Tricks, the easiest specialized event, generates speeds of 15 to 17 miles per hour, but in speed skiing you generate tremendous speeds. Donna Patterson Brice skied 111 miles per hour in 1977 to set the world's record. All jumpers and speed skiers should wear helmets to prevent head injuries.

If you fall while skiing at a high speed, spurts of water may shoot into your nose, mouth, ear, rectum, or vagina, rupturing or otherwise damaging your sinuses, middle ear, bowel, or vaginal wall. Although it is difficult to prevent most of these "douches," wearing wet-suit shorts will protect your vagina and rectum.

Weight Lifting, Power Lifting, and Body Building

Effects of Weight Lifting, Power Lifting, Body Building

Anaerobic
Strength: all over
Flexibility: hip, back, neck, shoulder

Weight lifting, also called Olympic weight lifting, is based on two over-the-head Olympic weight lifts: the snatch and the clean and jerk. In the snatch, you lift the barbell from the floor to a straight-armed position over your head in one uninterrupted motion. In the clean and jerk, you lift the barbell from the floor to the chest in one motion, and then from the chest to a straight-armed position over your head in a second movement. Weight lifting requires agility, coordination, speed, and timing in addition to strength.

Competition in power lifting is limited to the three power lifts: the squat, the bench press, and the dead lift. In the squat, you take the barbell off its stands, rack (rest) it behind your head and across your shoulders, squat into a deep knee bend, stand up again, and replace the barbell on its stands. In the bench press, you lie on your back on a bench while straight-arming the barbell above your chest. You lower it to your chest and then return to the straight-arm position to complete the lift. In the dead lift, you bend over to pick up the barbell from the floor in front of you and then straighten up again until your legs are locked, your torso is upright, your shoulders are back, and the barbell crosses your upper thighs. Power lifting, as the name says, requires brute strength.

Body builders aim for muscle definition and symmetry of physique rather than performance or functional movement. At the beginning levels, their training sessions strongly resemble those of weight and power lifters, but eventually the workouts diverge as lifters focus on their specific lifts and body builders use a carefully designed sequence of submaximal lifts to define each muscle separately. Body building for women is a new sport. In 1980, there were less than 200 women competing in the United States. Uniform standards for judging the contests had yet to be codified, although all competitions consist of three events: relaxed standing, compulsory posing, and free posing, made up of an original routine of stances set to music. The predominantly male judges marked women down if they were "too muscular" or "too unfeminine." As more women judge these events, these prejudices will evaporate. Until recently, there were no age group divisions in physique contests: all ages competed together. Many male body builders won their international titles in their early forties, because it took years of workouts—two to five hours a day, five days a week—to reduce your body fat and grow the muscles necessary for world-class muscle definition. Current women body-building champions will continue to amass trophies into their forties and, if they wish, continue to compete at national and international levels through their seventies and eighties.

Although these three sports are distinct and separate forms of competition, they are discussed together because their physical effects and training requirements are similar.

Evaluation.   Weight trainers and body builders have notoriously low oxygen uptake and very poor aerobic capacity. Weight training is an anaerobic activity, requiring great bursts of effort for a very short time. You perform one, two, or three lifts using the most weight you can lift ten or twelve times. Then, you rest for five to fifteen minutes until you have the strength to work on another area of your body. Only circuit training has aerobic potential (see chapter 6), but it is rarely used by weight lifters, power lifters, or body builders. Circuit training is usually reserved for other athletes aiming at working on sport-specific or generalized strength training.

All three sports strengthen every muscle in your body and get rid of body fat. Contrary to popular belief, lifting weights does not necessarily make you stiff. If you move the weight through your muscle's full range of motion, each exercise maintains or increases your flexibility. "In order to be a weight lifter," says Mabel Rader, national chairwoman for the first annual women's weight-lifting championships, May 1981, in Waterloo, Iowa, "you have to be very, very flexible, especially in the shoulders, back, and hips. Otherwise you can't get under that weight quickly and get it to the arm's length. Power lifters don't have to be as flexible, because their lifts rely mostly on power. Body builders are the most agile of all."

Training.   Although you can begin training at home with calisthenic-type resistance exercises and lightweight dumbbell lifts, for full-fledged heavy barbell workouts you must learn the proper lifting techniques from a qualified coach or teacher. At a gym, you receive instruction, careful spotting (helping you position the weights), and the camaraderie that weight lifters need. After all, more than 75 percent of every lift is psychological.

Few male body builders do any sort of aerobic work, but women body builders, because they are younger and more aware of modern trends in training, conscientiously run or do some other form of cardiovascular exercise at least three days a week. Swimming, cycling, and rope jumping are as useful as running as long as you work at your target heart rate for at least fifteen minutes.

Before and after each weight-training workout, perform at least one lap of the concentrated stretching circuit to lengthen the muscles you contract during each different lift. This warms up your muscles and prevents injury.

Injuries.   Hand blisters are so common among lifters and body builders that no one considers them an injury. All accomplished weight lifters have bad knees, usually suffering medial ligament injuries during the squat phase of the clean and jerk. Straight-backed dead lifts cause hyperextension of the lower spine and may lead to spondylolysis in power lifters. However, the safer round-backed lift is prohibited in competition. Other injuries are "uncommon, very uncommon" according to Mabel Rader, and most are due to inadequate warm-ups and stiff muscles.

Wrestling

Effects of Wrestling

Anaerobic
Strength: all over
Flexibility: all over

Wrestling is one of the oldest sports known to human beings. Two hundred and fifty wrestling positions are illustrated on the walls of Egyptian tombs built from 3000 to 2000 B.C., and organized competition was well established by the time it was recorded in 1788 B.C.

Nonetheless, the women's wrestling movement is just getting under way. A few schools in Texas, Kentucky, and Pennsylvania have girls' wrestling teams, and some competitive wrestling groups have sprung up in New England, North and South Carolina, California, and Great Britain. At this stage, most of the non-scholastic matches are held in the competitors' living rooms. Wrestling is particularly suited to women because it uses the legs as much as or more than the arms, and women are 60 percent stronger in their legs than their arms. Wrestling, says Dorothy Harris, director of the Center for Women and Sport at the Pennsylvania State University, has great therapeutic value for girls and women who are insecure about their bodies. "You get to know your body and its capacities," she says, "but that's true for any sport. In wrestling, though, you also get sensory input and feedback all over. It improves body awareness for those who have real gaps in that area."

Strategy is as important as brute strength because the athlete must be aware of what her competitor is doing, react to it, and take the initiative, says Mildred Burke, women's world champion wrestler from 1937 to 1957. "You can't learn wrestling overnight," she says, "because you must keep adding knowledge. At the same time, you're constantly building up your body, so you stay in top condition longer than in almost any other sport." A wrestler doesn't reach her peak, Burke believes, until she is forty or forty-five. Burke retired undefeated after 6,000 matches, the first 200 against men.

Evaluation.   Wrestling, Dorothy Harris says, is not an aerobic sport. "It is primarily an anaerobic sport, with sustained intense isometric effort over a short period of time. It builds strength and flexibility throughout the body because you use every muscle, even those in the fingers and toes, to apply force to your opponent, and you use every joint to get out of every conceivable position."

Training.   A wrestler needs aerobic and anaerobic fitness in order to wrestle an entire match at full speed. In addition to wrestling practice sessions, run two or three miles a day, three days a week, and add some sprints or interval training to develop your anaerobic capacity. Many wrestlers also run stadium steps carrying dumbbells or wearing a weighted vest to develop leg strength and stamina. Bicycling or riding a stationary bicycle will also build your legs. An overall weight-training program such as the circuit-training program in chapter 6 builds strength in every muscle of your body. However, do each exercise as slowly as possible to simulate an isometric effect. After all, most wrestling moves involve pushing against an immovable object. Slow-motion push-ups and pull-ups are especially useful. In addition, practice isometric resistance exercises throughout the day by pressing your hands or arms against a doorway, trying to lift a heavy desk with your forearm, or trying to raise a couch with your foot and ankle. Hold each isometric contraction for six seconds. Strong ankles, wrists, and hands are crucial for good wrestling performance. In addition to these isometric ankle lifts, strengthen your ankles with ankle inversion and eversion exercises. For your wrists, do wrist curls and grip-strength exercises.

In order to get in and out of wrestling holds, you need extremes of flexibility in every joint, but particularly in the Achilles tendons, hamstrings, hip flexors, groin, lower back, and shoulders. Concentrate on Achilles and calf stretches, gravity toe touches, towel stretches, runner's starts, wall splits, wasp waisters, plows, posture clasps, birds, and door leans.

Complementary sports. Any strength or endurance sport improves your physical condition for wrestling. In addition, Harris suggests doing gymnastics or gymnastic-related exercises to train yourself to get into and out of all positions. She says the two sports are comparable in their strength, flexibility, and agility demands.

Injuries. Wrestlers cut, scrape, and bruise themselves constantly. They tear and strain their knee cartilage (meniscus) and medial collateral ligaments. If they don't wear knee pads, they are susceptible to prepatellar bursitis. If they fall on their shoulder points during a takedown, they may dislocate their shoulders. Many wrestlers have lower back problems which may be prevented by locusts, swimmer's kicks, killer sit-ups, twisting sit-ups, and dumbbell pullovers. Neck problems are also common, but neck-strengthening exercises, head twisters, plows, and king of Siam kowtows should prevent most of them. Wearing a sanctioned noseguard prevents most nosebleeds and broken noses. For wrestler's ear, see chapter 10.

III / THE INNER WOMAN

The first question I asked my obstetrician wasn't "When is the baby due?" but "Is it all right if I continue to dance?" She said yes. I nearly kissed her.

—A thirty-three-year-old ballet dancer

8 / Menstruation and Menopause

The interplay between menstruation and athletic performance is complex and individual. Some women are reduced to tears by premenstrual tension, while others barely know it's "that time" again. Some women can't play comfortably; others have won gold and silver medals in track and field events, swimming, basketball, skiing, skating, and gymnastics during their periods or the few days immediately preceding.

HOW DOES MENSTRUATION AFFECT YOUR EXERCISE PROGRAM?

Over the years, there have been so many myths about menstruation and deteriorating athletic performance that even women who breeze through their periods worry that they won't play as well during those few days and that they might hurt themselves if they try. However, recent research has shown that menstruation doesn't have to affect your game at all. Coordination *does* decrease in the few days immediately preceding menstruation and the first two days of menstruation, but actual performance, strength, work capacity, and aerobic and anaerobic capacities remain steady throughout the cycle. And contrary to popular belief, women are *not* prone to heatstroke when they are menstruating.

However, there is a difference between your physiological capacity and how you feel. Surveys asking menstruating athletes how they felt immediately before and during their periods reveal that women *feel* it is harder to do a set amount of work right before their periods than it is in the middle of their cycles. What's more, over one quarter of all athletes believe their athletic abilities decline in the week before their periods. Distance runners, dancers, rowers, other endurance ath-

---

SWIMMING MYTHS

Some of the most persistent myths about women in sports still linger around swimming.

Do you wonder whether swimming will bring on menstrual cramps? It's a slight possibility if you swim in cold water, but not if you swim in a heated pool or warm water.

Do you worry that your menstrual flow will contaminate the pool? Forget it. That's just an old lifeguard's tale. Water doesn't flow easily in and out of the vagina. In studies measuring the bacterial content of pool water after nonmenstruating and then menstruating women swam in it, the number of bacteria in the water depended on the number of bacteria on the swimmer's *skins,* not on whether the swimmers were menstruating or not. Even when women swam without any menstrual protection at all, the number of bacteria in the water didn't increase.

If you worry that scuba diving during your period—even with a tampon—will attract sharks to the smell of your menstrual blood, relax. There are no data indicating that women are attacked by sharks more frequently during their periods.

---

letes, and tennis players are most affected, while sprinters, track and field athletes, baseball players, gymnasts, bowlers, and other athletes using short spurts of energy fare better.

That leaves three quarters of all menstruating athletes who *don't* think their performance is affected. Some of these women simply have no premenstrual tension or cramps at all—about half of all adult menstruating women under the age of thirty-five don't. (The younger and leaner you are, the less likely you are to be affected by menstrual problems.) However, the other half of all menstruating women under thirty-five, and most women over thirty-five, have one or more symptoms as the result of the ebb and flow of their hormones, be it weight gain, depression, tension, anxiety, irritability, lethargy, heaviness or dull abdominal aching, nausea, constipation, head and backaches, breast pain, cramps, or the shakes. Many of these women still play up to par. They may be able to tolerate pain better than sedentary women; they may have the self-discipline and motivation to continue exercising and playing no matter what; they may be distracted by the rigors of their training; or they simply may not have as many symptoms.

The explanations depend on the person, but one thing is certain: Premenstrual tension and menstrual cramps have a real physiological basis. After centuries of dismissing menstrual complaints as psychosomatic, medical researchers have verified in the last few years that whatever happens to you at this time of the cycle is the result of biochemical changes in your body, not female hysteria. (Women and hysteria have been equated for thousands of years; the very word "hysterical" derives from the Greek word for uterus.) No wonder there was little biochemical research on menstrual problems until significant numbers of women became gynecologists, physiologists, and medical researchers. Says Clayton Thomas, M.D., vice-president of medical affairs for Tampax, Inc., and a member of the U.S. Olympic Council on Sports Medicine, "If men had had menstrual cramps for the last million years, there would have been a medical cure discovered for them a long time ago."

Whatever the cause, exercise may make your period more regular and easy. Active women suffer far fewer premenstrual and menstrual symptoms than sedentary women, and exercise makes the symptoms that do occur much milder.

TAMPERING WITH YOUR CYCLE

Women who are very concerned about competing in an important race or event at "the wrong time of the month" have resorted to inducing or delaying their periods with birth-control pills or other hormones. These drugs have all the usual side effects and potential dangers of birth-control pills (see the second half of this chapter) and may lead, at the very least, to bloating and nausea. As Dr. Forrest O. Smith asks, "Is it better to go through your period and have cramps, or to take birth-control pills all month long and have those side effects?"

Menstrual Discomfort (Dysmenorrhea)

Water retention causes many menstrual problems. Water held in and between your cells makes you feel stiff and heavy and accounts for much of the weight you gain before each period. It also presses on nerve tissue in your brain and spinal cord, giving you headaches, mood changes, and backaches. It makes your feet and breasts swell up and hurt and causes nausea, constipation, or diarrhea. No one knows for certain why you retain water. Estrogen, which peaks just before menstruation starts, makes you hold salt and therefore water, but progesterone, which also peaks immediately before menstruation, has the opposite effect. You would expect this progesterone to hold the estrogen in check, but it doesn't, so you bloat.

Exercise reduces the amount of water in your tissues by making you sweat away significant amounts of fluid and also by reducing the amount of excess salts in your system, because they are carried away in your sweat. Without these salts, the fluid around your brain, muscles, and digestive organs dwindles away, and you become less depressed, anxious, headachy, and nauseated.

TAMPONS AND TSS

For years, tampons have been the favorite type of menstrual collector for athletes because they are unobtrusive and don't rub or chafe. And then, in 1977, toxic shock syndrome was discovered. When it became clear that tampons were associated with TSS, all premenopausal women, and active women in particular, were faced with a difficult choice.

Tampons may be involved in one of several ways. Inserting and removing the tampon may scrape open the lining of the vagina creating an avenue for the offending bacteria, *Staphylococcus aureus,* to introduce its fever-producing poison into the bloodstream. Or soaked tampons may simply be an ideal medium for the bacteria to grow. Or tampons may promote the release of the toxin—or dam up the menstrual flow and encourage the absorption of the toxin from the vagina into the body—or stop up the vaginal outlet so that toxin-carrying blood returns to the body.

S. aureus is found in the vaginal tracts of 5 to 15 percent of all women, but no one knows why only three women in every 10,000—most of them under thirty years old—come down with TSS. (It's possible that women over thirty have been exposed to some disease that give them immunity to *S. aureus* or its poison, or that the *S. aureus* in TSS victims is a distinctive strain.) Symptoms of the vaginal disease are vomiting, diarrhea, high fever, sunburn-like rash with subsequent peeling of the fingers and toes, and rapid drop in blood pressure, leading to shock. Some women recover fully, about 30 percent have recurrences, others are left with numb fingers or arms, and some die. (*S. aureus* also causes nonfatal skin diseases such as infected toes, sore throats, and boils in women and men of any age.) There is no cure, so prevention is crucial.

1. The obvious solution is to give up tampons entirely and use only sanitary napkins—not a suggestion many athletes will take. But for a sport such as bicycling, where a pad doesn't rub or feel uncomfortable, you may be able to use napkins alone.

2. If you are a swimmer, a diver, or a gymnast, or play a game where napkins might show or chafe as you moved, be sure to change your tampon frequently—at least every six hours—and use pads at night and any other convenient time.

3. Avoid super-absorbent tampons. If your tampon is difficult to insert or remove, it is too big for you and may abrade your vagina. Do not use more than one tampon at a time.

4. Do not use tampons when you have itching, burning, or a discharge of greater than usual amount, particularly if it has an odor. These are symptoms of vaginal infection and may increase your chances of getting TSS. Wear napkins and see your doctor.

5. Keep exercising. Michael Osterholm, Ph.D., chief investigator of the Tri-State Toxic Shock Syndrome Study, told *the physician and sportsmedicine* magazine that women who had TSS in the Minnesota, Wisconsin, and Iowa study area exercised significantly less than their neighbors who didn't get TSS.

Exercise acts in other ways too. Strong supple muscles don't cramp readily when they are stretched by an enlarged uterus before menstruation; muscles weakened from lack of exercise or bad posture, on the other hand, cramp up quite easily. Exercise may cure cramps by warming up and stretching your abdominal muscles the way it loosens tight shoulder or calf muscles. And Harmon Brown, M.D., of Cal State Hayward postulates that exercise may inhibit uterine prostaglandins, the powerful chemicals which stimulate uterine contractions during childbirth and menstruation. "It's also possible," says Mona Shangold, M.D., assistant professor of obstetrics and gynecology at Cornell University Medical College in New York (City), "that the endorphins"—painkillers the brain manufactures for itself—"released during strenuous exercise mask the pain." Either theory explains why cramps sometimes eliminated by a heavy training schedule may return as soon as a woman returns to a normal lighter routine.

Exercises for Tension and Cramps

Many doctors believe that if you suffer premenstrual tension or menstrual cramps, do killer sit-ups and locusts every day of the month in order to strengthen your abdominal and back muscles and prevent cramping when your uterus expands. If you still get cramps, run through the concentrated stretching circuit in chapter 6 to warm up and stretch out the muscles in your trunk and upper thighs. King of Siam kowtows and wall splits may be particularly helpful. Or work up a sweat with some strenuous endurance exercise lasting at least thirty minutes to eliminate some of your excess salts and inhibit those cramping uterine prostaglandins.

Evalyn Gendel, M.D., director of the human sexuality program of the University of California at San Francisco School of Medicine, feels a combination of stretching and aerobic exercise is likely to help the greatest number of women. "Do both stretching-and-bending exercises and aerobics," she says. "You have to get your heart and respiratory rate up to target level for a half hour, but you've also got to build muscle strength and flexibility. Whatever you do, you've got to work up a sweat and build muscle tone."

Other Solutions

Unfortunately, exercise doesn't help everyone. If menstrual pain still cramps your style, you may have to look elsewhere for the cure.

Reduce salt intake. Eat less salt the week before your period. Salt encourages cells to hold water, and that extra water leads to bloating and pressure. Sugar and other carbohydrates also draw water into your cells. However, any fruit or vegetable high in vitamin C—such as watercress, cranberries, or oranges—or containing natural diuretic chemicals—artichokes, asparagus, eggplant—purge your system of extra fluids. So do vitamin C tablets. Vitamin C in fruits and vegetables or in tablet form also prevents menstrual-period bruises that occur because your estrogen level drops and your capillaries, the tiniest of all blood vessels, become fragile.

Improve your bowel function.   If constipation intensifies your cramps or backaches, eat fresh or dried fruit.

Take increased calcium.   A minor calcium deficiency can make you jumpy and give rise to menstrual cramps. It is normal for your calcium level to drop about ten days before the onset of your period, but you can counteract this by drinking a quart of milk a day throughout the month or by experimenting with calcium or dolomite tablets. Dolomite is easier to take because it provides you with the magnesium you need to balance the calcium. Six tablets are the average starting dose, but you may take more or less depending on your size and needs. If you take calcium tablets, be sure to take enough magnesium too. (See chapter 3.) To guarantee that your body absorbs the calcium, take 400 International Units of Vitamin D each day.

Get enough iron.   Premenstrual and menstrual weakness may be due to a low-grade undetectable anemia. Women in general need more iron than men, and women with heavy menstrual flows or women who use intrauterine birth-control devices need even more. Adding an iron supplement to your diet (see chapter 3) beginning about a week before your period is due will add, according to Joan Ullyot, "an extra 5 or 10 percent of hemoglobin," which "really makes a difference in performance."

Use acupressure.   Acupressure miraculously dissolves away menstrual cramps for many women. The pressure points are similar to trigger points (see chapter 10) and lie along your back between your waist and the crack in your buttocks (next to the eighth thoracic and third lumbar vertebrae and in your sacrum). Because the points run down your back, you can't administer this acupressure to yourself. You need a helpful friend with strong fingers.

Try heat.   Applying heating pads, drinking hot tea or soup, taking a hot bath, or having an orgasm may relieve that heavy, over-packed feeling in your belly. Some or all of these work wonders for some women, while others find that any kind of heat intensifies their cramps and any sexual encounter is extremely painful in the week before their periods.

ACUPRESSURE FOR CRAMPS

Lie face down on a firm surface. Your partner presses her fingers into the troughs or indentations on both sides of the ridge of your spine. Some of her fingers press into the troughs themselves, and the rest press the adjacent area, about an inch on each side. She starts at waist level and massages firmly for about thirty seconds, then moves down at half-inch intervals, pressing each spot for thirty seconds, until she comes to your sacrum, the flat, bony, fused vertebrae at the back of your hips. She massages that whole area, for thirty seconds or a minute, and then presses and massages the point at the top of the crack in your buttocks for another thirty seconds. Pressure should be firm—the equivalent of 15 pounds or more—but not enough to injure your spine. If you have trigger points along your spine, they will hurt when your partner presses them, but the ache and the cramps will disappear as soon as the massage is over.

Take ginseng. Barbara Seaman, in her book *Women and the Crisis in Sex Hormones*, says that ginseng has been used for thousands of years in China to get rid of the menstrual blahs. Seaman suggests that beginners buy Korean ginseng because its quality is strictly controlled by the Korean government. The capsules measure 8 to 10 grains, or about 500 milligrams, and you will need two or three a day, depending on your body weight, divided into two or three doses and taken on an empty stomach. Ginseng, it should be noted, is a powerful stimulant and induces nervousness, insomnia, and loose stools in some people.

See your doctor for medication. If your pain is severe or intractable, see your doctor. If you don't have a serious malfunction, an inhibitor can be prescribed to interfere with the prostaglandins stimulating your uterus to cramp up.

There are good prostaglandins and harmful prostaglandins in every cell of your body. Many are essential for life itself. These hormone-like chemicals help regulate blood pressure, blood coagulation, cell growth, metabolism, swelling, fertility, and the transmission of nerve impulses. Some cause inflammations, some reduce them. And some stimulate your uterus to contract during childbirth and menstruation.

"People say that menstrual cramps are due to excessive amounts of prostaglandins," says Mona Shangold, "but that's not true. Cramps are a *normal* response of the body to a *normal* amount of prostaglandins in the body. Menstrual cramps hurt when the strength of the uterine contraction exceeds the threshold of pain. They are very normal."

Prostaglandin inhibitors such as mefenamic acid (Ponstel), ibuprofen (Motrin), and naproxen sodium (Naprosyn) are a real breakthrough for women with painful menstrual cramps. These drugs, used originally as arthritis medications, are the safest of prescription treatments for menstrual cramps because you take the drug only when you expect or feel cramps. With other drugs, you take them all month long to *prevent* cramps. If you unknowingly become pregnant during the month, and you continue them, you are feeding your fetus drugs which may cause birth defects. Furthermore, most of the drugs you take all month long—such as natural progesterone or other hormones—have side effects that may impair your athletic performance.

In 1979, Penny Wise Budoff, M.D., at State University of New York at Stony Brook, reported great success using prostaglandin inhibitors on herself and three hundred of her patients over three and a half years. "Inhibiting prostaglandins in order to relieve menstrual cramps," Shangold says, "inhibits good prostaglandins too, but cramps are disabling. I recommend prostaglandin inhibitors to patients and I use them myself. Taking prostaglandin inhibitors also reduces the actual amount of blood loss, which might be an advantage for an athlete running a marathon because she wouldn't have to change her tampon as often."

However, prostaglandin inhibitors are not completely innocuous. Their effects on athletic performance haven't been studied yet. Researchers point out that they may aggravate asthmatic conditions and may make you nauseated or give you gas—problems that can be as incapacitating as the cramps themselves. They also can cause or aggravate peptic ulcers, unless you take them on a full stomach. If more than half of all women have high concentrations of uterine prostaglandins during their menstrual periods, and if these concentrations are normal, perhaps they perform an as-yet-unknown critical function in the body. What happens when you inhibit that function?

Menstrual Irregularity (Oligomenorrhea and Amenorrhea)

Probably the most publicized effect of exercise on menstruation is that of menstrual irregularity. Many popular magazine and newspaper articles warn that if you run long distances or dance or row too much, your periods will stop and you'll become infertile, "less of a woman."

Secondary Amenorrhea

Although secondary amenorrhea—a cessation of periods after you've menstruated regularly for a few years—does occasionally occur, it doesn't warrant the attention it has received. "Most of the women distance runners I know do not have amenorrhea," says Forrest Smith,

"and I know one hell of a lot of women because I'm a gynecologist."
Mona Shangold puts it another way. "In a study I did, the percentage
of women training for the 1979 New York Marathon who went from
irregular to regular periods," she says, "was greater than the percentage of women who went from regular to irregular. Among the women
I studied, most who had irregular periods before they started training
continued to be irregular during training. Most who had regular periods before training continued to have regular periods during training,
and most of the women who had amenorrhea before training had
amenorrhea during training."

Every woman sometime in her life misses a few periods when she
changes jobs, loses or gains weight, enters college, or flies across the
country. It is a normal harmless response to a shake-up in your hormonal cycles. Furthermore, some women naturally have only two to six
periods a year, and one estimate says that 70 percent of all women are
at least partially irregular a few months out of the year. Thus the medical definitions of amenorrhea (absence of periods) and oligomenorrhea
(scanty periods—four to eight periods per year) are pure abstractions
and inapplicable to many, many women.

It is true, nonetheless, that intense endurance exercise or physical
training does make some women's periods irregular. In general, women
who lose their periods run more than 30 miles a week or do equivalent
endurance exercises, weigh less than 115 pounds or lose more than 25
pounds after starting to exercise, are under twenty-five years old, and
have never had children. Why these factors should affect your periods
is still purely speculative.

Scientists have observed that many malnourished women (during
wars or famines) and about one quarter of all women athletes who
drop below 17 percent body fat either develop irregular menstrual periods or have only a few periods—or none—each year. At first, several
scientists, including Rose E. Frisch, Ph.D., lecturer at the Center for
Population Studies of the Harvard School of Public Health, postulated
that the loss of body fat triggered hormonal and metabolic changes
leading directly to a shutdown of the reproductive cycle: that nature
put the cycle in abeyance when there was no longer enough fat to
produce estrogen and maintain a healthy pregnancy.

Now it appears the explanation is much more complicated. When
women plebes at West Point were subjected to the same grueling physical training as men, 75 percent lost their periods within two months.
Three months later, although their training hadn't let up, only 45 percent still experienced amenorrhea. By the end of their first year, only 8
percent were amenorrheic and 23 percent were irregular. Throughout it
all, their amount of exercise—and their body fat (about 19 percent)—
remained the same. In another study, Michelle P. Warren, M.D., head

of reproductive endrocrinology at Roosevelt Hospital in New York, reported that ballet dancers often recommence menstruating during their vacations, although they gain neither weight nor body fat. "The evidence now," says Barbara Drinkwater, Ph.D., associate research physiologist at the Institute of Environmental Stress at the University of California at Santa Barbara, "is that body fat is only one factor." A second theory says the crucial factor is not the amount of fat itself but the body's ability to keep itself warm in cold weather. Since fat insulates you and keeps you warm, body fat does enter the picture, but indirectly. If you don't have enough fat, the theory goes, your hypothalamus goes haywire and loses its ability to keep you warm or cool and to regulate your periods.

If you lose your periods because of intense physical activity or emotional stress, don't worry. The effects are only temporary. As soon as you stop training heavily, you will begin to menstruate regularly again and will have as much chance of conceiving a normal child as you did before. In other words, exercise strenuous enough to halt your periods temporarily is not likely to leave you with permanent or serious hormonal imbalances. You don't become more masculine, grow more body hair, lose your sexual characteristics, or become infertile.

A few running-sports doctors say that secondary amenorrhea is entirely normal and healthy. One has even suggested that it may be the true female pattern, because through most of human history, women were more active and endured many periods of famine, and so were naturally lean. Ignore amenorrhea, and it will clear up by itself, they imply, unless you have one of the following danger signals: bleeding between periods, suddenly heavy periods (using, say, more than eight napkins or tampons a day), exuding milk from your nipples, or dropping large blood clots in your menstrual flow.

Shangold strongly disagrees. "Any woman who was once regular but whose periods become more than sixty days apart should be evaluated by a gynecologist, preferably one who specializes in reproductive endocrinology. No problem should be assumed to be exercise-related and not serious. The same serious problems affecting nonathletes also affect athletes—pituitary tumors, premature menopause, pregnancy—and can be identified only if they are looked for. Those people assume that a woman is not menstruating because she's not producing much estrogen because she's too thin. They say this low estrogen is all right; but estrogen has benefits, and we're still looking into what happens when a woman doesn't have enough of it."

Many doctors believe that if you have a thorough checkup and there is no organic reason for your irregularity, you can continue to exercise as before. (Your doctor may suggest fertility drugs, oral contraceptives, or other hormonal therapy to regulate or stimulate your periods. Take these drugs only if you have no other choice, for many treat the symptoms rather than the causes of amenorrhea and have emotional and physical side effects that may endanger your health. They also make you retain water and gain weight.) When you want to become pregnant, ease up on your training schedule, and your periods will probably resume within a few months. If not, see your doctor. If you don't want to change your training schedule, consult a fertility specialist or sports gynecologist who may be able to prescribe a treatment to counteract the effects of your exercise program. Meanwhile, don't rely on amenorrhea for birth control. You never know when your reproductive cycle will shift into gear again. Since you ovulate two weeks before you menstruate, and menstruation is the only outword signal that your cycle is resumed, you may have unprotected intercourse when you are fertile and only discover a few weeks later that you are no longer amenorrheic.

Primary Amenorrhea

Primary amenorrhea is a different story. If you are sixteen or older and have never menstruated at all, you have primary amenorrhea, the complete absence of periods. Girls usually start menstruating between nine and sixteen years of age. The average age of menarche (the onset of menstruation) is 12.2 years in nonathletes, 13.6 years for athletes, and 15.3 years for dancers. Again, no one knows exactly why athletes and dancers menstruate later. Perhaps heavy exercise and activity delay puberty for two or three years in the same ways they change already established periods. It's equally possible, however, that dedicated athletes would have menstruated at an older age anyway, and this delay gives them an edge—a year or two of additional growth and leanness before estrogen closes the growth plates and tells the body to accumulate fat. A late menarche doesn't affect a girl's ultimate reproductive ability. Once she starts menstruating, she will be as fertile as she would have been had she started earlier.

Before her period begins, a girl develops her secondary sex characteristics: breast budding, pubic hair, and underarm hair, usually in that order. The whole process is controlled by the hypothalamus in the floor of the brain. The hypothalamus controls body temperature, thirst, appetite, mood, and emotions; the increased flow of blood through the muscles during exercise; the function of the heart, abdominal organs, glands, and kidneys; and releases a brain hormone which stimulates the nearby pituitary gland to release chemicals to activate the ovaries. The ovaries then produce estrogen, which triggers breast and sexual organ growth and the laying down of body fat. At the same time, the girl's body produces testosterone, a male hormone all women have in small quantities. Testosterone stimulates pubic hair growth and teenage acne.

"A mother shouldn't rush her daughter to a gynecologist if she hasn't been menstruating by fourteen," says Michelle Warren, "particularly if the daughter is in a sport that involves low body weight. If a child shows no sexual development at all by age fifteen—no breast development, no pubic hair—that would be cause for concern. But if she looks normal and is not an athlete, you don't need to worry until she is sixteen, and if she is a ballet dancer (or gymnast or figure skater), I don't think there's any cause for concern until maybe seventeen or eighteen. When she does start menstruating, she'll catch up very quickly. There may be a process of selection going on here. There is some data that girls with the skeletal proportions most suited to ballet dancing may have a later menarche."

DANGER SIGNALS

If your periods stop but you have a discharge from your nipples, or intermittent staining (slight vaginal bleeding) or abdominal cramping, see your doctor. These are not symptoms of normal menopause.

If your periods resume after a year of amenorrhea, see your doctor quickly. Almost one third of all women of menopausal age who bleed in this way have cancer of the uterine lining.

HOW DOES MENOPAUSE AFFECT YOUR EXERCISE PROGRAM?

Menopause is the time when you stop releasing eggs each month, you stop menstruating, your ovaries stop producing estrogen, and your adrenal glands take over the production of your new reduced levels of that hormone. Life-cycle, or nonsurgical, menopause usually occurs between the ages of forty-six and fifty-two. Your periods become irregular, with longer intervals between them and scantier flow than before. You may have your usual premenstrual symptoms, minus the abdominal cramping when your period would have been due—a classic sign of menopause. The clinical definition is to go through one full year without a period.

Athletic Performance and Menopause

The physiological processes of menopause have no effect on your athletic performance. As the years march on, your reaction time and strength diminish slightly, but you can continue playing any sport you've been playing—including scuba diving—to the best of your ability, for the rest of your life. "Consider ballet performers, swimmers, and mountain climbers," says Evalyn Gendel, "who are well past 'menopausal age' and have endurance and performance levels equal to premenopausal younger women."

Symptoms of Menopause

Some doctors estimate that as many as 75 percent of all women going through menopause have one or more grossly uncomfortable complaints: hot flashes, chills, cold sweats, night sweats, insomnia, fatigue, anxiety, nervous tension, crankiness, crying, depression, occasional dizziness, headaches, swollen breasts, leg pains, weight gain or bloating, vaginal irritation or itching, or painful intercourse. Evalyn Gendel believes the figure is much lower. "Doctors simply never see all the people who don't have trouble," she says. "Attitude has a lot to do with it. We often create self-fulfilling prophecies. A woman who thinks she can't be active after menopause or won't be able to have sex is likely to do things that will ensure that happening. For women who are in good physical shape or who have been actively involved in some kind of exertion, or who come from some other culture, menopause is easier. It isn't so much that they may avert having those symptoms, but essentially they don't pay any attention to them.

"In England," she says, "you see women in their fifties, sixties, and seventies riding bicycles, very hardy, very in-shape because they don't know any other way to be. You hardly ever hear English women talking about menopause. Here, we treat menstruation and menopause as diseases. But every woman in the world begins to menstruate and every woman in the world stops."

Exercise and Diet During Menopause

Strenuous cardiovascular exercise is the most valuable ally you have during menopause. Exercising at your target heart rate for at least thirty minutes almost every day may minimize and even eliminate hot flashes while it helps you sleep better at night, relaxes you, makes you less anxious and less easily angered, prevents you from gaining weight, and improves your self-image. (As Rosetta Reitz points out in her book

Menopause: A Positive Approach, muscles make up about 40 percent of your total body weight, and, taken collectively, they make up the only organ easy to rejuvenate.)

Hot Flashes

Hot flashes are the most-complained-of menopausal side effect because they are visible to others and therefore embarrassing, a sign to all around you that you are getting old. For some women, the hot flashes are triggered by emotions—they may flash when they are startled or angry. If this is true for you, exercise, meditate, change your diet—do whatever you can to eliminate things that make you nervous. (One woman says that her hot flashes disappeared after she learned to acknowledge them in public without embarrassment. Perhaps when she stopped dreading them, she relaxed so they couldn't recur.)

Exercise may help diminish hot flashes and other side effects of menopause, because both exercise and hot flashes are controlled by the hypothalamus, a region on the floor of the brain between the two cerebral hemispheres. Among the functions of the hypothalamus are: controlling your emotions and moods; regulating your autonomic nervous system, the nerves that stimulate or suppress your heart and your digestive organs without your conscious control; regulating your body temperature; controlling how heavily you breathe during exertion; increasing the flow of blood to your muscles when you exercise; regulating your appetite and thirst; and controlling the pituitary gland, which in turn controls your kidneys and most glandular secretions, including estrogen output.

During a hot flash, your skin temperature rises between 8 and 20 degrees because the hypothalamus is sending irregular pulses of hormones into your bloodstream. As your blood hormone levels peak for a minute or two, the blood vessels in the skin open wide to release heat and perspiration the way they do in hot weather. In other words, your hypothalamus becomes irritable during menopause and reacts unpredictably and inappropriately to signals from the outside world. You feel hot or sweat in cool climates, or shiver in warm ones. (Because the hypothalamus also controls your emotions, you may also become testy, angry, anxious, and unable to sleep.) Exercise, it appears, calms down the hypothalamus and sets it back on the level. You should also avoid caffeine, nicotine, and other stimulants. Cut down on sugar and alcohol or eliminate them altogether, because they irritate the regulatory mechanisms in the hypothalamus. Sugar and alcohol also trigger a low-blood-sugar reaction which makes you even more irritable, anxious, and nervous than before. Breathe deeply and concentrate on relaxing during each flash—they only last a few minutes, after all—or cool your

cheeks with water or ice. (You flush where you blush. That's why cooling the forehead usually doesn't work.)

Your need for the B vitamins and vitamin E increases during
menopause. By eating more raw fruit and vegetables, and more whole-
grain bread and cereals, you may satisfy those needs and eliminate hot
flashes. Thirty to four hundred International Units of a vitamin E supplement taken with extra vitamin C each day may also relieve any
flashes or leg pains. Barbara Seaman, in her book *Women and the
Crisis in Sex Hormones,* says that ginseng sometimes prevents hot
flashes. Don't take these supplements, however, if you are allergic to
them, or if you have diabetes, high blood pressure, or a rheumatic
heart condition.

Osteoporosis

Osteoporosis, or thin, soft, brittle bones, is a serious problem in menopausal and post-menopausal women because your lower estrogen levels
make your body less efficient at absorbing calcium from the food you
eat. If you don't absorb enough calcium, your body steals it from your
bones in order to power your nerve and muscle cells, and if it's not
replaced, your bones lose 1 to 3 percent of their mass each year. If your
bones become thin enough, you can develop backaches, dowager's
hump, or wrist, hip, or vertebral fractures just from bumping up
against something, forcing open a window, or falling down. You don't
have to be a menopausal woman to suffer from osteoporosis. Alcoholics
get it, and so do aging men. Inactivity at any age will thin your bones,
because bones are stimulated to absorb calcium and other minerals
only when muscles pull on them. Therefore, wearing a cast, lying in
bed during a prolonged illness, or floating weightless during space
travel can cause osteoporosis. Women who undergo surgical menopause
before age 45, are more likely to develop osteoporosis within six years
of the operation than those who have surgery after forty-five.

Until a few years ago, osteoporosis was considered an inevitable
consequence of getting old, but now it appears that exercising against
the force of gravity and eating a good diet can forestall it. Physically
active women and women who do heavy labor have far fewer hip
fractures and other broken bones than do sedentary women. In a research project at Nassau County Medical Center in East Meadow, New
York, post-menopausal women who exercised for one hour three times
a week not only stopped losing calcium but actually regained some
they had already lost.

There have been so few studies done on menopausal athletes that
no one really knows what percentage of fully active women who have
been active for many years are nonetheless suffering from osteoporosis,

but it appears that anyone who has been active will have heavier bones than her inactive age mates. If you do have significant bone loss, however, you will be more susceptible to fractures on the playing field.

In other words, if you are active, stay that way. "Put your bones through the full range of joint and body movement each day," says gynecologist Sadja Greenwood. "Walk or jog for your lower body (and heart), and do push-ups, work with weights, saw wood, or do whatever lends itself, but exercise the upper body too." If you aren't active but want to start exercising, begin slowly and carefully. If you already have osteoporosis, begin even more gradually, with isometric exercises, and move on to isotonic ones only when you feel your bones and muscles are strong enough.

Make sure that part of your exercise is done outside each day. A University of Cambridge (England) study has shown that people who are exposed to the ultraviolet rays of the sun have high vitamin D levels in their blood. The more vitamin D you have in your system, the better you absorb calcium from the food you eat and the heavier your bones are. A biologically active hormone derived from vitamin D, in fact, is currently being tested as a treatment for osteoporosis in post-menopausal women at the Mayo Clinic, Creighton University in Nebraska, and the University of British Columbia in Vancouver. With an adequate amount of vitamin D, drinking an extra quart of milk each day, taking calcium supplements (1 to 1.5 grams per day), or eating sardines, salmon, chicken, collards and other dark leafy greens, cheese, and other calcium-rich foods may be enough to retard calcium loss.

Aluminum hydroxide antacids may cause bone loss. So may diets overburdened with protein. In 1974, Helen M. Linkswiler reported that people eating a moderate amount of protein and calcium (see chapter 3) maintained a healthy proportion of calcium in their bones. When these same subjects ate three times as much protein, they lost calcium even when they took three times as much of the mineral. Apparently the body uses huge amounts of calcium to neutralize the acidity of the protein waste products.

Depression

Only 7 percent of all women become depressed during menopause. This is only slightly more than the nonmenopausal women who suffer depression. Menopausal depression has nothing to do with the hypothalamus or hormones. According to several studies, this depression is the same sort of unhappiness men of the same age experience. It is caused by the fear of change. Women who center their lives around their children or who derive their sense of security from their femininity and their ability to bear children may lose their sense of self-worth and value during menopause. Here too, exercise helps, because it gives you a feeling of accomplishment and the knowledge that you can control part of your life and make yourself as attractive and healthy as it is possible to be. It also relaxes you so that you can release the anger hidden behind your depression. As the saying goes, depression is anger. You are angry at someone else, but can't express it, so you turn it onto yourself.

Insomnia

For insomnia, try drinking camomile tea, a popular sedative in Europe. Warm milk may also end your insomnia. The active ingredient in warm milk—L-tryptophan, an essential amino acid—calms you and works against depression, chronic pain, and insomnia. It doesn't actually make you sleepy; it just makes you ready to sleep, and, according to *The Medical Letter*, doesn't interfere with your dreams the way barbiturates do. A glass of warm milk thirty minutes before bedtime works for some people, but others digest the L-tryptophan and break it down before it reaches the brain. If warm milk alone doesn't help you sleep, drink a half glass of orange juice one or two hours before you drink the milk. The juice triggers an insulin response which carries the tryptophan to your brain. If that doesn't work, you might consider the 500-milligram L-tryptophan capsules sold without prescription at drugstores and health food stores. They are expensive, and you will need to take anywhere from one to six capsules on an empty stomach a half hour or an hour before bedtime. The dose depends on your weight and your insomnia. Don't take L-tryptophan capsules day after day for months on end because they must be balanced, over the long haul, with the other seven essential amino acids. An excess of one creates a functional, if not actual, deficiency in the others.

Vaginitis

If your vaginal tissues itch and you are susceptible to infections—or if intercourse is painful because your tissues are dry—regular orgasms, once or twice a week, may thicken and lubricate your tissues. Leisurely courtship and a harmless lubricator such as KY Jelly or cocoa butter also eliminates much of the pain. Taking 30 to 100 international units of vitamin E orally may also help. If these don't work, vaginal estrogen cream or suppositories will probably solve the problem and are relatively safe. A small amount of the hormone is absorbed into the system through the vaginal lining, but that amount does not appear to increase your chances for uterine cancer the way oral or injected estrogen does, according to a study by Drs. Ralph Horwitz and Alva R. Feinstein of

Yale University. However, without regular intercourse you may have to use the cream for the rest of your life. By the way, the fear that women lose their sex drive when their ovaries stop working is completely unfounded. The sex drive isn't dependent on estrogen at all. It is dependent on androgens, the male hormones all women produce in small quantities in the adrenal glands lying on their kidneys. Women who never enjoyed sex during their reproductive years sometimes use menopause as an excuse to become celibate, but the change isn't due to physiological causes. In fact, your sex drive may heighten because you don't have to worry about contraceptives or pregnancy anymore.

Estrogen Replacement Therapy

Doctors usually treat hot flashes, moodiness, and insomnia, the three most common menopausal discomforts, with tranquilizers, estrogen replacement therapy (ERT), or both. Tranquilizers are addictive and may dull your reaction time or stamina during exercise. ERT quadruples and sometimes even octuples your chances of getting endometrial (uterine lining) cancer, increases your chances of breast and liver cancer, gall bladder disease, high blood pressure, and blood clots may be physically and emotionally addicting, and has such side effects as bloating, weight gain, and allergic rash—all of which can throw off your game. The risks are higher for smokers and women with migraine headaches and women who already have blood clots or severe hypertension may even be endangered by estrogen creams.

Although it does stop hot flashes and vaginal dryness and *may* slow down the progress of osteoporosis—this is still under debate—ERT absolutely does not work for any other menopausal side effects. Furthermore, when you stop taking estrogen after menopause is over, your hot flashes will return. "Hot flashes," says gynecologist Sadja Greenwood, "are actually estrogen withdrawal symptoms. Not every woman gets hot flashes, but if you are one who does, and if you don't want to live on estrogen for the rest of your life, you are going to have to go through them. You can reduce their effect by healthy living, though."

Although ERT has risks, women entering surgical menopause may need it. "Women who have no uterus, and no ovaries," says Evalyn Gendel, "and have perfectly good physiological functioning, are good candidates for estrogen therapy, providing the uterus wasn't removed in treatment for endometriosis. There's no chance they can get uterine cancer because they don't have uteri." Women whose menopause is particularly unpleasant may also find it necessary. "A woman should take estrogen," says Greenwood, "if she is truly incapacitated by flushing and vaginal dryness, and if she's given a real try to healthy living and it hasn't worked, and if she doesn't have estrogen-dependent tumors to worry about, and if she takes it in a low dose under competent medical supervision." Recent research has shown that combining ERT with progesterone therapy reduces the incidence of endometrial cancer by two thirds.

For serious medical or emotional problems relating to menopause, refer to the menopause clinics at UCLA and University of California at San Francisco medical centers and at university medical centers in Dallas, Boston, and New York.

9 / Birth Control and Pregnancy

Everyone is aware of the physical changes in a woman's body when she becomes pregnant, but few know about the effects of various types of contraception on the female athlete's performance. This chapter examines the pros and cons of each type of contraception and shows that a pregnant athlete has much more freedom than tradition and overly protective doctors have dictated.

CONTRACEPTION FOR ACTIVE WOMEN

Every fertile woman from adolescence through menopause worries about contraception. Active women worry more. With each type of birth control, she risks the same side effects as any other woman—no more, no less—but what is acceptable to a sedentary woman is intolerable to her. A sedentary woman, for example, may be willing to endure the backache and heavier bleeding caused by an intrauterine device, but an athlete with a backache can't play at the top of her form, and if she menstruates unusually heavily she may become anemic and too weak to develop endurance or strength. A sedentary woman may be willing to risk the small possibility of a stroke in return for the convenience of birth-control pills, but an athlete doesn't need the day-to-day weight gain, nausea, and sluggishness the pills often bring with them.

Choosing a form of birth control is a lesson in risk-benefit analysis. The decision is complicated, individual, and highly personal. No one solution works for all women. Weigh the factors in this section carefully and choose the method most comfortable for you.

Birth-Control Pills

There are two kinds: a pill combining synthetic estrogen and progestogen (a hormone closer to the male testosterone than the female hormone progesterone) and a pill made up of progestogen alone. The hormones in the combination pill, taken daily for twenty days of each cycle, create a pseudopregnancy each month, thus preventing release of an egg and growth of the uterine lining where a fertilized egg would implant, and are 99.3 percent effective. The minipill of progestogen alone, taken every day without interruption, thickens the cervical mucus and makes it hostile to sperm and also makes the uterine lining unreceptive. Its reliability is 97 to 98.5 percent—if you miss a pill, there is a greater chance for pregnancy than with the combination.

Advantages.   Of all the nonsurgical methods, the pill is the most effective. It is convenient, usually reversible, permits sexual spontaneity, and cuts the risk of endometrial (uterine lining) cancer by half. It regulates periods so that you can schedule important competitions. If you are between the ages of eighteen and thirty-five, are white and middle-class, don't drink or smoke, and are restrained in your sexual liaisons, the risks from oral contraceptives appear to be negligible.

Disadvantages.   The pill depresses physical activity, slightly but enough to prevent peak performance. It may cause water retention, weight gain, headaches, and morning sickness. The intoxicating effects of alcohol last longer. There is an increased risk of high blood pressure. Smokers increase their risk of chronic heart disease, stroke, and lung cancer. Women with heavy exposure to the sun have an increased risk of melanoma skin cancer. Women who are very active sexually increase their chances of cervical cancer. Other potential side effects include: myocardial infarction ("heart attack" caused by the death of some heart muscle due to blocked circulation; this risk continues long after discontinuation of the pill), thrombophlebitis (an inflamed blood clot in a vein, especially after breaking or severely bruising an arm or leg), pulmonary embolism (blood clot in lung), change in sugar tolerance in diabetics *and* non-diabetics, change in liver function and growth of benign and malignant liver tumors, lowered convulsive threshold for epileptics, urinary tract changes and infections, growth of already existent estrogen-dependent tumors of breasts and uterus, visual changes and corneal swelling (making contact lenses uncomfortable), intensification of migraine headaches, increased pigmentation of skin (cloasma or "mask of pregnancy"), B vitamin deficiencies, acne or oily skin, absent or scanty periods, and breakthrough bleeding.

There is some concern that oral contraceptives may increase your chances of getting decompression sickness when you scuba dive because the pill encourages blood clotting, one of the symptoms of decompression sickness. Research on this is just beginning.

Cautions. Don't use the pill if: you are over thirty-five years old; you smoke; you are a DES daughter (your mother took diethylstilbesterol when she was pregnant); you have epilepsy; you are breast feeding; you have diabetes, liver or heart disease, a history of forming blood clots, high blood pressure, sickle cell disease, suspected or confirmed breast or uterine cancer; you are pregnant; you have severe headaches; you are planning surgery (stop at least four weeks before the operation to minimize the chance of blood clots forming); or you have varicose veins (because you have a greater chance of blood clots).

Cost. A pack for one month costs $5 to $6. Ask your doctor for free samples supplied by the drug companies.

Comments. If you want to get pregnant, discontinue the pill and then use some other form of birth control for at least three months. A baby conceived in those first three months has five times as great a risk of vertebral, anal, cardiac, tracheo-esophageal, kidney, and limb birth defects.

Withdrawal symptoms from long-term usage may range from erratic or absent menstrual periods to changes in skin, hair, sleeping habits, moods, and sexual appetite. They should all be temporary, especially for women who had regular periods before they went on the pill.

Monthly or semiannual injections, nasal sprays, capsule skin implants, some kinds of antipregnancy vaccines, and other similar forms of contraception are variations on the same synthetic hormone themes and have the same side effects.

The morning-after pill contains diethylstilbesterol (DES), a synthetic estrogen at fifty times the normal estrogen concentration put out by a woman's body, so its side effects are drastically intensified. Its risks are too high for routine birth control. It is reserved for emergencies, such as rape or incest.

Intrauterine Device

The IUD is a small polyethylene plastic device inserted into the uterus and left in place. A barium coating is present on all devices to make them visible to x-rays, and some also have copper or progestogen coatings. It is believed that IUDs prevent conception by stimulating an inflammatory reaction in the uterus, releasing large scavenger cells which destroy sperm or fertilized eggs. Copper or hormones in the device slowly leach into the uterus to immobilize sperm or prevent the egg from implanting. Because these chemicals steadily wear away, a progestogen device must be replaced every year and a copper one every three years.

Its reliability is second only to oral contraceptives among nonsurgical techniques, 94 to 99-plus percent. (Pregnancy rates are highest during the first year.)

Advantages.   An IUD is very convenient; there is nothing for the user to remember except to check her vagina after each period for the string or tail to make sure the IUD is still in place. It has a long-term, usually reversible, contraceptive effect and permits spontaneous intercourse. It does not disrupt normal hormonal cycles or prevent ovulation.

Disadvantages.   During the first few months after insertion (and, in some women, for as long as they carry the IUD) there may be pelvic pain and cramping which will interfere with your exercise, and vigorous running, jumping, or bouncing exercises or sports may induce or intensify this cramping. Increased menstrual flow and bleeding between periods in some women may lead to anemia and further impairment of performance. (Progestogen-impregnated devices reduce the amount of bleeding.) Women who do become pregnant while using IUDs, especially hormone-coated ones, have a higher frequency of ectopic or tubal pregnancies, which may lead to severe abdominal hemorrhaging and even death. Pelvic inflammatory-disease infections are four times as frequent in IUD users, leading to potential damage to reproductive organs, infertility, and occasionally death. Copper on devices may cause violent allergic reactions, including an agonizing recurring rash. There is a small chance that a baby conceived immediately after an IUD is removed may be born with malformations of the arms, fingers, and toes, so use another form of contraception for about six months before trying to become pregnant. The device may fall out, disappear into the uterus, or wander around. Migration or improper insertion may perforate the uterus or cause intestinal obstruction. If a pregnancy results while an IUD is still in your body somewhere, there is a much-increased chance of infection, miscarriage, birth defects, stillbirth, or maternal death. If you become pregnant, have the IUD removed.

Cautions.   Don't wear an IUD if: you have a history of pelvic inflammatory disease or ectopic pregnancies; you are anemic; you have cervical disease, abnormal Pap smears, or fibroid tumors; you have extremely heavy or painful periods; you have cancer of the uterus or cervix, undiagnosed vaginal bleeding, or leukemia; you are under continuous treatment with cortisone-type drugs; you are in your late teens or early twenties, have never had a child, and have more than one sexual partner (you are more susceptible to venereal infections with an IUD).

Cost.   The device itself costs from $5 to $30; insertion, $10 up.

Tubal Sterilization

This is a surgical procedure that prevents eggs from traveling through the fallopian tubes from the ovaries to the uterus. It is more than 99 percent effective, so tubal sterilizations (and vasectomies) have become the leading methods of contraception among American couples in their thirties.

Old-fashioned tubal sterilization involves cutting out or tying the tubes (ligation), or coagulating or burning them (no longer done). Newer techniques include blocking the tubes with clips or elastic bands. Some procedures are done with an abdominal incision; others go in through the vagina and cervix.

The minilap, or minilaparotomy, uses the best of both procedures. An instrument is inserted through the cervix to push the uterus up against the lower abdominal wall, and a one-inch incision is made through the abdominal skin to reach the tubes, which are then tied or cut. The surgery is performed under local anesthesia as an outpatient procedure (no overnight hospital stay).

Laparascopy, belly-button surgery, or band-aid surgery takes four to six hours from the time you walk into the hospital to the time you leave. The doctor injects two or more liters of carbon dioxide or nitrous oxide gas into your abdomen to move the intestine out of the lower pelvis. He then inserts through the navel a laparoscope containing cutting tools and a powerful light. When the procedure is completed, the gas is drawn off and the incision in the navel is closed with one absorbable suture. As the scar heals, it appears to be a mere fold around the belly button. At present, abdominal procedures are far safer than vaginal ones.

Advantages.   Once you have recovered, this is totally convenient and permits spontaneous lovemaking; there is nothing to remember or forget. It has the least effect on a woman's athletic performance of any popular method except vasectomy.

Disadvantages.   Tubal sterilization is rarely reversible (less than 40 percent), even with the skills of the best surgeons. Binding with the Falope, or elastic, ring seems to be most reversible. Ten percent or less of all tubal ligations may reduce the blood supply to the ovaries enough to cause irregular vaginal bleeding or hemorrhaging; in rare cases this can be remedied only by hysterectomy. Electrocoagulation (electrically cauterizing or burning the cut ends of the tubes closed) may lead to delayed heavy menstrual bleeding and cramping, both of which reduce your athletic efficiency. Other methods of sealing the tubes cause far fewer problems. Some women suffer mild to moderate abdominal cramping in the first two days after surgery. Because these are all surgical procedures, there is always the risk of anesthetic or surgical accident or complication—perforation, hemorrhage, fatal pulmonary embolism, even cardiac arrest. Women with Falope Ring sterilizations have an ectopic pregnancy rate of 0.2 percent. Vaginal tubal ligations present a higher degree of serious risk (3 to 13 percent), have a slightly higher failure rate, and have been abandoned by most doctors in favor of abdominal approaches.

Cautions.   Reject sterilization if: you are obese; you may want children later; you have had previous extensive abdominal surgery; you have an intestinal obstruction, extensive abdominal malignant tumors, tuberculosis, cardiac or respiratory disease, or inflammation of the abdominal cavity (peritonitis). If you have a hernia, your doctor may advise against tubal sterilization.

Cost.   Sterilization costs range from $400 at family planning clinics to more than $1,000 at hospitals.

Diaphragm

A diaphragm is a shallow wide dome of thin, rubbery material stretched over a springy flexible ring. You coat the inside with a spermicide and insert it into the vagina. The springy rim presses against the sides of the vagina to hold it in place, and the dome completely covers the cervix to prevent sperm from entering. The diaphragm must be inserted no more than two hours before coitus and remain in place for eight hours afterward. Used properly, it is 80 to 90 percent reliable. (The effectiveness rate depends on the user's experience and her determination not to get pregnant. Women who are improperly instructed in its use and women who are considering becoming pregnant have the lowest success rate.)

Advantages.   The diaphragm has no systemic side effects and has never been directly responsible for a single hospitalization. It is ideal for women who have infrequent intercourse, because they do not have to take the unnecessary risks of everyday birth control. It may reduce, although not eliminate, incidence of venereal diseases and cervical cancer. Since it temporarily catches the menstrual flow, it permits intercourse during menstruation for squeamish women or men. It is entirely reversible. The diaphragm is usually recommended for women in their late forties, because their remaining fertile years are too few to make the risks of sterilization worthwhile and IUDs and oral contraceptives are too dangerous for them.

Disadvantages.   An athlete who has to wear the diaphragm during training or competition a few hours after intercourse may be uncomfortable; some women complain that physical exercise encourages the draining or dripping out of the spermicide, which makes underwear or swim suits damp. A diaphragm must be professionally fitted and rechecked every year, because vaginal walls and supporting muscles often stretch, requiring a larger size.

In women who already lubricate well, spermicides may overlubricate and dull the sensations of intercourse. Insertion may be messy, and women who don't like to touch themselves may have trouble doing it properly. It may slip out of place during intercourse, especially in woman-superior positions, and may interfere with sexual spontaneity, although this problem is solved if your partner helps insert the diaphragm as part of foreplay. The rubber or the spermicide may cause burning or irritation in the man or woman, or may irritate recurrent bladder infections. May cause pelvic cramping, especially in women unaccustomed to sexual intercourse.

Cautions. Don't use a diaphragm if you have a severely tipped uterus, because the ring may not tightly encircle the cervix; if you have severe cystocele (protrusion of the bladder into the vagina) or rectocele (protrusion of the rectum into the vagina); or if you cannot be methodical in its use.

Cost. The cost of a diaphragm is $8 to $10; of the spermicide, $5 for approximately ten applications. You will also have an office visit to a family planning clinic or gynecologist for professional fitting.

Cervical Cap

A cervical cap is a small flexible rubber shield, much smaller than a diaphragm, which fits tightly over the cervix to prevent sperm from entering. It is held in place by suction and is usually used together with a small amount of spermicide. In England, where it has been used for decades, physicians insert it just after the end of a menstrual period and remove it before the next begins. Here, some family planning clinics teach women to insert the caps themselves. It may be left in place for a few days, with a small amount of spermicide inserted before you make love each time. Currently, the caps must be purchased from suppliers in England and come in only four sizes. However, Dr. Robert A. Goepp, professor of oral surgery at the University of Chicago, and Dr. Uwe Freese, chairman of obstetrics and gynecology at Chicago Medical School, have developed a new version which may be custom fitted, is held in place by a thin film of cervical mucus, is flexible, and has a one-way valve to permit exit of menstrual flow, so it may be worn for as long as a year. It is now undergoing large-scale tests.

The cervical cap is thought to be just slightly less effective than the diaphragm, although there are no official U.S. statistics on its reliability.

Advantages. The cap is smaller and more comfortable than a diaphragm; you can't feel it during intercourse or afterward. Since it may be left in place for several days, it doesn't interfere with sexual spontaneity. It may fit women who are difficult to fit for diaphragms and may not irritate women with recurrent bladder infections.

Disadvantages. Since the cervical cap hasn't been tested for efficacy in this country, it is not yet approved by the Food and Drug Administration. It is more difficult to insert than a diaphragm, and some women never get the hang of it. (Visiting a physician or clinic every time you must insert it is an impractical alternative.) Present British caps are available in only four sizes, so not everyone can be fitted. If the fit isn't exact, and if it isn't forced tightly against the cervix without harming it, the cap may become dislodged and permit sperm to enter.

Cost. The cost of a cap is $7; of the spermicide, $5 for more than fifteen applications. Add the cost of your office visit to clinic or gynecologist.

Condoms

A condom is a thin latex rubber or lamb-membrane sheath which the man fits over his penis to collect the ejaculate, so that sperm cannot enter the woman's vagina. Condoms are also called prophylactics, rubbers, safes, sheaths, and skins. Rubber condoms are stronger and stretchier; membranes permit greater sensitivity. They are 64 to 90 percent reliable depending on user care and motivation. When the woman uses spermicide at the same time, efficacy rises to 95 percent.

Advantages. There are no side effects for the woman at all, unless the man uses a colored condom, which may cause irritation and burning. It protects against the spread of venereal disease, vaginal infections, and cervical cancer. It is completely reversible, and no prescription or training is required to use one. A condom barely interferes with sexual spontaneity—simply open the wrapper at the beginning of foreplay and set it aside until the moment when one (or both) of you places the condom on the man. It is easy to use, readily available, and easy to carry.

Disadvantages. Some men in the United States claim a condom dulls their sensitivity, but in Japan, where 70 percent of all men use them, men say condoms enhance sex. Condoms may break or slip off during intercourse or, worse, after orgasm, when they are full of sperm-laden ejaculate. (If this happens, insert spermicide immediately. Do not douche, because the stream of fluid may force the sperm up the cervix.) Slippage may be prevented if the man holds the condom on with two fingers, or if he wears fitted or shaped versions. Breakage may be minimized by making sure the woman is fully lubricated before penile insertion, by wearing only freshly purchased condoms which were stored in a cool place, by wearing condoms with receptacle tips to catch the ejaculate, or by allowing some headroom. Some women are allergic to latex rubber condoms and suffer burning or itching afterward. Lamb-membrane condoms usually solve this problem.

Caution.   The penis with condom held firmly in place with fingers must be removed immediately after intercourse. Once the penis becomes flaccid, the sperm-filled condom may slip off and remain inside your vagina.

Cost.   Condoms cost between $2.50 and $14 per dozen, depending on material, shape, and whether they are lubricated.

Spermicides

Spermicides are chemical sperm-killing creams, jellies, aerosol foams, tablets, and suppositories inserted into the vagina within an hour before intercourse. Inert materials in the preparations also block entry of the sperm into the uterus. Foams, creams, and jellies may be used alone or with a diaphragm, cervical cap, or condom. Tablets and suppositories are simply foams in a solid state.

The effectiveness of a spermicide depends on motivation. The reliability, when used alone, of an aerosol foam is 71 to 98 percent; of jellies and creams, 64 to 96 percent; of suppositories and tablets, probably 71 to 98 percent; of suppositories and tablets, probably 71 to 98 percent (the data are inconclusive).

Advantages.   Spermicides need no prescription or fitting. They are simple to use and have no systemic side effects. They are suitable for women who have infrequent intercourse and don't want the unnecessary risks of day-to-day protection. Entirely reversible, they provide some protection from gonorrhea, syphilis, and trichomonas infections, although not as much as condoms or diaphragms.

Disadvantages.   Spermicides are messy. They often drip out, which may be embarrassing or uncomfortable during exercise. Since they must be inserted shortly before coitus, they interfere with sexual spontaneity. They taste bad. They may overlubricate women who already lubricate well, and dull sensation for one or both partners. They may cause burning or itching in one or both partners. Whereas foam is dispersed throughout the vagina as soon as it is inserted, creams and jellies are distributed partially by penile thrusting, so there is a greater chance of pregnancy if the male ejaculates quickly after penetration. Suppositories do not work until they melt in the vagina, and some take at least ten minutes to dissolve there. (In one test, Encare Ovals were still almost intact fifteen minutes after insertion in nine of twenty patients.) Effects last for only one hour, so a new application is necessary before each act of intercourse. They require motivation for successful use. Any type of spermicide may cause birth defects in a baby conceived ten months or less after its mother used one of these contraceptives.

Cost.   Foams cost $5 to $7 for about twenty applications; creams and jellies, $5 for about twenty applications; suppositories, $3.50 to $4.50 for twelve.

Sympto-Thermal Natural Birth Control

This is a new method, combining the observation and recording of changes in resting body temperature (Basal Body Temperature), cervical mucus, and other body signs to determine the seven or eight days surrounding ovulation when a woman is fertile. You may abstain from intercourse or use barrier methods to prevent pregnancy during that period, and use no contraception for the remainder of your cycle. It is considerably more precise than the old-fashioned rhythm or BBT methods used alone, with an effectiveness rate, depending on motivation, of 75 to 99 percent.

Advantages.   There are absolutely no side effects or allergic reactions, and anyone can learn the techniques. It is acceptable to women whose religious principles prevent other methods of birth control and makes a woman more aware of the changes and cycles in her body. Also, it involves the partner in the process of birth control. It may be applied at a later date to conception, for knowledge of your periods of fertility is as important in conceiving a child as in preventing a pregnancy.

Disadvantages.   The sympto-thermal method is time-consuming and requires total dedication on the part of the woman or couple. It requires classes or lessons in techniques and is best for a woman with one steady partner who is willing to abstain or use barrier methods during fertile periods. Even so, abstention may cause emotional distress.

Cautions.   Don't use this method if: you don't like touching yourself; you have irregular periods; or you have some illness—diabetes, thyroid disease, cancer—which alters your temperature patterns or mucus flow.

Amenorrhea from Strenuous Exercise

Amenorrhea is defined as absent or scanty periods for those who have already been menstruating normally (see chapter 8). Its reliability as a form of birth control is very poor. Even if you are menstruating, you may ovulate unpredictably.

Vasectomy

A vasectomy is a surgical procedure performed on men—the cutting of the vas deferens, the tubes carrying the sperm from each testicle. Its reliability is over 99 percent.

Advantages.   This simple procedure, often done with just a local anesthetic in the doctor's office, is much less hazardous and disabling for a man than tubal sterilization is for you, according to Barbara Seaman and Howard Shapiro. The death rate in the course of a vasectomy is zero. The man can bank his sperm, as insurance for future conception, if he chooses, and at least one quarter of the operations are reversible.

Disadvantages.   Vasectomy assumes you are permanently coupled and will make love to only this partner. The man may develop antibodies to his own sperm, and possibly this autoimmune response may lower his resistance in later years to arthritis, leukemia, lymphoma, and Hodgkin's disease. However, this theory is as yet unproven—and it is still a small risk compared to the well-documented ones women take when they use the IUD or the pill or undergo a tubal sterilization.

Cost.   A vasectomy costs $200 to $400.

Future Contraceptives

Before the end of 1983, several new nonprescription contraceptives will go on the market, assuming that the safety and efficacy studies now in progress satisfy the Food and Drug Administration. Milos Chvapil, M.D., of the University of Arizona College of Medicine has developed a collagen sponge to be inserted into the vagina like a tampon. Collagen, the three-stranded protein rope that is the primary component of all connective tissue, absorbs the ejaculate, while the acidity of the sponge destroys the sperm and glutaraldehyde in the sponge, kills foreign bacteria, including those from gonorrhea, syphilis, and, perhaps, toxic shock syndrome. The sponge may be left inside the vagina for up to 48 hours, allowing for repeated intercourse. It may be inserted and removed seven times before it must be replaced (at the cost of about half a pack of birth-control pills). Vorhauer Laboratories in Costa Mesa, California, is testing a synthetic Collatex sponge which is said to work on the same principles but costs less to produce.

Also in the works is a three-day vaginal spermicidal suppository, a spermicidal diaphragm which requires no fitting (and thus may be purchased, like condoms, over the counter), and a water-soluble condom that is absorbed by the woman's vaginal walls during intercourse to kill all sperm.

HOW EXERCISE HELPS DURING PREGNANCY

Active women generally have fewer backaches, cases of toxemia, and other complications of pregnancy than inactive women. They also have fewer premature births, shorter labor, and about half the incidence of Cesarean sections. Endurance athletes who continue to exercise throughout their pregnancy raise their work capacity in labor by 10 to 20 percent over what it would have been if they had rested for nine months. They tolerate the stresses of childbirth better with this extra energy and strength. Women who exercise have the same number of miscarriages as women who don't exercise. So much for the myth that vigorous exercise causes miscarriage.

Many championship-level women participate in sports throughout their pregnancies. "I played and taught judo," says Rusty Kanokogi, coach of the U.S. women's AAU judo team until 1980, "and did every phase of practice with the exception of competition all the way through both pregnancies. I stopped doing rollouts (forward rolls) in the ninth month because I had a hard time getting up." Cathy Rigby taught gymnastics throughout her pregnancy (although she did notice that her balance shifted as she got bigger) and was hitting tennis balls against a backboard up to the day before delivery; she delivered in a mere two hours and was back exercising in a few days. Jockey Mary Bacon rode when she was seven months pregnant. And Kathy Haddon, top shooter in the Tavern Pool League in St. Petersburg, Florida, won the league championship while she was in labor. When she sank the final two balls, her pains were less than three minutes apart.

It is next to impossible to jar the fetus loose, no matter what your sport or your everyday chores. The embryo lies inside a fluid-filled sac, which in turn lies inside the thick muscles of the uterus, which in turn lie inside the tough skin, muscles, and connective tissue of the abdominal wall. All of these absorb any shock to the abdomen. As long as you are comfortable, you can engage in basketball, field hockey, and other contact sports until you become really large.

Being active will *not* increase your chances of having a miscarriage. During the first trimester (three months), when your body is

making its most radical adjustments to carrying a baby, it may sponta-
neously abort the fetus. A miscarriage is nature's way of eliminating
imperfections. It is rarely caused by the mother's activities at the time.
Ellen Weber, in an article in *WomenSports* magazine, reported, "In
his book *Spontaneous and Habitual Abortion*, Dr. Carl Javert notes
that out of 2,000 cases of miscarriage, only seven occurred after a
woman had been in some kind of physical danger. Five of the women
had fallen; two were in minor car accidents. An examination of the
seven miscarriages revealed that in each case there was some problem—unrelated to the accidents—with the developing fetus."

For a while, there was a fear that exercise damages the fetus by
depriving it of oxygen or nutrients, but this turns out to be baseless.
After all, almost four million years ago, pregnant hominids were loping
across the savannah searching for food. If women, and other mamma-
lian females before them, hadn't evolved with the biological ability to
exercise without miscarriage, the human race wouldn't have survived.
Tests on human beings have shown that even when a woman exercises
at 80 percent of her maximum heart rate, the fetus's heart rate doesn't
speed up much—it stays within its own normal range. Animal studies
at Loma Linda Medical School and elsewhere have shown that when
pregnant sheep and other animals go into oxygen deficit, their unborn
babies are unaffected. The body makes sure that the fetus has enough
oxygen, even if it means depriving the mother of some of her share.
The minute the mother's oxygen level goes down, she automatically
starts panting to draw in more air for herself and her baby. The fetus is
also protected from the accumulation of lactic acid and any other
chemical waste products in the mother's blood because no actual blood
passes between the mother and her baby. The umbilical cord transfers
oxygen and nutrients to the baby after they have been screened from
the blood by the placenta, a thick disk attached to the lining of the
uterus. The mother's waste chemicals do not pass through the placenta
to reach the baby.

The First Five Months

The general rule is: If you've been doing something athletic, you can
continue to do it as long as you're comfortable and as long as you have
no complications of pregnancy, but cut back on intervals and other
intensive training toward the end of the second trimester.

Swimming, Evalyn Gendel says, is "the greatest" because your increasing bulk doesn't get in your way; you've gotten rid of gravity. Old
husbands' tales to the contrary, swimming during most of your term
will not infect your uterus because (1) no water gets into the vagina
unless it is forced inside when you fall or jump into the water with

---

WARNING SIGNALS

If you feel any of the following symptoms before, during, or after exercise, stop and call your doctor:

- bleeding
- severe pain
- abdominal cramping
- leaking amniotic fluid

If you become light-headed, or if your lips or fingertips become numb, or if you become very short of breath, slow down—you are too low on oxygen.

---

your legs spread wide open (as you might in a waterskiing fall); and (2) the cervix (the neck of the womb projecting into the vagina) is closed up tight and smooth and sealed with a mucus plug. During the last six weeks, however, the cervix begins to open, especially in a woman who has had previous pregnancies, so you may want to curtail your swimming then.

As your pregnancy proceeds, you gain weight and your breasts become heavier. Even if you've never needed a sports bra before, you will probably have to use one of the highly supportive models whenever you do any kind of bouncing exercise (see chapter 5).

When you are pregnant, you have an increased risk of accident in some sports because your balance is off. Gendel advises testing your balance after the first trimester. For example, "You may be an expert skier," she says, "and have never had an accident, but if some idiot on the slopes hits you and your balance is off, you could fracture your pelvis." She suggests discussing with your doctor the risks of doing extremely jarring sports exercise—such as the takeoff in a surfing stunt, horseback riding, or waterskiing over jumps.

Very serious traumatic injuries during pregnancy are particularly complicated because not only do you risk initiating early labor, you also endanger the baby with diagnostic x-rays and painkilling drugs. X-rays are known to cause birth defects. "If possible, try to avoid x-rays and radiation," says Gendel, "but if a woman is seriously injured—in sports or in an automobile accident or just crossing the street—you have to take x-rays because you have to know her condition. When you talk about birth defects, you're talking about long-time exposure, and one x-ray, or even a limited series, doesn't make any difference. Besides, if the injury is to an extremity, the abdomen will be shielded by lead screening, and the x-rays won't harm the baby."

However, some doctors routinely take x-rays not because they need them to diagnose what's wrong with you, but because they want the x-rays as back-up evidence in case they are sued for malpractice later on. Before you agree to an x-ray, ask your doctor whether you can be treated without one. It may be possible to diagnose your injury by palpation (touching) or other means. Or the treatment may be the same whether you have a sprain, say, or a break. In these cases, you won't have to risk x-ray damage to your baby.

"Breaking an arm or a leg is a big deal," says Gendel, "and wearing a leg cast or an arm cast when pregnant isn't very comfortable. Whether a woman should take a painkiller depends on her tolerance to pain. Aspirin helps some people, but others need a painkiller for a brief amount of time. The least amount of medicine you take, the better it is for the baby. If you need painkillers, ask your doctor about the side effects of a short-term dose."

The American Academy of Pediatrics has stated that no drug has been proven safe for the fetus or nursing baby. RICE (see chapter 10) takes care of most injuries, except the most serious. Steroids for ankle and knee sprains are inadvisable at any time, but during pregnancy or nursing they may damage your baby by causing abnormal bone growth and irregular sexual development. If you break your leg or dislocate your shoulder or otherwise put yourself into excruciating pain, weigh the consequences of any drug against the severity of your pain: Is a lifetime of possible birth defects in your child worth masking your pain for two or three days?

Even aspirin may cause birth defects or may make newborns bleed easily. It may also increase your gestation period (the time you are pregnant) or complicate your delivery. However, a couple of aspirins once in a while probably won't hurt you or your baby.

The Last Four Months

As your pregnancy proceeds into the later stages, you will find that you become slower as you become more ungainly, and that you get winded sooner. Your blood pools in the farthestmost veins of your arms and legs and doesn't return as easily to your heart because your enlarged uterus is in the way. Don't push yourself beyond your new—and temporary—limits. If you are too slow to play satisfactorily in a stop-start sport such as basketball or racquetball, or if it hurts to run, switch to a non-weight-bearing sport such as bicycling or swimming. As far as judo goes, Rusty Kanokogi says that you, as a pregnant woman, shouldn't do some of the falling techniques or let an opponent or partner come in repeatedly to throw you. "You may come in on them," she says, "and practice your throwing techniques because you're using your legs, hips, and behind, and these are very strong parts of your body not affected by the pregnancy."

To be on the safe side, avoid exercising so strenuously that you raise your body temperature above 103 degrees Fahrenheit or collapse of heat exhaustion. There have only been a few animal studies done on overheated pregnant mothers—and none on human beings—but it appears that animals taxed beyond their limits develop temperatures well above their safe limits, and these elevated body temperatures cause fetal deaths or defects in the fetuses' spinal cords. Take adequate precautions when exercising in heat or humidity (see chapter 10) and use the talk/sing test to monitor your target pulse level.

Scuba diving poses special problems of its own. There has been very little definitive research done on whether pregnant mothers and fetuses are more susceptible to decompression sickness, or whether fetuses develop birth defects from breathing oxygen under pressure or from breathing extra oxygen, extra carbon dioxide, or nitrogen. According to Kenneth W. Kizer, M.D., past president of the Hawaii Undersea Medical Association, writing in *the physician and sportsmedicine*, there is a chance that human fetuses may be susceptible to the bends, and that the bubbles forming in the bloodstream may not be screened out by the liver and lungs the way they are in more mature individuals. This means an air bubble (embolism) could clog an artery within a vital tissue in the fetus. The pregnant mother may also be at increased risk of developing the bends if she is holding any extra fluid in her tissues (as most pregnant women do), because fluids pass into her blood vessels differently now, as do molecules of various solids and gases. The extra body fat a pregnant woman carries slows down the amount of nitrogen she eliminates. All of this skews the standard decompression tables.

There is a small chance that the extra oxygen the mother and fetus absorb when a woman dives on compressed air may cause birth defects. There is no evidence one way or the other about the effects of the extra carbon dioxide divers retain when they dive at depth, but Dr. Alfred P. Spivack, clinical professor of medicine at Stanford University Medical School, writing in the *Stanford M.D.*, says that nitrogen builds up in the bloodstream when the mother breathes compressed air. Nitrogen is a known narcotic and can depress the development of the fetus's brain and central nervous system.

This suggests that a pregnant woman shouldn't scuba-dive. However, many women have scuba-dived well into their pregnancies and delivered normal babies. Discuss this problem with an obstetrician well versed in diving medicine. For pregnant women who refuse to limit their diving to snorkeling along the surface of the water, Kizer says, "They should be advised to limit their dives to less than thirty-three feet of water (at which point atmospheric pressure doubles), to avoid repetitive dives, to avoid becoming chilled or unduly fatigued, to not

dive when size becomes a problem (generally late in the second trimester), and to otherwise dive conservatively."

Exercises for Delivery

If you weren't athletic before your pregnancy, don't suddenly take up
some extremely strenuous sport, such as judo or trick waterskiing or
horseback riding, now that you're pregnant. However, beginning some
form of exercise will make pregnancy and childbirth much easier. Exercise during pregnancy strengthens muscles stretched and weakened
by the pregnancy itself, increases your flexibility, counteracts the fatigue you may feel during the later stages, builds stamina and endurance for childbirth, and sets you up for a quicker recovery. Start out
slowly, with a light aerobic exercise, such as walking or bicycling or
swimming, and increase your workout only as much as is comfortable.
In addition, add exercises to strengthen your abdominal, buttock, outer
thigh, and pelvic floor muscles.

Killer sit-ups strengthen your overworked abdominal muscles,
asked to both stretch and support the added weight of your gravid
uterus. What's more, as you become bigger, your back will become
more swayed if your abdominal muscles are weak, and you may develop serious backaches. Side leg lifts strengthen your inner and outer
thighs to prevent the typical waddle of advanced pregnancy. Front leg
lifts strengthen your buttocks, which helps support your back and prevent pregnancy swayback.

Kegels strengthen and tighten the muscles of your pelvic floor.
These muscles run under the uterus like a hammock and are stretched
out by the weight of the baby. Jarring exercises and running with a
heavy uterus may stretch them even further, and childbirth certainly
does. If you practice Kegels religiously, before and after delivery, you
will recover much more quickly from the rigors of childbirth and have
fewer complications, such as urinary incontinence.

If you take pregnancy preparation classes, the instructors will
teach you exercises for conditioning, relaxation, and helping you
through the delivery. None of these conflict with your normal sports,
or with killer sit-ups, front or side leg lifts, or Kegels. Sometimes, however, prepared childbirth instructors advocate some unsafe exercises,
such as duck walks and full (deep) knee bends, which are very bad for
your knees, and straight leg lifts while lying on your back, which are
very hard on your back. Don't do anything now you wouldn't do at
any other time.

As a general rule, labor is shorter for women in top condition.
Strong abdominal muscles, elastic pelvic floor muscles, and strong cardiovascular endurance make childbirth easier. As one gynecologist said,

KEGELS

The first step is to find your pelvic floor (pubococcygeus, or PC) muscles. They are the muscles that contract or flutter during orgasm. Try to move those muscles in an imitation of an orgasm. If you are moving your abdomen or buttocks, you are using the wrong muscles. Another way to find the muscle is to spread your legs apart while you are sitting on the toilet. Try to shut off the flow of urine. The muscles you are moving are the PC muscles, because they are the only ones which can stop the flow of urine in that position.

Kegel 1: Sitting, standing, or lying down, contract the PC muscles, and hold for three seconds. Relax for one rep. Do not suck in your gut or tighten your buttocks. Start out with twenty reps, but work up to at least 100 reps per set. Do at least one set a day.

Kegel 2: Sitting, standing, or lying down, contract and relax your PC muscles very quickly for one rep. Do as many reps per set as you can at first, but work up to two or three hundred flutters per set, two or three sets per day. If you flutter your abdomen or your buttocks, you are probably not using your PC muscles.

This may seem like a lot of Kegels in a day, but it's not: 100 three-second contractions, with two-second relaxation periods between each one, take only eight and a half minutes; 300 flutters takes about five minutes. Since no one can see your PC muscle contracting, you can do Kegels anywhere—watching television, typing in an office, or waiting for the bus—without adding to your already busy schedule.

"When these women bear down, they really bear down." However, top-level physical fitness isn't a guarantee of speedy, effortless labor. One cyclist writhed through twenty-six hours of labor before finally undergoing a Cesarean section. "After having my son," she says, "Suicide Hill in the Coors Classic is easy."

Diet During Pregnancy

A normal healthy baby is born with about 16 percent body fat. In order to provide your baby with enough calories for bones, muscle, and fat, you must gain more than the twelve or fifteen pounds your baby and the afterbirth will weigh. What's more, you need extra body fat of your own to breast-feed your baby, because subcutaneous fat is used for milk production. If you are particularly lean, you can afford to gain thirty to forty pounds. This weight will probably be gone six months to a year after your baby is born. If you carry normal weight and body fat, twenty-four pounds should be enough, and if you are already overweight, fifteen to twenty should be fine. Put the weight on gradually, adding two to four pounds during the first three months when the fetus is small, and then laying down slightly less than a pound a week for the next six months.

All this weight gain is going to wreak havoc on your game, but Grandma was right: You are eating for two. If you hold your weight down, you endanger yourself and your baby. You may suffer high blood pressure and convulsions during delivery, and your baby may be born in distress, or weakened, or defective, or unable to survive beyond a few days or weeks.

The "average" woman, who is five feet five inches tall and weighs 125 pounds, should increase her caloric intake by 300 to 500 calories per day, drawn from a balanced diet of protein, carbohydrates, fats, vitamins, and minerals to give her fetus all the building material it needs. If your body doesn't find the building materials it needs for the fetus, it will rob your own tissues. If you don't have them available, the fetus's development will suffer. You also need extra fluids to increase your blood volume by the necessary 40 percent it takes to support a healthy pregnancy. However, if you suddenly put on a startling amount of weight, you may be holding water—a sign of toxemia of pregnancy. See your doctor.

Foods and Drugs to Avoid

You must be particularly careful now about what you put into your body. Many things cross the fetal membranes and affect your baby's growth. Consider eliminating or cutting back on tea, coffee, cola drinks, cocoa, and chocolate. The FDA says that the caffeine and its relatives cross the placenta and cause birth defects and delay skeletal development. They may also enter the mother's milk and slow the newborn baby's growth.

Don't drink alcohol while you're pregnant. Not only are the infants of alcoholic mothers born addicted to alcohol themselves, but 30 to 50 percent are born with small heads, mental or physical retardation, or deformed faces, eyes, ears, and joints. Those who appear to be normal have a much higher mortality rate during the first weeks of life. Fetal alcohol syndrome, in fact, is the third largest cause of congenital mental deficiency in the United States—and entirely preventable. Scientists now believe that even light drinking significantly endangers your baby. In July 1981 the Surgeon General warned that a group of women who drank as little as 1 ounce of alcohol twice a week had significantly more miscarriages than nondrinkers and that women who drank as little as two highballs a day (about 1 ounce of alcohol) during their pregnancies bore babies with significantly decreased birth weights. A March 1980 report in the *Medical Tribune* states that 1 ounce of alcohol a day may subtly change the neurological development of the fetus so that it will be born more irritable and less sensitive to light and visual images. Alcohol also severely damages developing fetal muscles, causing the fibers to become frayed and entangled instead of lying smooth and parallel. The results are heart disorders and inability to breathe. In fact, says Edward Adickes, M.D., who co-authored a study on fetal muscles with Robert Shuman, M.D., many of the defects once thought to be based in the central nervous system appear to be caused by the muscles themselves. (Both Adickes and Shuman practice at the University of Nebraska Medical Center in Omaha.)

Many women smokers give up cigarettes when they become involved in sports because smoking interferes with their performance, but a pregnant smoker has a double reason. Nicotine and carbon dioxide from cigarettes retard the development of her baby and may even cause the baby to be premature or stillborn or to die within the first few weeks of life.

If you can't kick the habit while you're pregnant, give up smoking for at least forty-eight hours before the baby is due. This will increase the supply of oxygen during those all-important hours of delivery and give your baby a chance for a normal, safe birth.

Smoking marijuana also threatens your baby. Moderate to heavy use of the drug, which may cause temporary infertility and shorter menstrual cycles in unpregnant women, may cause miscarriages in pregnant women. It may also reduce the amount of estrogen in the placenta, which in turn reduces the amount of oxygen to the fetus, theorizes Sandra R. Stevens of Baylor College of Medicine in Houston, Texas. She and her colleagues are now conducting experiments to explain the exact biochemical interactions of marijuana and estrogen. And according to Ethel N. Sassenrath of the University of California, babies born of regular marijuana users do not learn as quickly or adjust to social situations as well as the offspring of nonusers.

CHILDBIRTH, MOTHERHOOD, AND EXERCISE

After delivery, breast-feeding your baby hastens your recovery because the same response which releases milk from the breast stimulates the uterus to contract and expel excess uterine material. Nursing has little effect on your training, but your training may increase your flow of milk. At least it does in cows. A USDA study in 1979 discovered that forcing dairy cows to walk one or two miles a day for several weeks prior to delivery boosted their milk production by about three quarts a day. (The cows also calved easier and with fewer complications.)

Vaginal Births

Following an uncomplicated vaginal birth, you can return to sports as soon as you feel like it, says Darlene Lanka, M.D., obstetrician and gynecologist at Kaiser Hospital in Walnut Creek, California. If you reduced your activity gradually, cutting some sports out as you became bigger and clumsier, return to them in the opposite order, playing the last ones first until you get into better shape.

Lamaze instructors tell you to start doing Kegels right away—on the delivery table. Lanka says that's all right, but "it really hurts, so I would wait a few days for comfort. This goes along with the general rule that if something hurts, don't do it." Do Kegels and killer sit-ups, she says, as soon as you can. She doesn't approve of groin stretches during the first three weeks, or any exercises involving standing up and pushing the leg out to the side to strengthen the inner and outer thigh. Both kinds of exercise may strain your episiotomy.

The episiotomy is an incision in the bridge of muscle and tissue between the genital organs and anus, performed in order to enlarge the outlet of the birth passage. It heals in two or three weeks, much more quickly than other sorts of incisions, because the vagina and vulva of a pregnant woman have extra blood vessels.

"Any sport," says Lanka, "is okay after the first week or week and a half. At first, you probably won't feel like doing sitting sports because your episiotomy will hurt. That lets out bike riding, but as soon as it doesn't hurt, you can do it. Swimming is safe, because the vagina closes up right away, but you're still bleeding and you can't wear a tampon for three or three and a half weeks. There's nothing dangerous about swimming before those three weeks are up, but you'll bleed into the pool. Basically, the rule for a mother after a vaginal birth is: If you have the energy, and it doesn't hurt, you can do it."

If you are a scuba diver who had a normal vaginal delivery, wait six weeks before getting back in the water because you want to be fully healed. If you aren't, you may become infected by a virulent marine bacteria. If you haven't dived for six or nine months and are out of condition, take it easy and be sure you are in good shape before you undertake anything exacting and strenuous.

Cesarean Sections

If you've had a Cesarean section—this also applies to hysterectomies and other abdominal surgery—your recovery will be slower. How soon you can return to exercise and athletics depend on your makeup. Fifty percent of all women are healed by six weeks, and 99 percent by eight weeks. Unfortunately, there's no way for you or your doctor to know whether you are in that remaining one percent who need more time.

"When we're talking about exercise after abdominal surgery," Lanka explains, "we worry about hernias in the incision in the fascia, the fibrous connective tissue sheath surrounding the muscles. The fascia is that thick tough inedible white stuff on the outside of chuck roasts and other meats. It's the strength that keeps the muscles and intestines in shape and holds everything together, but if there is a weakness in it, a hernia can develop."

In order for healing to occur, the old cells at the edges of the cut tissue are destroyed, and new tissue grows in its place. The cells making the new tissue are called fibroblasts. The incision in the peritoneum (the lining of the abdominal cavity) heals in three to five days—a week at the most. The skin is pretty well healed in two weeks. At five weeks, the suture material has dissolved, but the fibroblasts, which work relatively slowly in the fascia, have not finished their work. "At five weeks, the woman feels great," says Dr. Lanka, "but the fibroblasts are still not entrenching adequately. With the suture material gone, the incision at five weeks is as weak as it's ever going to be. For this reason, I tell women to wait eight weeks before doing abdominal exercise, just to ensure that the fascia has completely healed."

Cesarean Recovery Exercises

You can begin exercising in the recovery room after surgery as soon as you can feel your legs, says Barbara Swenson, a coordinator of the Cesarean Childbirth Trust in Lafayette, California, if you splint your incision. Simply interlace the fingers of both hands and press them over your incision when doing any of these exercises.

1. Toe flexers and ankle rolls while lying in bed. Repeat them several times during the following days to improve your circulation.

2. Leg slides. Lie on your back. Bend your leg by keeping your foot flat on the bed and sliding it toward your butt. Straighten your leg for one rep. Alternate with right leg. Do as often as is comfortable over the next several days.

3. Leg lifts. Lie on your back. Bend your left knee and keep your right leg straight. Slowly raise your straight right leg as high as you can off the bed, trying to point your foot at the ceiling. Slowly return your leg to the bed for one rep. Do five or ten reps. (Don't do this if it hurts.)

4. Pant in an open-mouthed, relaxed fashion, like a dog, to clear your lungs of congestion and prevent pneumonia.

5. Laugh. "Laughter is great abdominal exercise," Swenson says. "Take a joke book to the hospital. Laughter will keep your lungs going

---

BELLY BREATHING

Inhale deeply, feeling your belly bulge and your diaphragm sink. Then exhale, emptying your lungs from top to bottom and feeling your belly contract as the air leaves. Do this gently, once an hour, four or five times a day.

---

and strengthening your abdominal muscles. But be sure to splint your incision when you laugh."

6. Practice belly breathing. You should know that belly breathing after abdominal surgery is mildly controversial. Some doctors feel that even this small amount of pressure on the abdomen is too much. Others feel it is essential for getting rid of post-surgical intestinal gas.

As long as you rest your abdominal muscles, it's okay to exercise the other parts of your body almost immediately.

Lanka, a Cesarean mother and athlete herself, suggests the following guidelines for returning to your sport:

"Immediately after surgery, you are going to feel weak, exhausted, and almost fluish because your peritoneum has been cut. Don't push yourself. You should exercise, but stop before you become exhausted. If you are taking a walk, and you think you can walk two blocks, walk one, and turn around because you have to come back. If you overdo it, you will become so tired you won't be able to move for the next three or four days.

"Start walking in the hospital—it will reduce painful intestinal gas. Increase the length of time you walk each day until you're walking a mile or two.

"Bicycling is really good exercise because it places no stress on the abdomen. In fact, the bending-over posture favors the abdominals. If you're an experienced bike rider, you can ride the day you go home from the hospital. I had a woman go home from a hysterectomy and ride five miles the first day. That's great. I wouldn't advise riding if you're not familiar with it, because if you fall or jump off suddenly, you can hurt yourself.

"You shouldn't start jogging for two or three weeks. After that, try it. If the bouncing of the tissue bothers you, or if you feel pain, stop.

"If you're a swimmer, you can start swimming after two or three weeks because the incision is pretty well closed by then. Swimming doesn't put any pressure on your incision, so you can swim your head off. Even it you're not a swimmer, but know it a little, you'll find it a super toning exercise. People who go back to their swimming after surgery recover amazingly fast.

"Tennis is okay if you play a gentlewoman's game rather than a killer's game. It won't put that much pressure on your belly unless you're jumping. Doubles are good if you take the weaker side. I played tennis when I was five weeks post-C-sec, and I didn't have any trouble at all.

"Don't do any stretching or strengthening exercises using the abdominals before eight weeks: no rowing, no vacuums, no push-ups, sit-ups, chin-ups, or pull-ups. If you put pressure on the abdominal muscles, you may weaken the fascia and develop a hernia. Don't do anything which pulls the abdominal muscle tight."

Will motherhood slow you down? It doesn't have to. In fact, says Evalyn Gendel, many women feel stronger, have greater stamina, and give better performances after they have children. In July 1980, Evonne Goolagong became the first mother to win the Wimbledon singles title in sixty-six years, three years after her daughter was born. Skier Andrea Mead Lawrence's performance actually improved after she had her children. She became the first U.S. skier—male or female—to win two gold medals in the Olympics. (No male U.S. skier has ever won a single gold medal in skiing.) Diver Juno Stover Irwin became a legend in her own time by combining childbirth and athletic competition. Beginning in 1948, Irwin competed in four consecutive Olympic Games, carefully planning her pregnancies to occur during the four-year intervals. In 1952, she had one child and was pregnant with another when she won a bronze medal. In 1953, pregnant again, she competed in the Nationals. In 1955, she won the national title and placed second in the Pan-American Games. In 1956, after three children, she competed in the Melbourne Olympics and won a silver medal in platform diving. Three years later, in 1959, she was the mother of four and took a second-place medal at the Pan-American Games. Finally, in 1960, she placed fourth in the Rome Olympics.

IV/SPORTS MEDICINE

When I was fifteen, I hurt my knees playing on my mother's soft-ball team. My doctor gave me cortisone shots each time, but the knees kept getting worse. I finally went to another orthopedist, who had to operate twice in the same year. He says the cortisone shots weakened my knees, and I should have done exercises to strengthen them instead. If I had known about those exercises, I would have been saved from the pain and scars of the operations.
—A sixteen-year-old student

10 / How to Diagnose, Treat, and Prevent Injuries

Sports medicine is a new field in the United States. In 1955, when the American College of Sports Medicine was incorporated, bringing doctors, physiologists, and athletic trainers together, it was the first U.S. group seeking a total understanding of how the human body works during exercise. Everyone had been chugging along in separate narrow channels, talking to colleagues but not checking theories with people doing research in other disciplines. Cardiologists panicked whenever an athletic patient showed up with an enlarged heart. Orthopedic surgeons consigned patients to bed rest or prolonged immobilization for every kind of muscle or bone injury. Athletic trainers kept their players in action until they were so badly racked up they were permanently crippled. Physiologists said that sexual intercourse before competition had no effect on performance; trainers prohibited it. Physiologists said to drink water during strenuous exercise in hot weather to prevent heatstroke; trainers said no, drinking water during exercise would give their players stomach cramps; and emergency-room physicians continued to treat those players for heatstroke.

The ACSM broadened everyone's view by combining all the elements involved in sports: the value of exercise for promoting good health; the prevention of injuries; therapy and rehabilitation for the injured; and scientific research on the positive and negative effects of exercise, training, and competing, for both the healthy and the sick. In 1955 there was only one sports-medicine facility in the entire country; in 1970, about thirty-five; and by 1978 there were eighty-five.

WHAT IS SPORTS MEDICINE?

Sports medicine is a discipline combining family practice, pediatrics, obstetrics and gynecology, cardiology, orthopedic surgery, physical therapy and physiatrics (the medical specialty dealing with physiotherapy), athletic training and coaching, exercise physiology, biomechanics, podiatry, osteopathy, and chiropractic. Although it has been a recognized specialty in many countries of Europe for the better part of this century, sports medicine is unlikely to become a specialty here—on a par with cardiology, for example—for two reasons. First, many people feel that the twenty-two already recognized specialties have fragmented American medicine enough. Second, sports medicine treats not a single part of the body—such as the heart in cardiology or the bones in orthopedic surgery—but a single part of the population: the athlete at all levels of exercise.

American sports medicine in the 1980s has become an official subspecialty or field of competence or interest. A system of postgraduate courses, examinations, and certifications of competence from medical schools, residency programs, and professional societies such as the American Medical Association, the Society of Teachers of Family Medicine, and the organizations listed in Appendix A has developed to provide primary practitioners (family doctors and pediatricians) with the expertise to treat athletic injuries. There is enough communication now between the contributing fields to support several journals and millions of dollars in research. Sports medicine has become a growth industry.

Different Healing Methods

The revolution in sports medicine has brought with it another, subtler but more far-reaching change. Some sports injuries didn't respond to traditional medical treatment. They needed more than drugs and surgery. At first, athletes sneaked off to chiropractors, osteopaths, and podiatrists, and endured scorn and ridicule when their doctors found out. Gradually, medical doctors realized some of these nonmedical therapists succeeded where they had failed. General practitioners and orthopedic surgeons began to consult them on difficult cases—the first rapprochement in the United States in this century.

Allopathy

Allopathic medicine makes up most of western medicine as we know it today. It is founded on the idea that disease is caused by an outside agent. The doctor must attack this intruder and remove it from the body in order to heal the patient, using drugs that kill germs, scalpels that cut diseased sections out of otherwise healthy tissue, or casts that immobilize a muscle or bone so that it can't move and aggravate an injury.

Allopathy works wonders on appendicitis, heart failure, automobile accident injuries, and infectious diseases and is responsible for the major lifesaving advances of the last hundred years. Orthopedists have developed miraculous surgical procedures to save the knees and hips of severely injured athletes who, twenty years ago, would have been crippled for life. Physical therapists, working with orthopedists, teach athletes exercises to strengthen or loosen injured joints and muscles. However, most athletes' injuries come from using the body too much or in the wrong way. Modern medical science is virtually helpless to treat these overuse injuries—short of telling you to stop exercising—and can't prevent the damage you may do if your body is structurally imbalanced. Many doctors still cure a stress fracture by locking the leg up in a cast but don't correct the underlying cause—the fact that one leg is shorter than the other. And orthopedic surgeons still operate to cure the nagging pain of breaststrokers' knee, when proper technique and strengthening exercises would take the pressure off the knees and prevent recurrences.

Podiatrists. Podiatrists specialize in the investigation and treatment of foot disorders and of any leg, hip, and back problems caused by foot disorders. "Until the fitness craze began," says Tom Ferguson, M.D., editor of *Medical Self Care* magazine in Inverness, California, "podiatrists had terrible inferiority complexes. They were the invisible shadows of the health profession. They weren't really M.D.s, only people who knew about feet. It's strange, when you think about it, that feet were split off into their own field, largely to be ignored by the medical profession."

Podiatrists are highly trained professionals. They go through four years of podiatry school after a minimum of two years of undergraduate work; most of them have completed four years of undergraduate education with a B.A. or B.S. degree. (Physicians go through three or four years of medical school after a minimum of three years of undergraduate work.) Podiatrists treat complaints with exercises, mechanical devices—orthotics—inserted inside shoes, and surgery, when it is necessary. They are *not* chiropodists. Chiropodists treat very minor foot problems, such as corns and calluses, and don't need formal schooling or board certification before hanging out their shingles.

Legally, podiatrists are limited to medical and surgical treatment of the foot, below the ankle, and nonsurgical treatment of the muscles and tendons in the leg-controlling functions of the foot. There is animated debate about where the ankle starts and stops, but that debate is nothing compared to the warfare between podiatrists and orthopedic surgeons over who should have authority over the lower leg. Podiatrists say that orthopedic surgeons are too interested in cutting and in using restricting devices such as casts and braces to correct injuries and skeletal imbalances. They say that much of the damage to the muscles and tendons of the leg comes from biomechanical abnormalities in the foot—abnormalities correctable with exercise and shoe inserts of various sorts. Orthopedists say that podiatrists ignore the imbalances and diseases of the knee, hip, and spine and so neither cure nor correct many of the chronic aches, pains, and injuries of athletes.

Although the boundaries aren't clear-cut, podiatrists and orthopedists each have their contribution to make. If your pain is caused by disease or other lapse in your health—such as arthritis, a broken bone, degenerating vertebral disk, torn tendon, or prolapsed uterus—you need an orthopedist. Otherwise, continuing pain in your lower leg and foot may yield to the orthotic devices, exercises, and other ministrations of the podiatrist. Beware, however, of anyone who wants to operate before trying noninvasive solutions.

Osteopathy

Podiatrists are basically allopathic healers, just as medical doctors are. Osteopaths and chiropractors are not. Osteopaths believe that disease is caused not by an outside agent but by a musculoskeletal disorder. (Lately many osteopaths have combined this theory with the more traditional western model of disease, so the gap between physicians and osteopaths has narrowed.) Osteopaths prescribe antibiotics for bacterial pneumonia, for example, but also apply manipulative techniques to the chest to loosen the fluids there and thus hasten the patient's recovery. They are fully trained physicians who hold Doctor of Osteopathy degrees and are licensed to prescribe drugs, perform surgery, and administer the whole battery of diagnostic tests known to modern medical science.

Reliable sports osteopaths know more about treating sports-related muscle pulls, cramps, spasms, bursitis pain, and many back problems than most medical doctors and almost all orthopedists. They are particularly skilled at detecting injuries and aches caused by having one leg or arm shorter than the other. By massaging, pulling, pressing, and stretching muscles, joints, and bones, and then prescribing exercises for the patient to do regularly, they often cure some of the most stubborn of recurring athletic injuries.

Chiropractic

Some chiropractors believe that all disease is caused by spinal blockages and misalignments of the vertebrae, which, they say, disturb the flow of "nerve energy" to all parts of the body. Manipulating the spine, they claim, will cure everything from crossed eyes and acne to asthma and pneumonia. Chiropractors cannot prescribe drugs or perform surgical operations. They can, however, prescribe x-rays, and some of the less enlightened ones still give patients full-body x-rays to find "subluxations" (misalignments).

People who go to chiropractors for pneumonia or bladder infections may wind up sicker than before they went in. However, people who go to qualified sports chiropractors for stubborn overuse injuries caused by overstressing the muscles and tendons often obtain dramatic relief, for chiropractors, like osteopaths, perform much of their healing by manipulating parts of the body with massage and pressure. A good chiropractor can analyze weaknesses in muscles, leading to spasms in other overcompensating muscles, spot the effects of poor posture, and even analyze unproductive or injurious athletic style—and then massage, apply acupressure, stretch, push, prod, and prescribe exercises to ease pain and reduce nervous tension. Javelin thrower Kate Schmidt, runner Francie Larrieu, hurdler Patti Van Wolvelaere, skier Suzy Chafee, and pentathlete Jane Frederick have all relied on chiropractors, as have former National Football League player Alex Karras, decathlete Bruce Jenner, and baseball player Jim Palmer. And, in 1980, in a stunning show of acceptance, Detroit chiropractor George Goodheart was added to the American medical staff for the subsequently boycotted summer Olympic games in Moscow.

Choosing Your Own Specialist

To find a reputable sports medicine specialist in your area, contact one of the organizations listed in Appendix A. Or ask friends to recommend doctors who play your sport or doctors who have *successfully* treated them for injuries similar to yours. In the doctor's office, scan the walls for certificates of membership in sports-medicine societies or certificates of competence from a medical school or professional society offering courses and examinations in the field. Doctors do not need these certificates if they play your sport and understand the problems of athletes. However, those certificates show that a particular doctor has been specially trained and is likely to be abreast of the latest sports research. Family practitioners see 80 percent of all injuries to non-elite athletes, and yet only a few of them have been trained to treat these injuries and to know when to refer their patients to orthopedic surgeons, podiatrists, or physical therapists, let alone osteopaths and chiropractors.

What Treatments Are Used?

Sports medicine's biggest breakthroughs developed out of the pragmatic need to keep valuable college and professional athletes in action. Tendon transfers for polio patients were modified to repair the arms of major league pitchers. Once such a technique was perfected, it filtered down to the recreational athlete. Knee surgery for people who had suffered serious traumatic accidents became routine for ten-mile-a-week runners and weekend tennis players. Surgery is required for joint injuries more often than for any other type of injury. Knee operations are the most famous, because the highest paid athletes are usually in leg sports—football, baseball, and tennis—but shoulder injuries afflict tennis players, swimmers, and gymnasts, and hips degenerate as arthritis progresses. Twenty-five years ago, damaged joints were encased in plaster and braces and held immobile for six to nine months. Today, they are diagnosed and repaired so quickly that an athlete may be back in action in ten days or two weeks.

Arthrogram

The arthrogram speeded up diagnosis of joint injuries by making cartilage and other non-bony parts of the joint visible to x-rays. Until the arthrogram, a doctor either had to wait weeks, until the body revealed the nature of the injury, or cut the joint open; even if there was no cartilage damage, it took months for your muscles and ligaments to recover from the diagnostic surgery. Now, traceable dye is injected into the joint. The cartilage soaks up the dye and shows up on routine x-rays. If nothing indicates the need for rest or surgery, the doctor can prescribe a series of exercises and return you to your sport almost immediately.

Bone Scan

The bone scan is another noninvasive diagnostic technique in the sports physician's battery of tests. Also known as radionuclide imaging, a bone scan shows small cracks and stress fractures in bones that might not become visible on standard x-rays for weeks or months after the pain begins. It works because a newly cracked or fractured bone starts rebuilding itself immediately by sending in extra blood and laying down new bone cells. The doctor injects into the patient a radioactive substance readily absorbed by the new bone cells, then scans the bone with a computerized detector. If there is any damage, it will show up as a "hot spot" of white dots.

A bone scan shows damage immediately and is particularly useful for tiny breaks such as stress fractures; if you wait the three or four weeks for the injury to show up on conventional x-rays, the injury becomes worse, more stubborn, and you will need a longer recovery period. However, the procedure is expensive (about $200), and exposes you to the risk of full-body radiation. That radioactive tracer, after all, circulates throughout your whole system before some of it lodges in the target bone.

Arthroscopy

Arthroscopy is used as both a diagnostic and a surgical tool. The tube-like arthroscope, about as thick as a pencil, was first used by Japanese orthopedists in 1918 and works like a tiny underwater telescope. It is inserted into the joint through two small incisions, each so small it can be closed with one suture. The patient is placed under general anesthetic, and the doctor inserts the scope and its light source into one "portal" and an irrigation tube into the other. The doctor peers through the viewer and probes various structures inside the joint to see if they are still firmly attached to the bone. Diagnosis is almost 100 percent foolproof. If surgery is necessary, it may be the sort amenable to arthroscopic surgery, in which case the doctor will insert a miniature router to remove torn cartilage or bits of chipped bone. It may also be possible to pin parts of the bone together. The procedure lasts about an hour and a half, and the client leaves the hospital before nightfall. If the arthroscopy is purely diagnostic and turns up no damage, she can return to normal levels of exercise within a week or two—a much shorter period than if you had undergone exploratory surgery. If the arthroscopy is surgical, recovery is easier than it would be from full surgical opening of the joint.

DMSO

DMSO—dimethyl sulfoxide—is in a class of therapeutic agents all its own. Many doctors hail it as an exciting new medicine with great curative potential. In several European and South American countries, dimethyl sulfoxide has been approved as a prescription medication for shingles (a chronic herpes infection), scleroderma (a swelling and thickening of the skin), cystic mastitis (a benign though painful and chronic swelling and lumpiness of the breast tissue), and amyloidosis (kidney disease). However, in the United States, DMSO is approved only for veterinary use and for use against a relatively rare human bladder disease called interstitial cystitis. In Canada, it is used in patients with sclerodoma. Many professional and recreational athletes claim that "stuff," as they call it, almost instantaneously shrinks swelling, reduces pain, and hastens the healing of sprains, muscle pulls, bruises, tendinitises, shin splints, bursitises, and other musculoskeletal aches and pains, spurring a large black market in veterinary and industrial-grade DMSO. In fact, as lofty an authority as *The Medical Letter*, a highly respected pharmaceutical newsletter for physicians, says it *may* prove effective in reducing muscle spasms and swelling caused by muscle and skin injuries and some inflammatory diseases (exclusive of arthritis) and may also serve as a medium to improve the penetration of other topical drugs through the skin barrier. Researchers at Johns Hopkins say that DMSO may powerfully stimulate the immune system and so may be useful for treating rheumatoid arthritis and other immune-system diseases.

First synthesized in Russia in 1866, DMSO is a clear liquid or gel usually manufactured from lignin, a byproduct of wood pulp. It is used primarily as an industrial solvent, paint thinner, and remover of epoxy glue. It gives natural gas its distinctive odor. (Natural gas is odorless when it comes from the ground; utility companies add DMSO as a safety feature so that customers can smell gas whenever there is a leak.) Its most remarkable quality is the speed with which it is absorbed through the skin and into the bloodstream. It manages to penetrate the skin barrier with the efficiency of an injection and carries with it any other drug or chemical it touches. For this reason, athletes often mix aspirin, other painkillers, or hydrocortisone salve into the DMSO before they apply it. However, anyone who uses "stuff" must be careful to keep DMSO-coated skin clear of varnish, paint, epoxy glue, or even cosmetics, sunscreens, and residual soap film, because the solvent will dissolve the chemical, and DMSO's absorptive properties will carry it directly into the bloodstream.

An athlete using DMSO applies it as soon as possible after a sprain, pull, bruise, or other injury. She carefully cleans the area with plain soap and water, avoiding alcohol and other antiseptics because their residue will be absorbed into her bloodstream. She applies DMSO straight from the bottle or tube or dilutes it with one part distilled water to two parts DMSO, spreading the gel or liquid over the whole surface of the injury with cotton swabs. (Don't apply DMSO with your fingers because you may have undesirable chemicals lurking in crevices or under fingernails. One woman quickly stopped using DMSO when it melted off her nail polish.) Within a few minutes, her breath tastes and smells strongly of garlic or rotten oysters—the signal that DMSO has already permeated her system. She elevates her injured arm or leg for fifteen to thirty minutes, protecting it from furniture wax or varnish or any other chemical, for anything it touches will be dissolved and transported into her system. After thirty minutes, she wipes off the excess and continues to elevate the injury on and off throughout the day. She may apply DMSO again several hours later or the next day.

According to its principal proponent, physician Stanley W. Jacob, M.D., of the University of Oregon Health Sciences Center in Portland, DMSO probably blocks pain transmission through the nerve fibers, reduces inflammation, softens scar tissue, improves blood supply to the injury, and speeds healing. No one knows whether he is correct. DMSO's safety, according to *The Medical Letter*, is completely unknown. Some people have suffered severe allergic reactions, as well as blisters, skin rashes, headaches, nausea, diarrhea, burning on urination, temporary disturbances of color vision, and temporary sensitivity to light. Previous tests showed that the drug clouded the lenses of the eyes of monkeys, dogs, and rats after prolonged use and caused birth defects in several species of animals. No one knows whether these effects would also occur in humans. Finally, DMSO appears to weaken tendons and make them more prone to rupture. This effect disappears two weeks after treatment is discontinued. Black-market supplies of DMSO carry their own risks, for they may be contaminated with pesticides and other dangerous chemicals that are absorbed, along with the DMSO itself, directly into the bloodstream.

The FDA has demanded tests of DMSO's efficacy and safety before it approves its widespread use in this country. It wants to know if it works and whether there are any adverse short- or long-term side effects. Such tests are now under way at several universities, and the results should be published by mid-1982. This delay is extremely annoying to athletes convinced that "stuff" is a harmless miracle cure, but then Thalidomide, Bendectin, and seventy-three coal tar food dyes were said to be harmless too.

Rehabilitation

Sports medicine's greatest contribution by far is its focus on rehabilitation. Over the years, sports doctors have discovered that carefully stressing a bone or a muscle actually makes it heal faster than just immobilizing it.

Exercise: To speed your recovery by as much as 50 percent, you can exercise an injury while it is inside a cast on an isokinetic Cybex machine, which maintains a constant speed throughout the whole range of motion. (A Nautilus machine, in contrast, maintains a constant amount of weight.) Each Cybex machine is specific for a part of your anatomy and is extremely expensive. The full array of machines is available only in professional athletic team training rooms and at sports-medicine clinics, although a few health spas also have them. However, sports-oriented physiatrists and physical therapists can prescribe exercises using surgical tubing (available to the public at any surgical supply store), rubber bands, or free weights to accomplish the same thing with almost the same speed. Your chances for full and speedy recovery are good as long as you are willing to do the work involved. Rehabilitation, says Billie Jean King, is "a pain, a huge mental and physical effort."

Sound waves: In addition to exercise, sound waves further stimulate regeneration of muscle, tendon, ligament, and bone cells. Ultrasound machines, originally developed for treating arthritis, send sound waves one to two inches into the body to stimulate blood supply and rebuild tissues in the area.

Electricity: With today's technology, ultrasound waves cannot penetrate more than two inches into your body. Many injuries, however, lie deeper. Electricity penetrates farther, to relieve pain and promote healing. For at least two thousand years, doctors have used electricity as a painkiller. Physicians in the time of Christ administered shocks of up to 220 volts (twice the voltage of normal American household current) from the torpedo fish to relieve joint pain, cramps, paralysis, and gout. Today, electricity has been scientifically proven to speed the healing of soft and bony tissues; to heal, regenerate, and prevent osteoporosis; to knit fractures in bones that don't meet (and would otherwise require surgical bone grafts); to eliminate phantom limb pain in amputees; to cut down postoperative pain after abdominal chest, bone, and back surgery; to reduce chronic low back pain; to relieve pain after breaking a bone, pulling a muscle, or tearing a tendon; and to exercise muscles (and thus prevent atrophy) while a part of the body is immobilized inside a cast or brace.

Electricity may be applied in many ways—with electrodes implanted in the brain or spinal cord, for example, or permanently or temporarily implanted through the skin and into the bone—but by far the most popular method of electrostimulation is transcutaneous electrical nerve stimulation (TENS), more commonly called transcutaneous nerve stimulation (TNS). With TNS, electrodes are placed *on* the skin near the injury (not in it), for pain relief, muscle stimulation, and healing. When inserted under a cast, they also reduce swelling and prevent muscle atrophy. For pain relief alone, however, some people clip them to points on the ear similar to acupuncture points. The electrical current scrambles the pain signals to and from the brain or stimulates the body to produce its own opiumlike chemicals called endorphins to block out the pain. It doesn't disappear; it just recedes into the easily bearable range for thirty minutes to several hours.

Occasionally, however, TNS users suffer a rebound effect; when they shut off the machine, the pain returns with a vengeance. Improperly used, TNS may cause skin irritations or burns. The technique should never be used by people with cardiac pacemakers, bladder stimulators, or other electronic medical regulators.

Compression devices: Instead of triggering your muscle fibers to fire and contract by electricity the way TNS does, intermittent compression boots and sleeves pump and press wounded muscles to speed the healing of bruises, sprains, and strains. This massage also minimizes swelling and can even push lactic acid wastes out of overtired muscles and back into your system for faster recycling. However, it is a passive massage rather than an active contraction, so it doesn't prevent atrophy in immobilized muscle or hasten the healing of broken bones.

Acupuncture

Although acupuncture has been used in China for some 4,000 years, and in Europe since the beginning of this century, it was greeted with disdainful skepticism when it was introduced into the United States a decade ago. However, now that research here and in Sweden, Austria, Canada, and the People's Republic of China has begun to explain how and when acupuncture works, many doctors are willing to try this controversial non-drug pain reliever on clients with intractable pain.

Acupuncture, says George A. Ulett, M.D., Ph.D., of St. Louis, Missouri, probably works either by blocking the pain by stimulating the area with another kind of sensation (much as clenching your jaw may make a headache more bearable) or by nudging the brain to produce endorphins, the brain's own painkillers. Whichever mechanism is operating—and it's possible that both do—it turns out that not all the traditional 400 Chinese acupuncture points are effective. The points that relieve pain when stimulated by manual or electric needles are those that correspond to points used in electromyography (a method of recording currents generated by a contracting muscle). Electrical stimulation is more effective than needle twirling, says Ulett, and needles must be inserted deep into the muscles for optimal painkilling and, sometimes, permanent relief.

Biomechanics

For years, orthopedic surgeons tried to diagnose the causes of chronic backaches and other skeletal pain by observing the walking style, or gait, of their patients, but their success was limited because so many essential movements of joints and muscles occur at the same time throughout the body. With sports movements, the problem was complicated even further by the speed with which each movement is made.

In the last few years, video and computer technology have become sophisticated enough to measure and analyze your stride, style, length of limbs, imbalances and overcompensations, and many other factors. As a result, there is a hot new specialty: biomechanics.

Biomechanics, a hybrid of mechanical engineering and biology, analyzes the human body as an assemblage of mechanical devices governed by the principles of fluid pressure, mechanical stress, friction, gears, and other engineering concepts. Biomechanics in general uses mechanics to explain everything from arterial blood flow to human motion in space, sports biomechanics covers the way the body moves mechanically, physiologically, and anatomically. It also studies the forces generated by that movement in order to design more efficient sports skills and equipment. The Sports Research Institute and the Biomechanics Laboratory, both at the Pennsylvania State University and foremost in the field, have turned out a pioneering body of work over the last ten years. The University of Massachusetts at Amherst, the University of California at Los Angeles, the School of Physical and Health Education at the University of Washington at Seattle, the University of Illinois, the University of Iowa in Iowa City, and Washington State University in Pullman also have laboratories in biomechanics.

Using video tapes or films and various other sophisticated telemetry tools, researchers can record an athlete exercising and then tell her to move her left foot two inches or lean a few centimeters forward if she wants to win a gold medal. They also look for generalized principles of technique, in order to avoid injury and improve efficiency. Is the swimmer's grab start the fastest way to begin a race? What is the most efficient pedaling stroke in bicycling? What is the optimal ratio of stride length to leg length? What are the sweet spots on a racket or the points of stress on ski poles or uneven parallel gymnastics bars?

In one type of analysis, for example, slow-motion videotape helps record your movements, while the Selspot isolates each part of each motion by sensing and filming tiny electronic pulsing lights attached to your body, lights which flash on and off at intervals of less than one one-thousandth of a second. Special high-speed cameras film the movement of target marks on your body at five hundred frames per second. This film is analyzed by a process called digitation, in which the targets are connected by a line and fed into a computer to draw a profile of the athlete's movement. Using this profile, the biomechanical engineer may discover, for example, that your sore knee is caused by rolling your ankle inward, your stride is too long for maximal endurance, or your wrists are too flexible for a powerful tennis serve. If your injuries are caused by a structural imbalance, it may be possible to prevent recurrences by strengthening or stretching designated muscles, retraining yourself to a new style, or placing a corrective device, or orthotic, inside your shoe. Biomechanical engineers also use data on the way the human body moves to design new equipment, playing surfaces, and springy, banked running tracks such as Harvard's tuned track, which cut seconds off the fifteen-hundred-meter and mile races and cut injuries by almost 50 percent.

HANDLING INJURIES YOURSELF

There were about 65 million sports injuries in 1981. More than 80 percent of them were minor—that is, not life-threatening, crippling, or excruciating. This is not to say they were a collective piece of cake. On the contrary, many such injuries were extremely painful and knocked their victims off their games, and their feet, for days or weeks unless they knew what to do about them.

Treating injuries is up to you. Using this chapter on sports medicine, you can care for them as well as—or better than—your doctor, because you apply the same general principles in order to diagnose what is wrong, choose the proper treatment, rehabilitate that part of your body, and prevent a recurrence of the same injury.

Basic Principles

RICE

The first thing to do for almost any injury is apply cold. Put cold on an injury for the first twenty-four hours, and perhaps longer. Never put heat packs, heating pads, infrared lamps, whirlpool baths, or anything else hot on an injury within forty-eight to seventy-two hours of the time you hurt yourself. Don't even soak in a hot bathtub. Heat encourages inflammation by increasing the blood supply to the area.

Cold is applied as RICE: Rest, Ice, Compression, and Elevation. *Rest* prevents further injury. *Ice* numbs the pain by slowing the conduction of nerve signals to and from your brain; it slows circulation and causes blood vessels to contract, thus decreasing the amount of bleeding and bruising; it prevents or reduces swelling because it slows down the flow of fluids through broken tissue membranes and lowers the temperature of the area. (Swelling is actually one of your body's healing mechanisms and is beneficial. It cushions and splints an injury, thus avoiding harmful motion, and contains antibodies and white blood cells to avert infection. However, the extra fluid presses on nearby nerves and is the major source of pain. Reducing the swelling relieves much of your discomfort and muscle cramps.) *Compression*, or pressure on the injured area, inhibits swelling by pushing fluids out of the injured tissue. *Elevation* of the injured part above the level of the heart allows gravity to drain fluids away from the site, thus further limiting swelling.

When you hurt yourself, apply ice packs to the injury as soon as possible. Store-bought commercial ice packs, available at surgical supply houses and kept in the freezer for just such a contingency, work fine, but so do polyethylene food storage bags filled with crushed ice. (Ice cubes are okay, but they don't conform well to the shape of your body.) Drape the ice bags on and around your injury and hold them firmly in place with an elastic bandage. (Don't apply enough pressure to cut off your circulation, or you'll cramp or become numb.) Prop up the injured part of your body on pillows so that it is higher than your heart, and rest it there for ten minutes. Then remove the ice pack, rebandage the injury, and elevate it again for another ten or fifteen minutes. Repeat the ice, with pressure and elevation, for another ten minutes; then pressure and elevation alone; then ice, pressure, and elevation; then pressure and elevation alone—for a total of three or four rounds. Repeat the whole procedure every four hours for the next day or two.

If the ice packs burn your skin, wrap them in towels. Unless you have exceptionally poor circulation, ice cannot actually freeze your tissues because its temperature is 32 degrees Fahrenheit, and living tissue freezes at temperatures below 25 degrees. As long as the ice and its melted water hover around 32 degrees Fahrenheit, you're safe. (In other words, don't add salt to the ice to make it colder. You're not making ice cream.) Restrict the time you wear the ice pack to ten minutes, because after that time, the cold triggers an anti-freezing reaction in your tissues—it opens blood vessels in the area and speeds warm blood from your chest to your injury. This makes your skin turn red, itch, or burn, and heightens the swelling instead of reducing it.

Use cold packs. Don't just stick your sprained wrist or sore ankle into a bucket of ice water. Not only does the bucket force your poor arm or leg into a painful, artificial, constrained position, but it holds your injury well below your heart. The fluids pool down there, and you swell more than if you had done nothing at all.

Don't use cold therapy if you have a severe allergy to cold, Raynaud's syndrome, any rheumatoid disease, or paroxysmal cold hemoglobinuria.

Aspirin

If you wish, take a couple of aspirin every four hours to limit the swelling and cut the pain. Plain old aspirin is a powerful anti-inflammatory drug because it stops tissue membranes from breaking and leaking their contents into surrounding tissue, thins the blood, and inhibits prostaglandins. Prostaglandins throughout your body cause swelling and cramping. Tylenol and other acetaminophen aspirin substitutes don't control swelling because they don't have the same anti-inflammatory and anti-prostaglandin properties. They simply mask some of the pain.

Aspirin has been used for more than one hundred years and has been proven by long use to be one of the safest drugs on the market. Nonetheless, it does have side effects if used over long periods of time or in high doses: stomach bleeding or ulcers; indigestion, nausea, or vomiting; allergic reactions; ringing of the ears; and, in extremely high doses, poisoning. You can minimize the stomach irritation by grinding up your two aspirins and dissolving them in milk, chocolate pudding, applesauce, or whatever disguises the sour taste. (Milk or milk products are best because they buffer or coat your stomach and neutralize the aspirin. Orange juice and other vitamin C-rich foods are verboten, however, because vitamin C magnifies the bleeding effect of the aspirin.) If grinding and milk don't work, try Ecotrin, a coated aspirin, which passes through the stomach untouched, eliminating stomach irritation, and dissolves in the intestine, where it is immediately absorbed.

Some athletes take a couple of aspirins before every workout to prevent the swelling and pain from a chronic injury. Since aspirin doesn't cure the cause of the swelling, and since long-term use may cause ulcers and make you bruise and bleed more easily, it makes much more sense to find out why you hurt, and correct the problem, than to pop aspirin for the rest of your athletic life.

Heat

Use heat to rehabilitate an injury, starting the third or fourth day, after the swelling or acute stage of the injury are past. Heat hastens the healing process at this point by increasing the blood supply to the area, widening your blood vessels, bringing in white blood cells to carry away byproducts of the damaged tissue, and reducing any remaining swelling. Best of all, heat relaxes muscle spasms and eases pain.

Moist heat packs, such as hydrocollators (available at drugstores), infrared heat lamps, whirlpool lamps, heating pads, and moist towels all work well. (If you use an infrared lamp, cover the exposed skin and injured area with continually moistened towels, station the lamp two feet away from you, and use it for less than twenty minutes per treatment.) Hold the temperature below 100 degrees Fahrenheit, for your skin burns or cooks at 113 degrees and above. The heat should feel pleasant and warm, and loosen up the tissue. If it hurts, it is too hot. Lower the temperature of the bath or heating pad to 102 to 110 degrees, or insulate yourself by inserting dry towels between you and the moist heat packs. You get the maximum effect in fifteen or twenty minutes.

Warning Signals

You can't handle every injury. See your doctor if:

- You have any of the danger signals listed at the end of chapter 2
- You have severe pain from a blow, fall, or other trauma (you may have broken a bone or dislocated a joint)
- You have any injury that looks deformed (don't try to push anything back into place yourself)
- You have very marked, very quick swelling
- You have an injured part that won't function properly (you can't bend your elbow, for example)
- You have any traumatic injury to the neck, head, or back
- You have numbness, tingling, burning, or marked weakness **(burning pains in the hands and arms are a sign of spinal-cord injury)**
- You are bleeding profusely
- You feel disoriented, dizzy, uncoordinated, nauseated, headachy, have pupils of two different sizes, can't keep an outstretched arm steady with your eyes closed, lose your memory, or lose consciousness, especially after a blow to the head
- You can't see clearly, especially when you look upward, as the result of a blow to your eye
- You hear a popping noise accompanied by unbearable pain when you try to extend your limb (you may have ruptured a tendon)
- You have pain in a joint, bone, or muscle that lasts for more than two weeks
- You have an injury that doesn't heal in three weeks, assuming you've rested it and given it ample opportunity to mend
- You have an infection in or under the skin showing pus, red streaks, swollen lymph nodes, or fever

---

Exercise

Stay in shape while injured by practicing another aerobic sport which doesn't use your injured part. If, for example, you have a leg injury from a running sport, try swimming—you can even run laps in midriff-level water. If you have swimmer's shoulder, try cycling. Exercising at your target pulse rate not only maintains your stamina while you are healing but also speeds your whole recovery, by improving your circulation, metabolism, and oxygen uptake.

Resume exercising slowly and gingerly. Unless otherwise instructed, wait until the pain is gone and the swelling is down. The injured part should be able to support your weight and move in all directions. If it is too stiff to bend in one direction, too weak to support you for at least twenty seconds, or feels very soft, it isn't healed enough to retrain.

When you no longer hurt at rest, start gently moving. As long as nothing hurts, keep going, but stop if you feel pain. When you can move carefully through your full range of motion, start increasing the intensity of the exercise and the workload by 10 or 15 percent *maximum* per week. Stretch and strengthen the injured joint or muscle with specific daily exercises listed under your injury. Stretch again after each workout and ice the injured area for ten minutes, even if it is free of pain. Continue the ice until you are back to your pre-injury training level.

HOW TO USE THE *SPORTS MEDICINE GUIDE*

First, rule out all aerobic warnings and other danger signals. If you have any of the symptoms just listed, call your doctor immediately. If your injury is not an obvious emergency, find your symptoms in following the appropriate section on the outline that follows to look for your symptoms. (Problems are grouped by body system and then by body area, from bottom to top.) Read about the injury to confirm that you actually have it and then treat it as suggested. Note any warnings included and do not attempt self-treatment if you have any doubts. In addition to the treatment suggested, you will also find hints for speeding your return to normal, as well as advice and suggested exercises to keep from hurting yourself again. You can locate any exercise quickly by looking it up in the separate Exercise Index in the back of the book. If you have more than one symptom, you may have more than one injury. Look them up in order of severity.

For some problems, home treatment will be your only choice. It is the same therapy your doctor would provide. If you follow the directions conscientiously, you should solve the problem. An injury requiring home treatment is not necessarily trivial. It may simply be the type of problem for which you can do as much as a doctor can. For this reason, take your home therapy seriously and minister to yourself with as much attention as you would expect from a doctor.

For other injuries, home treatment is a stopgap measure, or a first step. If your symptoms disappear, fine; if not, see your doctor. But even when you have to see a doctor, read the description and appropriate therapy and rehabilitation in this section first so that you are armed with as much information as possible.

To ensure accurate diagnosis and effective treatment, give your physician the following information:

- Precisely how and when the injury occurred
- Whether the injured part is stiff, sore, or numb when you first wake up in the morning
- What kinds of movement aggravate the pain
- Whether the pain intensifies or disappears during a workout and at what point (if it gets worse, stop exercising)
- How the injured part feels after the workout—if it hurts, note when the pain starts, how severe it is, and how long it lasts
- What sort of home treatment you've applied

NOTE: Many of the exercises suggested for treating, rehabilitating, or preventing injuries are used in other parts of this book for sports conditioning. During training and conditioning, you build muscle and stamina by performing exercises quickly and aggressively. However, for therapy you recover lost strength and mobility by doing each exercise slowly and deliberately (unless otherwise noted); otherwise you may aggravate rather than relieve your pain. And remember: Don't force anything. It takes three days to rebuild the strength in a muscle for every day you wear a cast or brace.

SPORTS MEDICINE GUIDE

Contents

Head *(cont.)*

Black Eye
Eye Guards
Subconjunctival Hemorrhage
Corneal Abrasion
Sunburned Eyes
Swimmer's Ear
Diver's Ear
Surfer's Ear
Ruptured Eardrum
Runner's Ear
Wrestler's Ear
Sinus Squeeze
Nosebleed
Broken Nose
Runny Nose
Cuts and Scrapes Inside the
    Mouth
Toothache
Tooth Pain
Tooth Knocked Out
Tooth Pushed Out of Line
Tooth Cracked or Broken Off
Tooth Bumped

Skin   390

Abrasion
Blister
Bruise

Laceration
Bicycle Burn
Saddle Sores
Chapped Lips and Skin
Cold Sores
Herpes Rash
Nighttime Hot Flashes
Bites and Stings
Poison Ivy, Poison Sumac, or
    Poison Oak Rash
Sunburn
Sun Poisoning

Heat   395

Heat Cramps
Heat Exhaustion
Heatstroke
Hitting the Wall
Hypoglycemia

Cold   399

Frost Nip
Frostbite
Hypothermia

Altitude   402

Altitude Sickness
Acute Altitude Sickness

CIRCULATORY SYSTEM

Pseudoanemia

Description: Also called runner's anemia. Lower-than-normal red blood cell count in endurance athletes, detected during routine blood tests. A low blood cell count usually indicates that you are anemic or that you are losing blood by bleeding through an ulcer or other lesion in your intestinal tract. If you are an endurance athlete, however, your exercise may simply have increased the volume of liquid in your blood. You have the same number of red blood cells you had before, but you have more liquid to dilute them. This is a completely harmless condition, but it is important to be certain that you have pseudoanemia rather than true anemia. Thus, if you show a low red blood cell count during the standard finger prick test, ask your doctor to perform a blood volume test. If you test within normal ranges, ignore your pseudoanemia; it will have no effect on your health or performance. If you still test low, more tests are in order.

Shock

Description: Failure of blood circulation due to a sudden drop in blood pressure and consequent ineffective heartbeats. Can be fatal because not enough fresh, oxygenated blood reaches the brain.

Often present with severe injury or trauma or bleeding.

Home Treatment: None. Keep the victim warm enough to prevent shivering, but don't move her. Get medical help immediately.

DIGESTIVE SYSTEM

Exerciser's Diarrhea

Description: Also called runner's diarrhea. Diarrhea, gas, or stomach cramps during or after strenuous exercise, but none of the signs of ulcers: no burning pain relieved by eating, no sour taste, no problems between workouts. These symptoms are relatively common during endurance exercise and have a wide variety of causes. Some are heat cramps caused by lack of fluids, some are genuine digestive disturbances, and some are cramps in your abdominal muscles. To test whether the symptoms are caused by cramps in your abdominal muscles, lie on your back and lift your straight legs about six inches off the floor. This tightens your abdominal muscles. (Don't do this test if you have back problems. It is actually a double leg lift and strains your lower back.) If the pain and tenderness persist when you press with your hands on the sore area, your abdominal muscles themselves are weak and aching. If the pain disappears, it probably comes from your stomach and intestines.

If your problem is digestive, you will have to find the cause—and cure—by a trial and error. No one knows for certain why strenuous exercise irritates the gastrointestinal tract. It may increase the gastrointestinal movement in your body. It may restrict the functioning of your intestines by drawing blood away from the gut and into the muscles, thus reducing the blood supply necessary for digestion. It may make you much more sensitive to food allergies, so that foods you can tolerate when sedentary you can't tolerate during exercise. Allergies produce prostaglandins, the same family of chemicals that cause menstrual cramps. Therefore, you can test for allergy-induced exerciser's diarrhea by taking an anti-prostaglandin drug such as aspirin or Motrin (see chapter 8). If the medication prevents the gas, diarrhea, or cramps, you have an allergy. If it doesn't, you probably don't. However, this test has a few flaws. First, the prostaglandin inhibitor may itself cause diarrhea. This is certainly true for aspirin. Second, the medication may not be strong enough to counteract the quantity of prostaglandins you produce.

Home Treatment: If your cramps are due to muscle pain, treat as for side stitch. If your problems are intestinal, there is very little you can do for them during an attack. The symptoms clear up by themselves within a few hours after you stop exercising.

Prevention: If your cramps are due to muscle pain, strengthen your abdominal and back muscles with killer sit-ups and locusts. Try piston breathing. If you have intestinal distress, eliminate one food at a time from your pre-exercise meals. Milk in any form is the most frequent culprit. Many people are allergic to it, and even more people do not have the enzyme necessary to break down milk sugar. If your diarrhea disappears when you abstain from milk products, you can determine whether you have a milk allergy or a milk intolerance (absence of the enzyme that breaks down milk sugar) by reintroducing *cultured* milk products to your diet. Unpasteurized yoghurt, cultured buttermilk, and most cheeses do not aggravate a milk intolerance because the bacteria in the culture breaks down the offending milk sugar, called lactose. Wheat is another common allergen, as are oranges, beef, shellfish, chocolate, nuts, and eggs. Raw fruits and vegetables sometimes cause diarrhea if eaten within a couple of days of a particularly strenuous race. Exercise on an empty stomach and bowel. Drink at least two glasses of water before you exercise and cut down or eliminate sugar before your workout to reduce your chances of heat injury. Don't take anti-diarrheal medications unless you are really desperate. The side effects of the drugs, including drowsiness, last far longer than the diarrhea and cramps themselves and may adversely affect your performance for the next day or two.

Cotton Mouth

Description: Painfully dry mouth, occasionally accompanied by gagging or dry heaves during exercise. No nausea, dizziness, or weakness (These are signs of heat injury). Caused by anxiety or exercising with a dry mouth.

Home Treatment and Prevention: Suck on hard candy or gum while you exercise to start your saliva flowing. Drink water before and during your workout.

Giardiasis

Description: Also called traveler's diarrhea (one form). Bulky bloodless diarrhea with extreme flatulence (gas); no fever; occurs one to three weeks after returning from a backpacking or mountain climbing trip; contracted by drinking supposedly clean water contaminated with the intestinal parasite *Giardia lamblia.*

Home Treatment: Drink fluids. Stay off solid foods for a day or two; drink clear liquids, chicken soup, and rice gruel or congee prepared by simmering one half cup of rice in six cups of water for an hour or two. (The Chinese call this *juk* and have used it for centuries as a cure for diarrhea.) Alternatively, take four to eight tablespoons of Kaopectate (depending on your height and weight) after each bowel movement. The clay-like kaolin and the gelling substance pectin combine to solidify stools in cases of mild diarrhea and appear to have no side effects. See your doctor if the condition doesn't clear up after two days or if your diarrhea is severe.

Prevention: Even the clearest, cleanest-looking mountain streams contain *Giardia,* for it is transmitted by dogs, beavers, deer, coyotes, and bears. Before you drink any such water, add five to ten drops of iodine tincture per quart and let stand fifteen minutes.

Hemorrhoids

Description: Also called piles. Sharp, burning, or dull pain in the rectum; itching; occasional bleeding during exercise. Hemorrhoids are dilated varicose veins in the rectum. The blood vessels fill with blood, the surrounding muscles are too weak to push the blood out again, and the veins enlarge and bulge into hemorrhoids. Exercise does not cause hemorrhoids. Straining during bowel movements does.

Home Treatment: Lubricate them before each workout with a bit of petroleum jelly. Lubrication relieves most of the symptoms because it prevents friction when you move, and petroleum jelly works as well as most of the over-the-counter hemorrhoid ointments you can buy. You may find temporary relief from ointments containing the local anesthetics Benzocaine or pramoxine hydrochloride; the anti-swelling agents ephedrine sulfate, epinephrine hydrochloride, or phenylephrine hydrochloride; or the anti-itching agents menthol, calamine, Hamamelis water, zinc oxide, aluminum chlorhydroxy allantoinate, or resorcinol. Suppositories inserted into the rectum, above the anal sphincter, can't stop the pain and itching because only external hemorrhoids lying on the outside skin of the rectum hurt.

Prevention: Exercise is extremely important in preventing and controlling hemorrhoids. If the external muscles around the rectum are lax and weak, they can't push the blood back to the heart, and the veins dilate into hemorrhoids. Cardiovascular exercise of any sort prevents constipation and straining during bowel movements. Vigorous lower body exercises such as running and bicycling strengthen the seat muscles. Bumps and grinds specifically strengthen your buttocks muscles, while flutters strengthen the internal rectal muscles.

Flutters: Suck in your anal muscles, the opposite of bearing down during a bowel movement. Release them for one rep. Do not move any other part of your body. Since no one can see you do flutters, you can perform them at work, while waiting for the bus, or while watching television. Do two hundred to six hundred a day.

If you do Kegels, you can perform them at the same time as flutters. Improper lifting techniques increase the pressure inside the abdomen and on the rectal veins just as childbirth and straining during bowel movements do. If you have hemorrhoids, ask your sports doctor about the advisability of lifting very heavy weights. If it's okay, wear a lifting belt to support your abdominal muscles. Eat a diet high in raw fruits, vegetables, and bran and other cereal fibers. Drink at least eight glasses of water a day to moisten your stools. Do not become constipated, and do not strain when you go to the toilet.

If you start bleeding for the first time, don't ignore it or assume you have a hemorrhoid. Rectal bleeding is one of the early warning signals of cancer. See your doctor.

Pseudohepatitis

Description: Liver enzymes present in your bloodstream after strenuous exercise, detected during routine blood tests. Occurs after strenuous pounding or pummeling exercise. No history of trauma or liver disease. Ordinarily, the presence of these enzymes in your bloodstream indicates that some cells in your liver are damaged. However, these same enzymes are released by your muscle cells during exercise. Routine blood tests can't determine the origin of these chemicals. The condition is harmless and does not indicate liver damage.

Home Treatment: None. If your doctor tells you that your tests show abnormal liver function, abstain from exercise for forty-eight hours. Then take the same blood test again. The enzyme levels should be back to normal. If not, further tests are in order.

MUSCULAR SYSTEM

Trigger Points

Description: A trigger point is a particularly irritable point in a muscle which sets off a painful muscle spasm when stimulated. The pain may surround the trigger point or be referred to another distant area of the body. Headaches, low back pain, stiff necks, muscle spasms (including shin splints), bursitis, tendinitis (including tennis elbow), and many other types of chronic pain may be caused by trigger points. Usually, you have more than one trigger point, and they are stationary. They remain latent in your muscles, and fire only when irritated.

For this reason, once you have found your trigger points, you can locate them again and again. Bonnie Prudden, whose book *Pain Erasure the Bonnie Prudden Way* builds on back doctor Janet Travell's work with trigger points, suggests mapping your trigger points so that you can always find them. (Travell treated President Kennedy's back.) Pressing these trigger points relaxes the spasm and relieves the pain.

If you have any sort of chronic pain, look for trigger points in the vicinity of the pain. Run your fingers firmly along the edges of muscles up and down the limb or body part affected. When you find a tender spot, press it firmly for seven to ten seconds (five seconds is enough for head and neck pain) and then move on and search for more trigger points. Mark the location of each trigger point on a chart of some sort so that you can find it again. When you have finished with the immediate area, extend your search to adjacent sections of your anatomy and to your back. Don't forget the bottom of your feet, your buttocks muscles, and any scar tissue from accidents or surgery. You may not be able to reach or press all of your trigger points yourself; ask a friend for help.

Press each point firmly, using the equivalent of about 15 pounds of pressure on an arm or back, about 30 pounds on very large muscles such as the gluteus maximus, and only about 5 pounds for spots on your face. (Get the feel for the right amount by pushing down on a bathroom or kitchen scale.) When you press a trigger point, the pain will be just short of excruciating. Press as hard as you can stand, but remember, this isn't an endurance contest. Don't be masochistic. When the seven seconds are up, ease off the pressure gradually. Your pain may be gone after you have pressed one trigger point, or it may leave only after you've pressed the whole series. Every three or four trigger points, stop and rub the edge of an ice cube (or spray on a coolant aerosol spray) along the line of the muscle, following the trigger points. Then gently stretch out that muscle with an exercise from the universal warm-ups or concentrated stretching circuit in Part Two of this book. (If your trigger points are particularly stubborn, TNS or other forms of electrical stimulation may defuse them.)

Cramp

Description: Also called by many other names depending on the part of the body affected. Painful, involuntary contraction or spasm of any muscle. Causes include depletion of the mineral salts in a muscle (heat cramps), reflex reaction to some trauma; or accumulation of lactic acid wastes from fatigue or overexercise or using out-of-condition or incompletely warmed-up muscles.

Home Treatment: Stretching and massaging the muscle at the very first hint of a cramp sometimes arrests it. If not, you'll probably have to stop exercising and apply RICE, massage, and stretching and relaxing exercises. Trigger-point therapy or acupressure may also relax the muscle and alleviate the pain (see **Calf Muscle Cramp**).

Prevention If a muscle cramps repeatedly, warm it up thoroughly, stretch it carefully and conscientiously, and then keep it warm during your workout with a sock or some other piece of clothing.

Tendinitis

Description: Diffuse pain along the line of a tendon; swelling; clicking or grinding noise when the injured part moves (crepitus); tender and reddened skin. As a general rule, the pain is most intense when you first get out of bed in the morning. It diminishes as you move around and warm up your body. The tendon is inflamed and irritated from stress repeatedly transmitted to it by the muscle. Possible complications: calcium deposits in the tendon, and binding together of membranes around the tendon (collectively called tenosynovitis).

Home Treatment RICE; trigger-point therapy. Don't do anything that hurts. When the pain stops, start rehabilitation by doing careful stretching exercises. Stretching is particularly important in preventing recurrences.

Muscle Pull

Description: Also called a strain. Sudden deep, persistent, localized tenderness and pain, especially when the muscle is stretched, moved, or tensed, accompanied by muscle spasms, swelling, and bruising. In serious cases, you may be unable to move the injured part. You have overstretched or torn some of the muscle fibers, or ruptured the entire muscle or tendon—muscle separates from muscle, or muscle separates from tendon, or tendon separates from bone. You feel a pull above or below a joint, not in the joint itself. This distinguishes a pull from a sprain, which involves ligaments and joints. Caused by trauma to part of the muscle from overuse or too much stretching. Possible complications: recurrences; tendinitis; permanent contracture of muscle; excessive scar tissue making the muscle inelastic.

Home Treatment RICE. In rehabilitation, stress strengthening exercise.

Muscle Spasm

Description: Also called a strain. Sudden, prolonged involuntary contraction of a muscle, accompanied by acute localized pain. Pain is rarely intensified by stretching. Pain may strike during exercise or several hours afterward. Usually caused by poor posture or overexerting weak out-of-condition muscles.

Home Treatment: Relax the muscles with massage and stretching. Look for trigger points. If none of this helps use RICE for a day and then, after forty-eight hours, massage the muscle in a hot bath or after heat treatments. If pain is unbearable or doesn't go away in a few days, see your doctor.

RESPIRATORY SYSTEM

Side Stitch

Description: Also called catch in the side and runner's ache. Stabbing, aching, or searing pain in either side; pain usually located along the upper abdomen but occasionally found in the middle or lower chest, the shoulders, and even the neck during or immediately after strenuous exercise. Symptoms disappear by themselves within an hour after the end of your workout. Causes vary with the individual: spasm of the diaphragm caused by heavy breathing and insufficient oxygen; spasm of one of the abdominal muscles owing to momentary lack of oxygen; constipation; stretching of the large intestine (colon) by pockets of gas accumulating during strenuous exercise; powerful contractions of the colon.

Home Treatment: One or more of the following suggestions may help. Bend over at the waist, raise the knee of the painful side, and press on the stitch with your fingertips. Or lie on your back and raise your arms above your head. Hold your nose and blow out steadily through pursed lips. Combine the pressing and blowing techniques. Stretch the stitch with reach for the sky or side stretches.

Prevention: Empty your bowels before you exercise. Don't eat beans, cabbage, or other gas-producing foods. Stretch your abdominal muscles with wasp waisters before each workout, and strengthen your muscles with killer sit-ups. When you inhale during a workout, piston breathe.

Piston Breathing: Fill your abdomen with air before you fill your chest. Raise your diaphragm to fill your abdomen, then let your diaphragm sink down like a piston, to push the air out when you exhale. Your belly protrudes on the inhalation and sinks in on the exhalation.

Uncomfortable Breathlessness

Description: Difficulty catching your breath after normally strenuous exercise; not associated with any of the warning signals listed at the end of chapter 2.

Home Treatment: Get down on your hands and knees, hang your head down between your arms, and pant like a dog.

Hyperventilation

Description: Dizziness and light-headedness not associated with trauma or any of the warning signals (end of chapter 2). Hyperventilating, or overbreathing, causes not an excess of oxygen in your blood but, paradoxically, a deficit.

Home Treatment: Stop exercising. Hold your breath. Scream or sing a long, sustained operatic note. Or hold a paper bag tightly around your mouth and nose and inhale and exhale into it for a minute or two. The carbon dioxide in your exhaled breath restores the biochemical balance in your bloodstream, and your body starts to absorb oxygen again.

Prevention: Breathe slowly. Relax as you work out. Breathe through your nose, with your mouth closed, until you can control your rhythm. Then return to the more efficient mouth breathing during workouts, but maintain your new breathing pace.

Exercise-Induced Asthma

Description: Coughing; rapid or difficult breathing; wheezing, intensified during exhalation; accompanied by tightness or aching in the chest or stitch in side; in serious episodes, sweating, flushed or pale of bluish complexion; occurs after at least six minutes of strenuous exercise at more than 65 percent of your maximum heart rate; sometimes occurs during exercise. (These symptoms are also the signs of some forms of heart disease. If this is your first episode—especially if it *hurts* rather than aches when you breathe—see your doctor immediately.) The word asthma describes heavy or difficult breathing caused by a spasm, a contraction of the smooth muscles around the small air tubes (bronchi) in the lungs. As a result, the inner tissues swell, and sticky mucus plugs the airways. The most likely cause of this mild form of asthma is breathing cold dry air, although the symptoms may also be triggered by an allergy to particles or pollens in the air or by cigarette smoke, colds, flu, nervous tension, or strained, irregular, fast breathing. For a definitive diagnosis, see your sports physician.

Home Treatment: You may be able to run through an attack by continuing to exercise for a few minutes after the wheezing begins. The bronchospasm usually reaches its peak within the first eight minutes of exercise. After that, the symptoms become milder. If, however, your symptoms are too severe to continue exercising, stop. Your symptoms will disappear by themselves after a few minutes of rest. Breathe slowly through pursed lips, as for **Side Stitch**.

Prevention: Warm up especially carefully for twenty minutes rather than the usual five or ten. This whittles away the spasm-inducing chemicals in your throat cells so they can't build up to a crucial threshold. Alternate five or ten minutes of stretching exercises with two- or three-minute bouts of jogging, jumping rope, doing jumping jacks, or riding a stationary bicycle. Breathe through your nose to bypass those touchy throat cells and humidify and warm the air before it reaches your lungs. (Doing the aerobic portions of this warm-up in a steamy bathroom humidifies your airways but is grossly uncomfortable.) Wear a surgical or mouthless ski mask, or a scarf over your mouth and nose, to filter out pollens and particles and to warm and moisturize the air your inhale. Do piston breathing. Don't hyperventilate; it may trigger an attack by blowing off the carbon dioxide you need to keep your bronchial tubes open. Aerobic exercise controls asthmatic attacks. The fitter you are aerobically, the less likely you are to suffer them; any attacks you do have are less severe and require less medication to control. In fact, during the first couple of minutes of aerobic exercise, your passages open wider than they were before exercise. For this reason, interval warm-ups and sports in which you alternate three minutes of intense exercise with three to five minutes of low-exertion exercise don't induce as many bronchospasms. However, they don't build cardiovascular conditioning either. If dry-land sports stimulate attacks (running and bicycling are the worst offenders), switch to swimming or some other water sports—even kayaking. Asthmatics rarely have attacks while swimming, possibly because they are breathing the warm, humid air just above the surface of the water. There is, however, a debate about whether asthmatics should scuba dive. Many doctors advise against it because they are afraid the change in air pressure and the mixture of gasses in the air tanks will bring on a dangerous bronchospasm. Others say that people with mild, controllable cases may be able to scuba dive without difficulty. If you never have asthma attacks when you swim, you may be able to dive. Ask your doctor. Even if you have chronic asthma, don't stop exercising unless you and your sports physician have failed in every attempt to control your bronchospasms during workouts. To prevent recurring exercise-induced asthma attacks, you can inhale the powdered prescription drug cromolyn sodium immediately before exercise and again about an hour into your workout. Cromolyn has few side effects because it is not absorbed into the body. You can also inhale salbutamol, terbutaline, fenoterol, or other beta-2 andrenergic stimulators to prevent attacks or to stop them once they start. The aerosol form causes very few side effects, whereas the oral form may cause tremors or shakiness. "With the new medications," says Simon Godfrey, M.D., chairman of the department of pediatrics at Hadassah University Hospital in Jerusalem, "there is no reason why an asthmatic has to worry about athletics."

UROGENITAL SYSTEM

Urinary Incontinence

Description: Involuntarily leaking a few drops or a steady stream of urine when you cough, sneeze, laugh, or do leg or abdominal exercises. This embarrassing condition afflicts about 40 percent of all women in the United States and, to one degree or another, almost all women runners and others who do pounding leg sports. It is most common in women who have had children because childbirth lowers the pelvic floor, stretches the perineal muscles around the neck of the bladder, weakens the valve muscle closing off the urethra, and makes the urethra's angle shallower. (The urethra is the tube carrying urine from the bladder to the outside.) Emotional stress can also make the bladder irritable and send it into a spasm. Exercise neither causes the problem nor makes it worse. However, it is embarrassing to exercise in public if your pants are wet. Furthermore, if you do any sort of leg exercises with damp thighs, the skin between your legs chafes.

Home Treatment: None. Although there are preventive measures you can take, there is no actual cure for urinary incontinence other than surgery. Surgeons eagerly promote either of two procedures to correct weakened urethral valves, a shallowly angled urethra, or an inadequately suspended bladder. If you have any of these problems, and you have never had this operation before, and you are middle-aged or younger, your chances for success are 80 to 90 percent. The younger you are, the easier the repair is. However, this is full-fledged surgery, and you run the usual risks of anesthesia and complications. Your urethra and surrounding tissues will be *very* sore for weeks. What's more, you will be hospitalized for ten days, won't be able to work for at least another three weeks, and will feel weak for a few months. Many women claim that the surgery has "changed their lives"; they now run and jump and dance the way they did when they were children. Others are reluctant to let a surgeon cut into a healthy body. After all, urinary incontinence is not life-threatening and causes no pain. It is not even a disease. When asked whether he recommended surgery for the condition, one urologist answered, "It's like cosmetic surgery. It makes a world of difference to some women, but to others it's not worth the pain. After all, no one ever died of wetting her pants."

Prevention: Your first line of defense is the Kegel exercise series described in chapter 9. Kegels, done for six months day in and day out without fail, have performed miracles for more women than surgery has. They strengthen your pelvic floor muscles, which consequently rise higher toward the bladder, elevate the angle of your urethra, and close around the urethra more tightly. As an added bonus, Kegels teach you to contract your pelvic floor muscles during intercourse, increasing your pleasure as well as your partner's. It takes a couple of months before you see small signs of improvement, and a full six months before you notice dramatic differences. Nonetheless, they're worth the patience.

In addition to Kegels, apply the law of specificity (chapter 2). Every time you urinate, cut off the stream of urine a few times to train your muscles to do the same thing while you are exercising. You can, in fact, tighten up your pelvic muscles

enough to shut off most or all of the drips.

Strengthen your abdominal muscles with killer sit-ups and twisting sit-ups. When your abdominals are strong and tight, they push your bladder into a better position. Empty your bladder before you exercise. Exercising with a full bladder not only increases the chances you will leak but aggravates your condition, because a heavy, full bladder is bounced and beaten more violently than a light, empty one. Avoid getting suddenly chilled, for that sends your bladder into spasms. Wear a stack of two sanitary napkins held in place by an old-fashioned sanitary belt as well as safety pins. (Double napkins stay in place better than single ones and are innocuous once you get used to them.) If your leg movements push the napkins out of place, try Ambeze, an adult version of Pampers disposable diapers (see Appendix II). They are comfortable, unobtrusive under clothes, and give you complete protection. Once you get over the stigma of wearing diapers, you'll discover just how useful they can be. Ambeze and other brands of disposable incontinent adult diapers are available at hospital supply houses. For some women, running and jumping rope actually tighten the pelvic musculature over time, but if nothing helps, or you lose patience, switch to bicycling, rowing, kayaking, swimming, or another non-pounding sport.

Runner's Hematuria

Description: Also called pseudonephritis. Bloody urine—red or wine-colored. Occasionally, urine does not have a red color, but red blood cells show up under a microscope during a routine urinalysis. Occurs after strenuous pounding or pummeling exercise. No history of trauma. Although an accumulation of red blood cells in your urine usually comes from your kidney and indicates urinary tract infection, tumor, kidney stone, or kidney disease, the blood in runner's hematuria comes from your bladder, does not indicate any disease at all, and disappears within two days.

Home Treatment None. If you notice red blood cells in your urine after a football game, running, or other strenuous exercise, save a sample and refrigerate it. Rest for two days, and see if your urine clears. If your urine is free of blood forty-eight hours later, you probably had runner's hematuria. If you want to check with your doctor to be on the safe side, take in that first urine specimen. If your urine still contains blood forty-eight hours after exercise, see a doctor familiar with the problems of athletes.

Jogger's Kidney

Description: Also called proteinuria. Protein in a specimen of your urine taken within a few hours of a strenuous workout. No trauma. Prolonged proteinuria is a symptom of kidney disease. However, Jogger's kidney, like runner's hematuria, is temporary and disappears within forty-eight hours. Pounding exercise loosens protein, white blood cells, and other particles from your kidneys which travel into your urine.

Home Treatment: None. Rest for two days and then present another urine specimen to your doctor. If there are no abnormal proteins in your urine, you do not have kidney damage. If there are, further tests are in order.

Bruised Vulva

Description: Soreness and swelling in the external genitals as the result of a blow, fall, or other trauma.

Home Treatment: As for any other bruise, RICE.

Ruptured Vaginal Wall

Description: Severe lower abdominal pain after a spread-legged fall off water skis (the "water-ski douche"). Water is shot with considerable force into the vagina and tears through one of the vaginal walls.

Home Treatment: None. See your doctor, because it may require surgical repair.

Prevention: Wear a wet suit whenever you water-ski.

Mid-Abdominal Pain and Fever

Description: Occurring a few hours or a few days after a spread-legged fall off water skis, this may indicate an inflammation or multi-bacterial infection in the lining of the abdominal cavity caused by water forced through the vagina, uterus, and fallopian tubes into the abdominal cavity.

Home Treatment: None. See your doctor.

Prevention: Wear a wet suit whenever you water-ski.

FEET AND ANKLES

Athlete's Foot

Description: White, soggy, blistered, scaling, burning, oozing, bad-smelling itchy sores between the toes and on the sole of the foot. Sores are sometimes open. Infection sometimes invades toenails. Initial infection is caused by the fungus *Tinea pedis* and is actually dry and scaly. This true athlete's foot is not uncomfortable, but when the infection is kept damp, bacteria start to grow, producing the symptoms described.

Home Treatment: For mild cases, try over-the-counter liquids containing tolnaftate, available under the brand name Tinactin. When the condition is under control, apply tolnaftate powders to finish the job and prevent reinfection. Benzoic and salicylic acid combinations also work. Wear sandals or well-ventilated shoes with white cotton socks. Athlete's foot is notoriously stubborn. If these medications don't work, or if you have weeping or open sores, see your doctor.

Prevention: Keep your feet cool and dry. Dust cornstarch or other absorbent powder in your shoes and socks and between your toes. Wear cotton socks; don't wear sweat socks or socks made of synthetic fibers.

Black Toenail

Description: Accumulation of blood or blood clots under a toenail as the result of a direct one-time trauma (dropping something on your toe) or continual and repeated jamming of the toe into the end of the shoe, as in fast stop-start games like tennis and basketball. If the jamming goes on long enough, the nail lifts up off the toe.

Home Treatment: If caused by a single blow, immediately press the nail and toe for five minutes to prevent pooling of blood. If the toe still hurts, the pain usually comes from a pool of blood pressing on the toe bone. Relieve this pressure by cleaning the nail thoroughly and then drilling a hole in the nail. This is a painless, completely safe procedure you can do for yourself in a few seconds, and it brings dramatic relief. Heat the end of a paper clip or thick needle in a flame until it is red hot. Before the paper clip cools, touch its tip to the nail, just above the blood, and melt a hole through the nail. Because nails have no nerve endings, you won't feel a thing—unless the metal sinks and touches the skin underneath. With a clean facial tissue, sponge up the blood spurting out of the hole and apply antiseptic to the area. (This also works when you smash your thumbnail with a hammer or slam your finger in the car door.) See your doctor if you notice any sign of infection. If the toenail is lifting off, trim it back to its point of attachment. Apply ice to reduce the pain and swelling.

Prevention: Cut nails short, wear cushiony socks, lace your shoes tightly enough to prevent your foot from slipping forward and jamming into the front of the shoe, buy shoes with a deeper toe box.

Ingrown Toenail

Description: Corner of a toenail turned under and digging into the flesh, causing exquisite tenderness, redness, and swelling.

Home Treatment: If you can pull the sore, puffy skin back, cut off the ingrown border of the nail. Try soaking your foot in warm sudsy water (use Dove, Ivory, or other mild soap) to soften the skin and nail and then numb the area with an ice pack before pulling the skin back. Don't leave any pointy fragments to push back into the skin. Keep area clean until it heals. If you can't get the skin back, or if the pain continues twenty-four hours after trimming, see your doctor.

Prevention: Cut your nails short and straight across. Wear wide shoes so that your shoes can't press the skin up against the toenail. One woman has successfully prevented ingrown toenails on her big toes by slightly shaving the center of each nail with the blade of her manicure scissors, working away from the cuticle toward the end of the nail to weaken the center of the nail so it makes a shallower curve.

Sprained or Fractured Toe

Description: Severe pain in toe or bones adjacent to toe; swelling, bruising; occasionally, crunching noise when you move the toe; result of trauma such as twisting, stubbing, or dropping something on it.

Home Treatment: If pain is bearable, splint the sore toe by taping it firmly but not tightly to an adjacent toe. Do not pull either toe out of place. If pain is unbearable, see your doctor, who will probably x-ray it and, if it's broken or sprained, splint it, as you would, by taping it to a neighboring toe.

Neuroma

Description: Stinging or aching pain between toes, or on top of foot near toes, without any visible sores or skin irritation. Pain usually intensifies when you squeeze the ball of your foot. This enlarged, inflamed nerve or growth on the nerve is a frequent problem for people whose second toe is longer than the big toe. May be caused by trauma, by narrow-toed shoes, or by anything that pushes the metatarsal or toe bones together.

Home Treatment: Place a pad of surgical felt or foam moleskin on the sore spot, or place two or more pads around the spot to stretch the ends of the bones away from each other. Lace your shoes loosely over the ball of your foot.

Pain Under Toe

Description: Pain, especially under the big toe, from continual irritation of a tendon caused by rubbing the metatarsal heads (ball of the foot) against the ridge of a shoe or the seam of a sock.

Home Treatment: Get a pair of shoes without a ridge of wear cushioned inner soles. If this doesn't help, you may have hallux rigidus.

Hallux Rigidus

Description: Arthritis or an arthritic growth in the big toe, affecting the joint where the foot and toe bones meet and restricting motion in that area.

Home Treatment: An orthotic or a sole that flares up from the joint to the toe box and helps you toe off to relieve the stress on the joint sometimes helps. If you have seriously restricted movement, or advanced bony growths, or gravelly noise when you move the joint, you may need surgery. However, surgery may only improve the condition for four or five years, and then the growth will recur.

Bunions

Description: Swelling, sometimes tender and painful, on one side of the first bending joint of the first or fifth toe. The bursa, or sac between the joints, may be inflamed. On the big toe, the bunion usually bends the toe sideways toward the little toe, a condition called hallux valgus.

Home Treatment: If it doesn't hurt, leave it alone. If it hurts, try cutting a slit in the tight area of your shoe. Put padding over the bunion to cushion it against the pressure of your shoe. Insert cushioned foam spacers between your first and second toes or your fourth and fifth.

Corns and Calluses

Description: A corn is a cone-shaped horny thickening of the skin, usually on the upper part of the small joints of a toe or between the toes at pressure and friction points. A callus is a flat, horny thickening of the skin anywhere that is constantly rubbed.

Home Treatment: If they don't hurt, leave them alone. Calluses, in particular, protect your skin from blisters and abrasions. (Rowers and gymnasts treasure their calluses because the thick skin eliminates most of the pain in their hands.) If the corns or calluses hurt, try padding *around* them or between your toes to relieve the pressure. Wear shoes that don't press on the affected areas. If the pain persists, the corn or callus may have to be trimmed by a doctor. Don't trim it yourself.

Nerve Inflammation

Description: Pins and needles or shooting pains or numbness in toes or feet after lengthy exercise involving repeated pounding. Nerves become inflamed, entrapped, or compressed by repeated shock impacts or swelling and by subsequent impaired circulation, in calf or shin muscles. If accompanied by pain and swelling along the inside of the ankle, it may be tarsal tunnel syndrome.

Home Treatment: Lace your shoes from the fourth hole up, leaving the bottom three holes untied. Install cushioned inner soles in your shoes. Wear a shoe with a higher and wider toe box. Wear heel lifts or arch supports.

Tarsal Tunnel Syndrome

Description: Pins and needles, shooting pains, or numbness in toes or feet after lengthy exercise involving repeated pounding. Top of the foot not affected. Pain and swelling along the inside of the ankle. If you tap the area when it's free of symptoms and elicit the same pins and needles or numbness, you probably have tarsal tunnel syndrome. Burning pain frequently happens at night and is relieved by hanging your leg out of bed or walking on the foot. Symptoms involve a thin band of fibrous tissue pressing on the tibial nerve running down the back of the leg, along the inside of the ankle, toward the sole of the foot. May be caused by abnormally tight ligaments squeezing the nerve on the inside of the ankle or by scar tissue from a previous injury or accident. May also be caused by trauma to the inside of the ankle, tendinitis, or overuse. People whose feet and ankles bend too far inward (over-pronate) are susceptible to tarsal tunnel syndrome.

Home Treatment: If caused by a biomechanical abnormality, built up the *inner* sole of shoe so that the ankle doesn't turn inward. Don't eliminate all pronation; some is necessary to absorb the pounding shock of each footfall. Or get yourself custom-fitted orthotics. If this doesn't work, and the discomfort or numbness is extremely annoying, see your doctor. Surgery may be advisable, to cut the fibrous band pinching the nerve.

Bone Bruise of Foot

Description: Also called stone bruise or periostitis. Pain, exquisite tenderness, reddened skin, muscle spasm, and pooling of blood between the bone and the tough membrane (periosteum) surrounding the bone. Caused by a blow to the bone, such as stepping on a stone. Occasionally also caused by strain of the muscle where it attaches to the bone. Possible complication: permanent thickening of that spot on the bone.

Home Treatment: Bone bruises usually heal by themselves in a few days and rarely need any attention. However, if the pain in your bone is intensified with exercise, see your doctor.

Dancer's Foot

Description: Also called metatarsalgia. Dull or burning pain in a localized spot on the ball of your foot, occasionally accompanied by swelling during exercise and for several hours afterward. Eliminate the possibility of other injuries by testing for stress fracture (localized pain, usually on the top of the foot; tenderness when tapped), neuroma (sharp pain on top of the foot between the bones of the ball of the foot), and bone bruise (exquisite tenderness in just one spot; red or bruised skin). Condition is usually caused by foot imbalances or pounding over long periods.

Home Treatment: RICE. Insert padded inner soles into your shoes or place moleskin or other adhesive padding directly on the sore spot. Stretch the plantar fascia (see **Arch Strain**) and extrinsic and intrinsic foot muscles.

If this doesn't work, try store-bought arch supports, or carve a depression out of the sole of your shoe immediately under your sore spot, and work out on wood, grass, or other surfaces with a little give.

Foot-stretching Exercises: To stretch the extrinsic or antigravity foot muscles, stand with your back against a wall and your legs straight out in front of you at an angle of about 45 degrees. Curl your toes up and lower them, for one rep. Do as many reps as you have patience for, as often as you can stand. To stretch the intrinsic foot muscles, pick up marbles or pencils with your toes.

March Fracture of Foot

Description: Also called fatigue fracture and stress fracture. Pain and tenderness at a specific spot on the ball of the foot (but may also occur on the top of the foot near the toes), sometimes accompanied by swelling and redness during jumping or pounding exercise. Tender or painful when tapped; hurts when pressed from above *and* below. Pain usually subsides with rest but flares up as soon as you resume exercise. Caused by repeated impact or shock, not sudden trauma (see **Tibial stress fracture**).

Home Treatment: RICE. March fractures usually heal by themselves after two or three weeks of rest. While resting your foot, stay in condition with some non-pounding sport.

Plantar Wart

Description: A wart deep in the sole of your foot. On first glance, it may appear to be a corn or a callus, but closer inspection shows that it has a clearly defined border and that the central core has brown or black spots of blood vessels and nerves. A corn hurts when it is pressed on its surface. A wart hurts when it is squeezed or pinched on its sides. Because a wart is a viral infection, it is contagious and may spread to other parts of your sole.

Home Treatment: If the wart doesn't hurt, leave it alone. If it does hurt, have your doctor remove it, especially if you have poor circulation, as diabetics and elderly people do. Over-the-counter wart-removing liquids are corrosive and may damage healthy skin. Warts are likely to recur, perhaps due to a failure of your immune system. To stimulate your immune system, take vitamin C or a total of nine dessicated liver tablets spread out throughout the day. Dessicated liver contains vitamins A, B, C, and D and the minerals iron, calcium, phosphorus, and copper. (See chapter 3.)

Arch Strain

Description: Also called plantar fasciitis or, inaccurately, heel spur syndrome. Pain beginning under the inner side of the heel and extending forward along the bottom of the foot into the arch; no swelling. Pain is intensified by pushing toes upward or by pressing on the area with your fingers, and often occurs after sitting for a long time or when you get out of bed in the morning. In downhill and cross-country skiers, pain is triggered by buckling down the ski boot. This is a partial or complete tear of the plantar fascia, the thick, fibrous, inelastic sheet running under the arch to connect the heel bone to each of the five toes. (Plantar means bottom of the foot.) May be accompanied by a heel spur, a small extra projection of heel bone where the plantar fascia attaches. Develops suddenly or gradually as the result of trauma, tight gastrocnemius and soleus muscles, repeatedly landing on the ball of the foot during jumps, wearing shoes with stiff soles that force you to do extra work to bend them across the ball of the foot or shoes without sufficient arch support, or rolling your ankle inward—over-pronating—when you stand, walk, or run (Ski boots often force you to over-pronate in order to control your inside edges.)

Home Treatment: RICE. Only mild to moderate causes respond to home treatment, and even these take months to heal. Stubborn cases require surgery. Gently stretch your gastrocs and soleus muscles, starting with toe flexers and then moving on to calf stretches, Achilles stretches, geisha kneels, and hunkers. These exercises indirectly stretch your plantar fascia because this band of connective tissue is a continuation of the calf muscle system. Directly stretch the plantar fascia with arch-stretching exercises.

Arch-Stretching Exercises: Place your arch on a beer can or soda bottle on the floor and roll the cylinder back and forth for five minutes at a time, three times a day, to relieve any muscle spasm and reduce swelling. As the pain subsides, progress to standing on a step with your heels hanging over the edge. Rise up on your toes, then lower your heels well below the edge of the stair, for one rep. Do as many reps as you can, as often as you can.

Wear shoes with flexible soles. Fit them with arch supports, heel lifts, a Sports Wedge to cup and tilt the heel, a "doughnut" to relax the fascia and relieve pressure over the tenderest spot, or custom-made rigid or semi-rigid orthotics. Adjust your style so that you never land directly on the ball of your foot. Ballet dancers, for whom this is a very common injury, should perfect their technique for leaps, beginning and ending in a demi-plié with their heels pressed into the floor.

Prevention: Use the same exercises, prostheses, and techniques to prevent recurrences.

Heel Spur

Description: Pain on the underside of the heel when you stand or walk on it, and when you press firmly over the base of your heel with your fingers. An abnormal pull by the plantar fascia (usually due to some biomechanical imbalance) causes a bony projection to grow forward from the underside of the heel. Frequently, a bursa (or lubricating sac) develops and a nearby nerve becomes trapped and pinched by continual inflammation. Occasionally, a person without symptoms discovers a heel spur when it shows up on an x-ray for some other problem.

Home Treatment: If it doesn't hurt, leave it alone. If it does hurt, use the same treatment as you would for arch strain: RICE, shoe inserts, exercises, and improved technique. Instead of arch supports, you may find a horseshoe-shaped heel insert relieves the pressure on the tender spot. Surgery is rarely necessary, and steroid injections, while they reduce the swelling and thereby temporarily end the pain, ultimately weaken the tendons and connective tissue and cause reinjury.

Black Heel

Description: Blackish color around heel. Repeated small bruises to the heel from constantly hitting the back of your heel against the back of your shoe cause small areas of bleeding.

Home Treatment: As for any other bruise.

Prevention: Pad your heel with adhesive foam bandages or moleskin. Pad the shoe with foam or felt inserts.

Heel Pain

Description: Soreness on the bottom of the heel during and after a long foot-pounding workout. Does not occur at the beginning of a workout. The shock-absorbing fat pad in your heel has thinned out because your shoes have loose or poorly supportive heel counters. If this condition continues, it may degenerate into a bone bruise or bursitis.

Home Treatment: Tape two strips of one-inch-wide adhesive tape around the base of the heel, just below the ankle bone, and two more strips under the foot just in front of the heel. Interlace the ends of the strips in a basket weave. The tape forces the fat pad to bulge and absorb impact. Pain should be gone with the first taping, but you will have to tape for several months, as well as wear a shoe with a supportive heel counter that cradles and cushions the heel, before the condition disappears entirely.

Numb Toes or Feet

Description: Occurs after long bicycle rides. Nerves are squeezed between the metatarsal bones of the foot and the pedals. (See **Ulnar Neuropathy.**)

Home Treatment: None. Goes away by itself as soon as you start walking around.

Prevention: Loosen your toe clips. Change the position of your toe clips. Install new pedals that apply pressure in different areas.

Achilles Tendon Rupture

Description: Also called skier's heel and pulled heel cord. Severe pain at the back of the ankle, ex-

tending up the calf; inability to lift your heel off the ground. Caused either by trauma or by ignoring Achilles tendinitis. Occasionally, you can rupture your Achilles tendon and still be able to lift your heel. For a precise diagnosis, perform the Thompson (also called the Simmonds) test.

Thompson Test: Place your knee and lower leg on a chair or bench. Let your foot hang over the edge. Squeeze your calf just below the widest part. If your foot doesn't plantarflex (point its toe and bring the sole of the foot parallel with the ceiling), you've ruptured your Achilles tendon and need medical care.

Home Treatment: If you can rise onto your toes, you have an incomplete tear. Use RICE and see your doctor for conservative nonsurgical treatment. If you can't rise onto your toes, you have a complete tear and will require surgery by a qualified sports orthopedist. The procedures used by sports physicians restore normal length and tension to the tendon complex more than 90 percent of the time. Other procedures may end your athletic career.

Ankle Pain Without Trauma

Description: Pain without swelling or tenderness anywhere around the ankle. No history of twisting, falling, or other trauma. In cyclists, this may indicate a tendinitis caused by riding in too high a gear, or pedaling with cold muscles, or moving your feet from side to side on the pedals. In athletes who do a lot of running, it may be caused by foot or leg imbalances.

Home Treatment: RICE, then treat as an ankle sprain.

Prevention: If you are a cyclist, warm up properly and use toe clips, cycling shoes, and cleats to fasten your feet to the pedals. If you are a running athlete, wear good shock-absorbing shoes and arch supports or heel cups. Play on level ground. Strengthen your gastrocnemius and soleus muscles with squats and heel and toes, and stretch the gastrocs, soleus, and Achilles tendon with baby foot flexers, towel stretches, geisha kneels, hunkers, calf stretches, or Achilles stretches.

Ankle Sprain

Description: Also called twisted ankle. Symptoms range from a mild ache a few hours after injury to immediate excruciating pain, swelling, tenderness in the joint, lameness, and bruising. Ligaments are overstretched or partially or completely torn, usually as the result of a sharp twisting motion, quick sudden turn, or fall. May also be caused by continuous stress on the joint without a sudden trauma. Possible complications: recurrences, stiffness, arthritis.

Home Treatment: RICE, with emphasis on compression. The moment you think you've sprained an ankle or other joint, grab it with both hands and squeeze it for about ten minutes. Elevate it at the same time, if possible. Then apply ice packs and another, more convenient form of compression (such as an elastic bandage). This should eliminate about 90 percent of the swelling. As soon as most of the pain and swelling are gone (one to three days), start moving the joint gently to stretch it and maintain full range of motion. Sprains heal much faster if you move that part of your body. In fact, if you use a device called an air splint, available from your doctor, you can return to exercise immediately. This U-shaped brace has a hard plastic outer shell and a soft inner lining with inflatable compartments. When you blow up the inner lining, it conforms to your ankle, knee, or other body part and eliminates almost all pain. Because you continue to move it, the sprain heals much faster than it would by taping or casting, and you never get out of condition.

If you do not use an air splint, start walking, with short, slow steps, in order to prevent further swelling and muscle atrophy. (If those ankle muscles do weaken, you will be susceptible to further sprains.) Walk barefooted on your uninjured as well as your injured foot to avoid a limp that throws your posture out of whack. Graduate to long quick walking steps, and then other exercise, as pain diminishes.

Rehabilitation and Prevention: Strengthen your ankle muscles with heel and toes and ankle inversion and eversion exercises. Whenever you are standing, rotate your ankles inward and outward, then rock back and forth from your heels to your toes to your heels. Repeat at least twenty times. The standing exercises use your weight for resistance. If you sprain your ankle over and over again, strengthen the outer muscles of your lower leg by repeatedly running a fifteen- or twenty-foot figure eight. Wear shoes with a solid heel counter and flared heel for stability. If your shoes are worn unevenly, have them resoled and correct the muscle imbalance with arch supports, varus wedges, or other shoe inserts. Flat feet and over-pronating (inward-rolling) ankles often cause ankle sprains. Strengthening your arch may help. Walk on tiptoes; walk on the backs of your heels; pick up marbles or pencils with your toes. High arches may also cause sprains. Here, arch supports or orthotics *encouraging* pronation are frequently helpful. Look for something that forces the outer edge of your foot up (the opposite of the normal arch support for flat feet). Even reversing your arch suports may help—put the right one in the left shoe and the left one in your right shoe. If you play stop-start sports such as racquetball or volleyball, buy shoes with basketball treads. Play or run on flat, smooth surfaces. Do not tape your ankles, for that makes them even weaker.

Weak Ankle

Description: Also called skater's ankle. Ankle gives out, twists easily, or wobbles from side to side. May be the result of injury or may be congenital. Do not tape unless absolutely necessary, for the tape, rather than your muscles, supports you, and your ankle muscles remain weak. Strengthen your ankle muscles with ankle inversion and eversion exercises. Buy a shoe with a wide base.

Achilles Tendinitis

Description: Also called Achilles tendon tenosynovitis. Pain running along the back of the leg anywhere between the lower part of the calf and the heel; tenderness and warmth at the point of the tear or swelling; occasional gravelly noise (called crepitus) when moved; pain may occur anytime or only during exercise or only when you jump barefooted. You may not be able to stand on tiptoes or to lower your heel to the floor. This inflammation of the tendon or its covering may be caused by repeatedly lunging or sprinting or by a single blow. In runners, Achilles tendinitis results from overused, over-strengthened, and over-shortened soleus and gastrocnemius muscles.

Home Treatment: If merely a dull ache, try preventive measures below. If you have swelling and crepitus and the condition is chronic, treat with RICE for two days and then use aspirin and moist heat packs to remove the fluid from the sore spot. Try trigger-point therapy.

Prevention: Much more effective than treatment. Work out on springy (though not soft) flat surfaces. If you are a dancer, avoid concrete floors. If you have high arches, try ¼- to ⅜-inch heel lifts to relax the tendons. If your shoes are worn unevenly, resole them and try to compensate for that biomechanical imbalance with better technique or shoe inserts. Wear shoes with sturdy heel counters, Achilles protectors, and flared heels. (*Note:* flared heels aggravate the problem for a few people.) Wear shoes with slightly lifted heels. If you are a dancer, put long heel lifts in your slippers. If you have flat feet, try store-bought arch supports before seeking out a podiatrist, and do arch-stretching exercises. Stretch your gastrocs with calf stretches, your soleus with geisha kneels, and your Achilles tendon with Achilles stretches. Achilles tendinitis often recurs because the inflammation leaves scar tissue, which impedes the smooth movement of the tendon within its sheath and causes further irritation.

Achilles Bursitis

Description: Also called heel bursitis, Achillobursitis, retrocalcaneal bursitis, and superficial calcaneal bursitis. (The calcaneum is the bone of the heel.) Bursitis is caused by a blow or fall or by continual irritation. There is pain inside the bump at the back of the heel about the level of the ankle bones, intensified when you press it, and redness and irritation even though your shoe isn't rubbing up and down on your heel, but no particular pain when you jump barefooted. (This distinguishes it from Achilles tendinitis.) A bursa is a lubricating fluid-filled sac located at points of considerable friction. Inflammation of the two bursae just above the insertion of the Achilles tendon into the heel is often caused by walking around too much in cleated shoes or by pressure on the bursae from the heel counter. High-arched people are most susceptible because their heel bones protrude.

Home Treatment: RICE to reduce the swelling if present. Eliminate the pressure from the shoe with a heel lift. Cushion the heel with a thin, soft pad until the irritation subsides. Try trigger-point therapy.

Prevention: Heel pads or custom orthotics.

Posterior Tibial Tendinitis

Description: Aching pain and swelling on the inside of the ankle bone; pain may run up the leg. Crepitus (gravelly noise) sometimes present. Often caused by slightly pigeon-toed gait or playing on uneven surfaces or banked tracks.

Home Treatment: RICE. Try trigger-point therapy.

Prevention: Work out on flat surfaces. If you must work out on banked surfaces, reverse your direction halfway through your session so that each foot is inverted only half the time. A heel wedge, arch support, or orthotic may prevent excessive pronation.

Diabetic Foot Care

Even the most minor injury or infection can become gangrenous in a diabetic. The diabetic athlete punishes her feet more than a sedentary diabetic and must be obsessive about foot care. Do everything you can to avoid even the slightest break in your skin. Prevent blisters by wearing properly fitted shoes with good toe room, soft, clean, dry socks, and moleskin or Spenco Second Skin. Powder your feet to keep them dry (see **Blister**). Don't cut corns, calluses, or other skin growths or remove them with skin removers. The acids in corn removers, wart or ingrown toenail removers, as well as in iodine and strong antiseptics, may burn your skin and lead to infection and, eventually, gangrene. Cut your toenails after a bath, while they are still soft.

If you come down with athlete's foot, your problem is complicated by the fact that many athlete's foot liquids are absorbed into the skin and can cause their own infection. Try to arrest it in its earliest stages. If you wait six months or so, the fungi and bacteria may spread throughout your body and lead to serious complications. Tinactin, available without a prescription, is probably your best bet if you catch the infection early. If it involves your nail or otherwise becomes serious, try Fulvicin, available by prescription through your doctor.

When you buy a new pair of shoes, break them in gradually by wearing them thirty minutes on the first day, thirty to sixty minutes on the second, and so on. If your circulation is poor, as it is for many diabetics, don't wear garters or socks with tight elastic tops. Don't sit with your knees crossed or with one leg bent under you. You can stimulate your circulation by lying with your feet propped up higher than your hips for thirty seconds, then hanging them over the side of the bed for sixty seconds, for one rep. Do several reps several times a day. If your feet swell, prop them on a footrest.

Diabetes is no deterrent to an active, sports-filled life, but diabetic athletes must attend to foot care, exercise routines, diet, shifting insulin dosages, and much more. *The Diabetic's Sports and Exercise Book* and *The Diabetic's Total Health Book* covers every aspect of the topic (see Selected Reading). One of the two authors, June Biermann, is herself a diabetic.

LEGS AND HIPS

Leg-Length Discrepancy

Description: One leg shorter than the other. There are two types. In the first, one leg actually measures short. (Measurements are taken from the bony protuberance at the top of the side of the thigh and measured all the way down to the outside ankle bone.) This anatomical discrepancy affects only about 3 percent of all people with leg-length discrepancies. In the second type, the legs measure the same, but the pelvis is tilted so that one leg is lifted higher off the ground than the other. This functional discrepancy may be caused by having one arch higher than the other, bad posture,

abnormal range of motion in any of the joints of your leg or hip, or weak muscles in one leg.

Leg-length discrepancies cause a flood of aches and injuries: foot or ankle pains and sprains; shin splints; knee pain; sciatica (pain in the buttocks and down the back of the thigh produced by inflammation of the sciatic nerve); hip, low back, upper back, and shoulder problems (you tilt your shoulder up on the side of your shorter leg); headaches; and even tingling or numbness in the hands or arms. If you repeatedly pull the same muscle, you may have a leg-length discrepancy.

If your legs measure the same but you have any of the above complaints, test yourself for the second, or functional, type of discrepancy. Lie face down on a bed or bench with your feet and ankles hanging over the edge. Wear shoes because they have flat soles. Your feet bottoms are rounded and harder to compare. A friend can judge whether one leg appears to be longer than the other. Now bend your knees up to a 90-degree angle. If you have an anatomical discrepancy, the same leg will appear longer. If you have a functional discrepancy, your legs will appear even or the shorter leg will look longer. Your friend may also see evidence of a discrepancy by observing your naked back. If one of your legs is shorter than the other, your posture and shoulders will compensate. One hip will appear lower or stick out slightly, your spine will have a side-to-side S curve, one shoulder will be lower than the other, or your head may be tilted for balance.

Home Treatment: Balance an anatomically short leg by inserting a heel lift in your shoe. Correcting a functionally short leg is much more complicated because you must pinpoint the cause first. Once you know the cause, you can correct the imbalance with shoe inserts or by exercises to stretch or strengthen your arch or the involved muscles.

Varicose Veins

Description: Symptoms range from unsightly purple veins with absolutely no pain, through mild nagging aching or itching in the legs and muscle fatigue, to swelling, discoloration of the skin, continual pain, and even ulcers from poor circulation. Varicose veins are stretched, distended, dilated blood vessels with weak walls. These veins have weak valves that don't close tightly enough to prevent the blood from flowing backward and downward under the pull of gravity, so the blood pools in your legs, stretches out the veins, and causes pain and pressure. About 40 percent of all women, and a smaller percentage of men, develop varicose veins. They run in families—you simply inherit the weak valves or the thin-walled inelastic veins. Thus, if your mother or grandmother had varicose veins, you probably will, but you may prevent or at least minimize them by vigorously exercising your legs every day. As you exercise, your leg muscles contract and squeeze around the veins to keep them firm. The muscles also pump or milk the blood back to your heart. This prevents the overstretching that comes from increased amounts of blood pooling in your legs.

If you have a tendency to varicose veins, they can develop from a variety of causes. Standing for long periods draws the blood down into your legs and keeps it there to pool, thus stretching your veins. Wearing garters, girdles, or other constricting garments around your groin or legs forces your muscles to work harder to push the blood back to the heart. Obesity, pregnancy, or sitting for long hours all increase abdominal pressure on the groin veins and improve your chances of pooling blood in your legs. Exercise does not cause varicose veins.

Home Treatment: If you already have varicose veins, exercise won't correct the varicosity, but it may alleviate the pain by reducing the amount of blood pooled in your veins. Wear support stockings or elastic bandages all day, but particularly when you exercise. The stockings compress the walls of the veins and divert blood into deeper nonvaricosed veins. Support stockings are particularly important when you lift weights. In addition, expressly strengthen your leg and thigh musculature for added support when you strain to pick up heavy weights. If you play contact sports, avoid blows to your legs: A sharp blow to a large varicose vein may break the vein wall and cause a hemorrhage. If you bicycle, don't bend over your bars far enough to cut off the circulation in your groin. If it hurts to exercise on land, try swimming. The horizontal position of your legs and the buoyancy of the water take away much of the pressure, and kicking relieves the rest.

With any exercise, your legs will tire and ache sooner than they would without varicose veins because the pooled blood does not carry away lactic-acid muscle wastes or return to the heart for oxygen, leaving your muscles with less than the optimal amount of oxygen.

At the end of a workout, keep moving slowly until your pulse is down below 100—walk if you've been running, ride at a leisurely pace if you've been cycling, but don't just stop and rest. An athlete's cool-down is designed to prevent the pooling of blood in the legs, a problem you already have. When your pulse is down below 100, sit or lie down with your feet elevated to drain the rest of the excess blood from your legs. Don't just stand around after exercise.

Standing or kneeling for extended periods is terrible for your varicose veins, even if you wear support hose. Straining during bowel movements also aggravates your condition, as do obesity and pregnancy. At night, sleep with your feet elevated to drain the blood back to your heart.

If your varicose veins are particularly painful, your doctor may recommend surgically removing them, using a procedure called stripping. Until a few years ago, this operation required a three- to six-day hospital stay. Now, most surgical stripping is done on an ambulatory basis. Surgery is performed in the morning, and you walk out of the hospital that afternoon; most people return to work the next day.

Calf Muscle Cramp

Description: Also called charley horse. (This is one of two usages of "charley horse." The other refers to a bruise in the quadriceps, the muscle on the front of the thigh.) Sudden grabbing pain, sometimes preceded by a growing tightness in the muscle; may be caused by insufficient oxygen and buildup of lactic acid from overstress or an inadequate warm-up, by the sheath of connective tissue strangling enlarged well-developed muscles and cutting down on their blood supply (posterior compartment syndrome), by the loss of mineral salts and water in hot weather, by exercising (or even resting) with your toes gently or aggressively pointed, by leg-length discrepancy (the cramp is usually

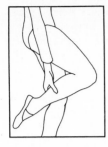

ACUPRESSURE FOR LEG CRAMP

in the shorter leg), by over-pronation (rolling ankles inward), or by irregularly worn shoes.

Home Treatment: As for any cramp, stop immediately and try to massage it away. Straighten and stretch the muscle. Stand on that foot or pull the toes upward. If that doesn't work, hobble over to the nearest ice pack and apply it to the cramp for ten minutes. (Or use the ten-minutes-on, fifteen-minutes-off technique you use for RICE until the cramp is gone.) Stretch out the muscle slowly and deliberately with calf stretches and Achilles stretches. Use acupressure to relieve the pain. You have a choice of two points: the web between your thumb and forefinger, and your upper lip.

Acupressure for Cramp: To use the first pressure point, firmly pinch and push on the web of the hand on the same side of your body as the affected leg—if, for example, you have a cramp in your left leg, squeeze the thumb web on your left hand and hold for twenty or thirty seconds. To use the second point, press the V in your upper lip with your forefinger, or pinch it by placing your thumb inside your lip and your forefinger outside your lip, and hold for twenty to thirty seconds.

Acupressure performs miracles on cramps. If your cramp does not let up, and the pulse in your foot and ankle is weak (indicating that the popliteal artery in the back of your knee and into your calf is constricted), you probably have a posterior compartment syndrome. A fasciotomy, a surgical procedure in which the fascia is slit, will relieve the pressure and permit you to return to full and pain-free activity.

Prevention: Everyone gets a cramp once in a while. However, if you get them frequently, they are probably interfering with your workouts and cutting down on the time you can exercise each session. Prevention for you is more important than cure. Stretch very thoroughly to warm up your muscles before your workout. If you already warm up conscientiously, change your pattern. Warm up as usual, then do a light cardiovascular warm-up (jog a mile or two, cycle slowly for ten minutes, or swim a few laps at a leisurely pace—whatever gets your heart rate up or makes you sweat). Then stretch your calf muscles again with calf stretches and Achilles stretches and with heel and toes. This increases the blood flow to your muscles. Start your regular workout, but stop every ten or fifteen minutes for stretching. Cool down thoroughly. Strengthen your shin muscles to balance your scrupulously stretched calf muscles. Keep your muscles warm by wearing high socks or dancing tights. Add a heel lift or arch support to each shoe, or remove it if you already wear one. Wear shock-absorbing shoes. Change your kicking flutter during swimming. Apply heat before exercising to warm your muscles and start the blood flowing. For properly functioning muscle fibers, eat foods rich in potassium (bananas, tomatoes, oranges, potatoes), magnesium (beans, peas, nuts, green leafy vegetables), and calcium (dairy products, broccoli, beans, oysters, and turnip and mustard greens). Many of these suggestions apply to night cramps. If you don't have circulatory problems, stretching before bedtime, wearing socks to bed, replacing potassium, magnesium, or calcium lost during the day (especially if you are taking diuretic medication), eliminating coffee, tea, cocoa, chocolate, cold soft drinks, and any other caffeine relatives from your diet (they make your muscles contract) may help. In addition, put a pillow or footboard under the covers at the foot of the bed to raise the covers off your feet. Blankets sometimes press your feet so that you point your toes.

Shin Splints

Description: Hot searing pain and tenderness on your tibia or shinbone along its inner, outer, or front side, or deep inside the shin at the back of the bone. Pain may occur just above the ankle or run all the way up the shin. It diminishes within an hour or two of rest. Stretching the shin during a shin splint sometimes makes it worse. If the pain is along the inside of the leg, you may have a stress fracture, especially if the sore area is only an inch in diameter and tender to the touch. Shin splint is a wastebasket term for several overuse syndromes: swelling of the periosteum, the lining of the tibia; swelling of the tendons that anchor the muscle to the bone; or enlargement or swelling of the shin muscles inside a tight and restrictive tube of connective tissue (anterior compartment syndrome). This constriction reduces the blood flow the leg muscles need to contract smoothly. Figure skaters, dancers, race walkers, and runners are particularly susceptible, as is anyone who walks or runs on hard surfaces. Frequently, the muscles running down the inside of your shin, past the inner ankle and into your inner arch, are overtaxed, because they and their tendons must maintain your arch while you walk, run, or jump. Over-pronation (rolling your ankles inward), coupled with exercising on too soft a surface, may be another cause.

Home Treatment: RICE and calf and Achilles stretches (actually stretching the shin muscles may make a shin splint worse). While resting your shin splints, ride a bicycle or swim to stay in shape. If the outside of your calf swells up or becomes hard, or if the pain persists or intensifies after two hours, you may have an anterior compartment syndrome, a fairly common injury in distance runners and cross-country skiers. A fasciotomy, or surgical decompression (see **Calf Muscle Cramp**), relieves the pressure very effectively.

Prevention: Shin splints are very stubborn. Experiment with some or all of the following: Stretch your calf muscles with calf and Achilles stretches and heel and toes. Wear heel lifts. Strengthen the shin muscles by performing ten-pound kiddie kicks, which work your shin muscles while they strengthen your quads. If you have chronic fatigue, aching, or stiffness in your legs, cut back your workouts *before* you develop shin splints. If one leg is longer than the other, build up the short leg. Wear full shoe inserts to cushion your feet during impact. Wear heel lifts or heel cushions. Work out on wood or otherwise springy (not soft) surfaces. Wear high socks to keep your muscles warm. Run backwards or climb stairs backwards steadily for ten or fifteen minutes every day. This reverses the effects of forward motion—strengthening the muscles you usually stretch, and stretching the muscles you usually tighten.

Tibial Stress Fracture

Description: Deep pain at one spot along shinbone. Spot very tender to the touch. Very common among ballet dancers and runners.

Any stress fracture, also called fatigue fracture or march fracture, is marked by sudden or gradually building, often excruciating, localized pain, sometimes accompanied by swelling, tenderness and reddening of skin, all somewhat alleviated by rest. Pain increases with activity. The pain, located at one easily identifiable spot, usually hurts when you press on it from above and below. (Tendon and ligament injuries, in contrast, usually are sensitive only on one side.) If you have a particular circumscribed spot that swells up and hurts when you tap it with your fingers, you probably have a stress fracture. These hard-to-detect tiny cracks in the surface of your bones—most frequently the ball of the foot, hip, thigh, and lower leg, but occasionally even the ribs and pelvis—only show up on x-rays about half the time. They show up on bone scans almost 100 percent of the time. Stress fractures are caused by repeatedly overloading the injured part against some firm resistance, such as running on a concrete track. They may also be caused by biomechanical abnormalities such as bones with pronounced curves, over-pronating (inward-rolling) ankles, or muscle imbalances; they are *not* caused by trauma. Women suffer stress fractures of the lower leg ten times as frequently as men. This may be due to their relative lack of training or to their wider hips. It may also be due to wide hips, bowlegs, and an inward bend of the thigh bone where it attaches to the hip socket. Possible complications: recurrences; complete break.

Home Treatment: RICE. With rest, stress fractures usually heal themselves; casts are rarely necessary. You don't have to turn into a marshmallow, however. Substitute another aerobic exercise—swim, cycle, run in water while wearing a life jacket—as long as it puts no weight or pressure on your stress fracture. Because strong muscles absorb shock, begin non-weight-bearing strengthening exercises for the area almost immediately. Exercise both members of a muscle pair equally—quads and hamstrings, for example, or biceps and triceps. If one muscle is tighter than the other, you set up an imbalance. For that reason, stretch out both members of the pair equally too. Wear store-bought arch supports, heel lifts, or custom-made orthotics if they are appropriate. Gradually return to your sport after your symptoms are gone.

Prevention Do not work out on hard surfaces; wear shoes with cushioned soles or springy innersoles; strengthen and stretch the entire leg, front and back.

Fibular Stress Fracture

Description: Deep pain at one spot along lower outside edge of calf. Spot very tender to the touch. See **Tibial stress fracture.**

Catch in the Calf

Description: Sharp pain in calf muscle (gastrocemius) as the result of a scar forming over a tear in the muscle fibers.

Home Treatment: Massage it away. Apply ice.

Prevention: Stretch the calf and shin muscles thoroughly during your warm-up. Add a small heel lift or sponge heel insert to relax the gastroc. Wear ripple-soled shoes and avoid hard surfaces.

Trick Knee

Description: Also called locked knee, weak knee, collapsing knee. Knee either gives out or locks in spasm. Usually caused by torn ligaments or cartilage combined with weak knee muscles. Injury occurs from any jumping, pivoting, or start-stop exercise and from skiing.

Home Treatment and Prevention: For locked knee, shake it, try to extend it suddenly, or let the leg dangle so that gravity helps you realign it. For all types, strengthen the muscles around the knee

with kiddie kicks, hamsters, run-'em-out-of-gym-class sprints, and dumbbell lunges. Severe cases may require surgery.

Water on the Knee

Description: Large, puddly swelling and accumulation of synovial (lubricating) fluid under the muscles and skin of the kneecap or inside the joint (under the cap itself). Not an injury, this is a symptom of infection, strain, trauma, or arthritis, and a signal to see a doctor.

Pain Around the Kneecap

Description: Minor ache without history of trauma. A form of bursitis caused by excessive rotation of the knee during bicycle pedaling.

Home Treatment: RICE.

Prevention: Wear cycling shoes and cleats to affix the shoe to the pedal.

Runner's Knee

Description: Also called basketball knee. Pain behind the kneecap during exercise. This is a catch-all term for a variety of tendinitises, tenosynovitises, bursitises, torn cartilages, and more. It usually results from backpacking or running downhill or from excessive pronation (rolling your ankle inward) which forces your lower leg to turn in while your kneecap is pulled outward by three of the four muscles of the quadriceps.

Home Treatment and Prevention: RICE, if pain is severe enough. Kiddie kicks and hamsters to strengthen the quads and hamstrings and stabilize your knee. Stretch the calf muscles and hamstrings. Wear arch supports or heel wedges to prevent overpronation.

Kneecap Chondromalacia

Description: Also called runner's knee and chondromalacia patellae. Mild to excruciating pain behind or around kneecap when walking downstairs (or, less frequently, upstairs), getting out of a deep chair, going downhill, kneeling, or doing activities involving knee bends. Stiffness, creaking or grinding noise and gravelly feeling or popping (crepitus), occasional knee weakness or locking, stiffness and pain from sitting or otherwise bending knee relieved by straightening the leg. No history of trauma. Involves softening or fraying of the cartilage on the inner surface of the kneecap, owing to misalignment of the leg or foot, overweight, or weak ligaments around the knee. Exists to some extent in everyone over thirty. In the general population, twice as many women as men suffer from chondromalacia, but among athletes the incidence is about equal between the sexes.

Home Treatment: RICE. Stretch the calf muscles and Achilles tendon with calf stretches and Achilles stretches and the hamstrings with gravity toe touches, towel stretches, and runner's starts. Strengthen the quadriceps to stabilize your knee by doing kiddie kicks. If your knee hurts too much to do kiddie kicks, start out with isometric quads.

Isometric Quads: Sit on the edge of a table or high bench and straighten your leg in front of you. Hold for ten seconds, then lower it, for one rep. Do ten reps, and repeat as many times during the day as you can. When these become easy, add a pound or two of ankle weight and build up to ten or twenty pounds per leg.

When your leg is stronger, advance to kiddie kicks, using as much weight as you can handle without pain. Do the same exercises on the uninjured leg so that you know how much weight your injured leg will be able to handle when it is healed. Strengthen your hamstrings with hamsters, run-'em-out-of-gym-class sprints, or dumbbell lunges to avoid a muscle imbalance that will lead to a hamstring pull. Wear arch supports, orthotics, or other shoe inserts to prevent over-pronation (inward-rolling ankles.) Work out on surfaces with some give. Don't run on banked tracks; or, if you must, keep your sore knee downhill. Avoid jumping and stop-start sports such as tennis, basketball, and volleyball. Chondromalacia comes and goes. Continue with your quad and hamstring exercises after the episode is past, to prevent recurrences.

Most cases respond to some combination of these nonsurgical therapies. However, if your pain is intense and isn't relieved by any of these mea-sures, see your doctor. If surgery is recommended, first get a definitive diagnosis by arthroscopy. There are about 150 different surgical procedures for correcting chondromalacia, a sure sign that doctors don't really understand the problem yet. So far, the most successful are performed using the arthroscope and involve releasing the tight lateral structures forcing your knee out of line. Less successful is shaving the underside of the knee to make it smoother.

Osgood-Schlatter Disease

Description: Also called football knee, rugby knee, osteochondritis, osteochondrosis of the tibial tubercle, and tibial tubercle apophysitis. Pain between kneecap and shinbone, often accompanied by swelling or tenderness about an inch below the kneecap (the area of the tibial tubercle, the bony bump below the knee). Aggravated by kneeling, running, climbing, jumping, and forceful straightening of the knee. Often affects both knees. Occurs only in adolescents. The tibial tubercle is pulled free away from the shaft of the tibia at the weak, unossified (not yet bony) growth plate by direct or indirect trauma, or by the pull of the strong quadriceps on the weak growth plate at the top of the tibia or shinbone. Some physicians believe the injury is an overuse syndrome and is caused by heavy exercise; others believe that a sudden contraction of the quadriceps pulls the tendon attached to the tibial tubercle and yanks the tubercle free.

Home Treatment: RICE for pain. Because the condition is self-limiting, ending when the growth plate turns to bone, surgery and casts are indicated only in the event of excruciating pain or the development of an ossicle, a separated bonelet.

Jumper's Knee

Description: Also called basketballer's knee, placekicker's knee, runner's knee, or patellar tendinitis. Pain immediately below the kneecap, at the point where the patellar tendon from the tibia (shinbone) attaches to the lower part of the patella (kneecap); less frequently, pain just above the kneecap at the attachment of the quadriceps tendon. Small area inflamed and tender to the touch just below the kneecap; crepitus on movement may also be present. Hurts only during or after jumping. This form of tendinitis is caused by the stress of a strong impact traveling up the leg to be absorbed by the knee and may come on gradually. Frequently seen in basketball and volleyball players, and in long and high jumpers, but does occur in some runners.

Home Treatment: RICE. When the pain is gone, carefully stretch your quads, hamstrings, and calf and shin muscles with storks, towel stretches, calf stretches, and geisha kneels. Strengthen the same muscles with kiddie kicks, hamsters, and heel and toes.

Prevention: Wear shoe inserts or orthotics to correct any biomechanical imbalances and to absorb some of the impact. Wear cushioned shoes. Play on springy surfaces. Land on the balls of your feet.

Torn Knee Cartilage

Description: Also called medial meniscus tear or lateral meniscus tear, depending on location. Acute and sudden pain often accompanied by popping noise; knee gives out; after a while, it may support you enough to walk on it. Pain may be due to immediate twisting trauma or to previous trauma which degenerates over time. You probably have torn or separated one of the cartilages lining the thigh or shinbone. It is possible, however, that you have torn one of the semilunar cartilages (menisci) cushioning the knee joint, but women have far fewer of these tears than men. If a doctor says you have a meniscal tear, request arthrography or arthroscopy for verification.

Home Treatment: Rest, for mild cases; see a doctor for acute cases. Once you have torn a cartilage, it will pop in and out of place each time you rotate your knee. This causes a small amount of wear-and-tear damage to the joint, perhaps leading to a degenerative form of arthritis. However, arthroscopy or the surgical removal of the offending piece of cartilage will probably lead to an early bout with the same type of arthritis, so surgery is indicated only when the pain is persistent or the knee repeatedly locks or gives way.

Prevention: Strengthen your quadriceps with kiddie kicks and your hamstrings with hamsters to stabilize your knee.

Wrestler's Knee

Description: Also called housemaid's knee or prepatellar bursitis. Swelling on top of the knee as the result of a blow, fall, scrape, or other trauma. Caused by the accumulation of fluid or blood under the loose skin over the kneecap—a minor though grotesque injury.

Home Treatment: Clean and disinfect all abrasions, apply ice, and protect the knee from further bumps with some sort of pad. Swelling should go down within two weeks. If the swelling is severe, or if there is evidence of infection from the abrasions, see a doctor.

Overuse Knee Sprain

Description: Also called swimmer's knee or collateral ligament syndrome. Pain along the inside or outside of the knee without any history of trauma. Little or no swelling. In breaststrokers, the pain runs along the inside of the knee because of overuse stress on the medial collateral ligament stabilizing that part of the knee. In freestyle swimmers, soccer players, and dancers, pain may be on the inside or outside. Pain on the outside indicates overuse stress on the lateral collateral ligament. (There are other causes of swimmer's knee, but they are treated the same way.)

Home Treatment: Ice packs or RICE.

Prevention: Apply ice packs for fifteen minutes immediately after every workout. Swimmers: Correct your technique during the frog kick (see chapter 5); alternate with other strokes. Dry-land athletes: For inner knee pain, wear arch supports to prevent over-pronation (ankles rolling inward); for outer knee pain, wear heel wedges to raise the outside of your heel.

Sprained Knee

Description: Pain along the inside or outside of the knee, with or without swelling, as the result of a twisting trauma or of being hit on the outside of the knee (as during football, hockey, basketball, or soccer contact).

Home Treatment: As with all sprains, RICE for one or two days, until swelling and pain subside. Then start moving your knee gingerly, beginning with easy stretching exercises and working up to full use of the leg. If pain has not subsided significantly within twenty-four hours, see a doctor. If the injury is serious and requires surgery, any delay will allow the ligaments to shrink and weaken, which drastically reduces your chances for full recovery.

Prevention: Don't wear cleats during contact sports because they anchor your foot to the ground, exaggerating the twisting force on your knee when you are hit. Strengthen your quadriceps with kiddie kicks and your hamstrings with hamsters to thicken the ligaments. Jack Rockwell, who designed the universal warm-up program, suggests that people who damage their knees by being hit at high speeds should do their strengthening exercises at high speeds to train their muscle fibers to absorb such impacts.

Iliotibial Band Syndrome

Description: Pain anywhere along the outside of the knee and down the outside of the tibia (shinbone). This overuse injury develops as the tendon-like iliotibial band rubs over the side of your thigh bone. The iliotibial band extends along the outside of your thigh from the gluteus muscles attached to your ilium (hip bone) to the outside of your tibia. Your knee aches because the iliotibial band helps stabilize your knee. Iliotibial band syndrome is a sign of training too far and too fast. It particularly afflicts bowlegged people.

Home Treatment: Treat as for tendinitis, with RICE. When the pain is gone, stretch the iliotibial band by doing calf stretches while jutting your hip out to the side. Check your shoes for worn spots. Repair the soles and wear shoe inserts or orthotics to correct your bowlegs or the imbalances indicated by uneven wear. If you run, avoid downhills and speedwork. Shorten your stride.

Charley Horse

Description: Also called quadriceps contusion. (There are two kinds of charley horses. The other is a cramp in the calf.) Pain in the front of the thigh, accompanied by intramuscular bleeding and swelling as the result of a direct blow. The blow pushes one or more of the four muscles of the quadriceps into the femur (thigh bone). The injury is more severe if the quads are relaxed.

Home Treatment: Stretch the quads by bending your knee in order to minimize the intramuscular bleeding and swelling. Apply RICE to the fully flexed knee at least twice. For the next two or three days, use ICE frequently, with or without the rest, then decrease to once or twice a day. When the pain and swelling are down, stretch the quads slowly by bending the knee through its full range of motion. Graduate to storks. You can continue to play with a mild charley horse, but you should wait three to seven days with a moderate one. If you have a severe case, with extreme pain and a large amount of hemorrhaging, see your doctor.

Sciatica

Description: Also called sciatic neuralgia or sciatic neuritis. Severe searing, stabbing, or throbbing pain along the back of the thigh buttocks, thigh, and, perhaps, down the calf into the foot. Not an injury but a symptom, sciatica may be caused by pressure on the sciatic nerve (running down the back of your thigh into your lower leg) from an intervertebral disk, by a leg-length discrepancy that tilts your pelvis, or by pressure on the nerve from the thigh muscles caused by bad sitting posture or a poorly designed seat.

Home Treatment and Prevention: Find the cause of the symptom and eliminate it. Strengthen your abdominal muscles with killer sit-ups to correct your posture. Strengthen your gluteal muscles with run-'em-out-of-gym-class sprints and your lumbar muscles (the back muscles between your ribs and your pelvis) with locusts. (*Note:* Locusts may aggravate the condition in some people with low back problems. Test yourself with an easy locust or two before you do them wholeheartedly.) Keep your lower back and hamstrings flexible with plows. If plows hurt your back; substitute towel stretches and wasp waisters or king of Siam kowtows. Do not hyperextend your back, as in back arches or back bends. While running, tilt your pelvis forward and keep your lower back straight. Wear cushioned shoes, shoe inserts, or orthotics to correct any structural imbalances. Do not overstrain. You are more susceptible than most to the effects of trying to go too far too fast. Don't lift and carry heavy packages, and don't lift weights with exercises that strain your lower back. Keep your own weight hovering around its ideal percent of fat.

Irritation, Rash, or Rawness Between the Thighs

Description: Comes from rubbing your sweaty legs together during exercise.

Home Treatment: Coat the area with petroleum jelly (Vaseline) before beginning your workout. Wear tubes of cloth fashioned from pantyhose, long cotton underwear, or sewn-together elastic bandages. (Put the seams on the outsides of your legs.) Lose weight or firm up your inner thighs with groin squeezes, side leg lifts, or front leg lifts.

Groin Pain

Description: Sharp or dull pain, running in any or all of several directions: down the inside of the thigh from the crotch to the middle thigh; up from the crotch toward the bladder; or curving from the crotch to the hips and around to the sacrum, the part of the spine just above the buttocks. Moving your thigh and knee outward aggravates the condition. Rest relieves or eliminates the pain. May develop gradually or suddenly, as the result of tendinitis, bursitis, or leg-length discrepancies; or myositis (inflammation of a muscle). A traumatic groin injury is usually provoked by a sudden thrusting overstretch of the leg and thigh—kicking outward to the side while rotating your foot outward during a soccer game, for example. It may also be caused by gripping something very broad, such as the back of a rodeo bull, between your thighs. If there is a point of tenderness anywhere in the area, you may have a stress fracture. If the pain travels down the back of your leg toward or beyond your knee in a sharp line, you may have sciatica.

Home Treatment: RICE for a few days will handle a mild injury. However, moderate and severe groin pain is very stubborn and may require six to eight weeks of rest and a few months to recover before you can start rehabilitation exercises. Because this miserable malady has diffuse causes, one or more of the following suggestions may help. After three days of RICE, use warm sitz baths, electric heating pads, or moist heat packs. As soon as the pain is tolerable, start stretching as far as you can, lying on your back and moving the leg out and in through its full range of motion, rotating your foot in every direction. When the pain has subsided further, perform these same exercises standing up, adding increasingly heavy ankle weights to the affected leg to strengthen your hip abductors and adductors. Apply a heating pad to the area every night. Every day, ice down the affected area for ten minutes, then massage it, perform your range-of-motion exercises as above, and ice it down again for another ten minutes.

Prevention: Check for leg-length discrepancies or other structural imbalances and correct them with shoe inserts or orthotics. Unevenly worn shoes suggests a structural imbalance. Do not wear worn-out shoes. Strengthen the inner thigh muscles with a slow-motion version of groin squeezes, taking twenty seconds to push in, and twenty seconds to push out, for one rep. When these become easy, graduate to split shifts. Strengthen your lower back with locusts and your abdominals with killer sit-ups. Stretch these same muscles with runner's starts, wall splits and hunkers, wasp waisters, and king of Siam kowtows. Also stretch your hamstrings with gravity toe touches and towel stretches. Run backwards or climb stairs backwards at least ten or fifteen minutes every day. This reverses the effects of forward motion, strengthening the muscles you usually stretch and stretching the muscles you usually strengthen.

Numb Groin

Description: Numbness or pain and tingling anywhere around the groin after long bicycle rides. The nerves running from your spine to your legs are squeezed between the seat and the bones in your bottom and upper thigh.

Home Treatment and Prevention: Stop riding and walk around until sensation returns. Tip your seat *slightly* forward. Raise the handlebars so that you put more weight on your hands and less on your buttocks. Use a wider seat.

Hernia

Description: Deep-seated, wrenching pain in the groin, at the top of the thigh, or at the margin where the abdomen meets the thigh. Usually followed by a bulge. A loop of intestine breaks through a congenital or traumatic weak spot in the muscle wall when you lift or move something very heavy, or after continual or repeated straining. Inguinal hernias occur in the fold in front of the hip joint, where the abdomen and thigh meet, and strike men more frequently than women. Femoral hernias occur in the upper thigh, just below the groin, and strike more women than men.

Home Treatment: None. Even if the pain is not excessive, see your doctor, for the loop of intestine can become trapped and strangulated in the small opening, cutting off its blood supply—a condition as life-threatening as a ruptured appendix. Trusses may ease the pain, but they can't prevent this incarceration, as doctors call it.

Prevention: Don't move or lift weights significantly heavier than you are accustomed to. Warm up your muscles before lifting heavy objects, and then lift by squatting close to them, holding them against you, and straightening your knees while keeping your back straight. Strengthen your abdominal muscles with killer sit-ups.

Hamstring Pull

Description: Also called hamstring strain. Sudden yank or gripping pain, or definite feeling of tightness at the back of the thigh. Usually excruci-

ating—frequently the victim pulls up lame and can't even walk on the leg. Pain is caused by anything from a slight tear to a full-fledged rupture of any of the three hamstring muscles running down from the rump bone (sacrum) across the hip, down the back of the thigh, to the back of the tibia or shinbone. If you strengthen and shorten the hamstrings, as in distance running, without strengthening and shortening the quadriceps at the same time, you are likely to tear some hamstring fibers. Conversely, if you strengthen and shorten the quadriceps while ignoring the hamstrings, as in sprinting, you are also liable for tears. A sudden lunge, shift of direction, or high kick with inadequately stretched and warmed muscles may pull the muscles, as may simple muscle fatigue.

Home Treatment: RICE, as for other strains and pulls. It may take eight to ten weeks to heal.

Prevention: Strengthen your quads with kiddie kicks and your hamstrings with hamsters. Ideally, your hamstrings should be able to lift about 60 percent of the weight your quads can. Stretch your quads with storks and work toward exaggerated flexibility in your hamstrings with gravity toe touches, towel stretches, runner's starts, and plows.

Buttocks Pain

Description: Sharp or dull pain during exercise in the upper half of the buttocks, sometimes followed by a dull ache in the hips. This inflammation of the top of the hamstring muscle where it inserts into the pelvis is usually due to an overstrengthened, and thus overshortened, hamstring muscle.

Home Treatment: Pain rarely persists after exercise, so no treatment is necessary.

Prevention: Stretch your hamstrings with gravity toe touches, towel stretches, runner's starts (which also get your iliopsoas), and plows. Stretch your calves with calf stretches.

Snapping Hip

Description: Also called clicking hip. Noise or feeling of something snapping on side of hip when knee is bent and hip moves inward. Fibrous bands of connective tissue slide and snap over the protuberance on the side of the femur (thigh bone). Hip does not actually dislocate. May be caused by hip bursitis or other unknown stimuli.

Home Treatment: None, if painless. If it hurts, treat as for Hip Bursitis.

Bowler's Hip

Description: Also called gluteus medius tendinitis. Pain, sometimes accompanied by tenderness deep inside the side of the hip joint, above the trochanter of the femur (the bony side of the hip). Pain sometimes radiates to the front of the hip above its bony protuberance (the iliac crest). Although it may result from any running movement, this inflammation of one of the tendons of the hip joint is most frequently caused by twisting the low back while extending one leg, as in the bowler's lunge.

Home Treatment and Prevention: RICE, as for any tendinitis. When it stops hurting, stretch the area with wasp waisters. Correct your form.

Hip Bursitis

Description: Also called golfer's hip or trochanteric bursitis, depending on location. Severe pain on the outer side of the hip (trochanteric bursitis), or over the bony protuberance at the front of the hip, or in the upper rear hip and lower back. Tenderness over any bony protuberance and the feeling that the hip and thigh bones are grating together. Hip may pop out of joint. May be aggravated by moving your thigh *toward* the midline. May be caused by overuse; imbalanced gait; blow to the bone; or infection. Location depends on which bursa (sac or pad of lubricating fluid) is inflamed, but treatment is similar for all.

Home Treatment: As for any bursitis, RICE. (For mild pain, reduce activity for a few days or until pain leaves; for severe pain, rest completely.) Look for trigger points. If one leg is shorter than the other, put a heel lift in the shoe of the shorter leg. If your foot pronates too much, use arch supports or custom-made orthotics. Correct your technique to minimize or eliminate excessive twisting

of your body. (Keep your rear leg flexed, for example throughout your entire golf backswing.) Stretch your hip muscles with wasp waisters.

Hip Muscle Strain

Description: Also called runner's hip. Tenderness and diffuse pain in the front of the hip, or in the middle or lower part of the rear hip and buttocks and/or in the lower back, especially after extended use or when the thigh is extended out to the side. Caused by overuse or overtraining, leg-length discrepancy, flat feet, or high arches. If your abdominal muscles are weak, your iliopsoas (hip flexors) may have shortened, tilting your pelvis forward.

Home Treatment: As for any muscle pull, RICE. Strenghthen your abdominal muscles with killer sit-ups to balance your hip flexors. Stretch your hip flexors with runner's starts; stretch the backs and sides of your hips with wasp waisters. Place a heel lift in the shoe of your shorter leg, or use arch supports or wedges to correct other structural imbalances. Exercise on surfaces with some give.

Hip Pointer

Description: Also called iliac crest contusion. Pain and sometimes disabling tenderness on the bony protuberance at the upper front of your hip, on each side of your belly. Pain often shows up when you cough and may last for a few moments or for hours. Tingling or burning in some part of the leg of the injured side may also occur, as may an inability to lift your thigh. A direct blow during contact sports or when casting on the gymnastic uneven parallel bars crushes one or more of the nerves, veins, or muscles in the area against the bones of the front hip. Rare in women playing contact sports, because they have deposits of body fat to protect their hips. However, gymnasts and skinny girls are susceptible to this injury.

Home Treatment: Assess the severity. If pain gradually subsides within an hour, and if you can lie down on your back and lift your leg so that your foot points to the ceiling, *and* if you can hold your leg straight out in front of you while you sit in a chair, you have a mild hip pointer. Cold compresses and pressure applied on and off (as in RICE) for an hour should relieve the initial pain. Repeat the cold and compression several times over the next day or two to reduce the swelling and black-and-blue color. If your leg below the bruise is numb, or if you can't pass both of the above diagnostic tests, or if the pain is severe after an hour of cold and compression, you may have partially or completely damaged a nerve or ruptured a muscle. See your doctor.

Prevention: Use properly fitted hip pads designed for gymnastics or contact sports.

BACK

Back problems are very complicated. See your doctor if you have:
- severe upper or lower back pain unresponsive to aspirin or aspirin substitutes
- pain lasting more than three days
- upper back pain along your spine
- lower back pain, worse at rest or at night, accompanied by pain or weakness in your foot or leg or by pain radiating down the back of your leg, or by difficulty urinating or moving your bowels; pain accentuated by coughing, sneezing, straining or standing, all signs of a degenerating or rupturing disk, a stress fracture (spondyloloisis) or vertebral dislocation (spondylolisthesis)

Lower Back Pain

Description: Moderate in intensity, on one or both sides; aggravated by the twisting movement of a tennis serve, golf swing, cross-country ski poling, the hyperextension of back bends, or the butterfly stroke. Pain eases when you rest and diminishes within two or three days. You may have a degenerating vertebral disk (the padding between two vertebra); a pinched lining between some of the small joints in your spinal column; a pinched nerve; a small stress fracture (called spondylolysis); a forward slippage of the entire spinal column; leg-length discrepancy; or excessive stretching of the ligaments stabilizing the spine.

Home Treatment: Cold packs and rest; aspirin or aspirin substitute for pain. If it doesn't hurt try pelvic slants.

Pelvic Slants: Lie on your back on the floor, legs flat. Keeping your trunk and legs on the floor, point your toes while you tighten your buttocks (gluteus) muscles and suck in your gut. Hold for five to ten seconds, then flex your feet so that your toes aim at the ceiling while you relax your gluteus and abdominal muscles, for one rep. Perform as many as you can before fatigue or boredom sets in, and do these four to six times a day. This exercise realigns your pelvis and takes the pressure off the nerves in your lower back.

Prevention: Eighty-one percent of all backaches are caused by weak muscles or nervous tension. Relax and stretch your back several times a day with birds, king of Siam kowtows, or, if you feel very flexible, plows. If you have weak abdominal muscles—and most people do—your lower back will curve too much and give you a chronic backache. Strengthen your front and side abdominals with killer sit-ups and twisting sit-ups. If they don't hurt your back, do twenty locusts every day to strengthen your back extensors. If these do hurt, avoid them and any other exercise that forces your back to arch markedly (hyperextend)—don't do back bends, pole vaulting, or the butterfly stroke until you are entirely free from pain. If you are a weight lifter, lift with a round back, which pulls the posterior spinal ligaments to their full length and supports and straightens your back as you lift. Don't use the Olympic-style straight-back lift. Don't wear high heels. They shift your center of gravity forward the way pregnancy and overweight do. Your back arches to compensate and gives you a chronic backache. Correct your posture. Military posture, with your shoulders back, your chest out, and your pelvis back, is hard on your back. Instead, stand or sit with the slight slouch of a fashion model, with your pelvis tilted forward, your buttocks tucked under, and your abdominal muscles pulled up rather than sucked in. If your legs are uneven, they throw your whole posture out of whack. Your pelvis tilts to compensate for the shorter leg, making the longer leg functionally shorter. Insert a heel wedge into one of your shoes to balance your legs. Placing the wedge in the shoe of the shorter leg works for some problems, and placing it in the shoe of the longer leg works for others. Experiment.

Cracking Noises

Description: If there is no pain, the noises are as harmless as cracking your knuckles. Neither cracking your back nor cracking your knuckles will lead to arthritis. The noise is simply the sound made when pressure is suddenly released, or when a tendon or ligament snaps across another tendon, ligament, or bone.

Home Treatment: None, as long as there is no pain or swelling.

Prevention: Warm up gradually to make your ligaments elastic before you stress them.

Upper Back Pain

Description: Moderate, not along the spine. Usually a muscle pull caused by inadequate warm-up before swimming, tennis, baseball, football, or other arm strength sports.

Home Treatment: RICE.

Prevention: Proper warm-up.

SHOULDERS

Stitch

Description: Stabbing, aching, or searing pain in the top of the shoulder and neck in the midst of huffing and puffing exercise. Disappears when exercise ends. This is probably the most common cause of shoulder and neck pain during exercise and is the same sort of pain you get in your side or rib cage. It is a spasm of the muscles in your diaphragm caused by heavy breathing. You feel it in your upper shoulder and neck because the nerves controlling the diaphragm come from the neck region of your spinal cord.

Home Treatment: See **Side Stitch.** Press on the stitch with one hand, hold your nose with the other, and blow out forcefully but slowly through pursed lips. Even without any home remedy, the pain will go away by itself within an hour.

Prevention: See **Side Stitch.** It is possible that you feel the stitch in your shoulder instead of your side because the straps of your bra are pressing on your shoulders and against the nerves running down to the diaphragm. Release the tension on your bra straps or find another brand.

Low-grade Muscle Pain

Description: Appears toward the end of long bicycle rides. No history of trauma.

Home Treatment: If annoying, treat with cold packs, rest, posture clasps, and head twisters. Look for trigger points.

Prevention: Strengthen your trapezius muscles with shoulder shrugs.

Shoulder Separation

Description: Also called acromioclavicular sprain. Sharp, persistent, sometimes searing pain and tenderness at the point where the collarbone (clavicle) attaches to the shoulder blade. Tenderness may extend behind the joint. Sometimes accompanied by swelling. Extreme pain when you try to raise your arm to shoulder level or higher. (See **Ankle Sprain.**) This partial or complete tear of the ligament connecting the bony prominence on the point of your shoulder (acromion) with the collarbone is caused by a fall or collision (including running into a wall). In the most serious cases, the ligament connecting the front of the shoulder blade (coracoid process) with the collarbone is also torn. If a part of your collarbone seems to be sticking up, or if pain is severe, you may have fractured your collarbone or dislocated the acromioclavicular joint. See your doctor.

Home Treatment: RICE for the first twenty-four hours. To take the weight off your shoulder, carry your arm in a sling until your shoulder doesn't hurt when your arms hang loose. Exercise is important in minimizing the effects of a sprain. Begin to move your arm gently through its full range of motion as soon as pain and swelling have partially subsided—within a week or ten days for a mild sprain.

Rotator Cuff Strain

Description: Sharp or mild pain in the back of the shoulder where it meets the upper arm, sometimes accompanied by weakness or spasms in the midpoint of the movement when you move your shoulder outward. Tenderness in the upper end of the humerus (upper arm bone). Occasionally accompanied by gravely noises or sensations (crepitus) when you move your shoulder. You have pinched or torn the tendons of the rotator cuff, made up of the teres minor, supraspinatus, infraspinatus, and subscapularis muscles. These muscles stabilize and rotate the shoulder joint at its junction with the upper arm. Caused by a trauma—a fall onto your outstretched arm, for example—or by overuse, swimming long distances, or repeatedly swinging a racket, bat, or other piece of equipment upward with your arm and shoulder extended. (See **Muscle Pull.**) If you have swelling, heat, or persistent pain at rest, see **Shoulder Bursitis.**

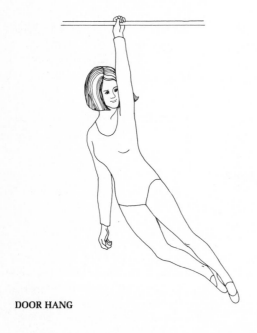

DOOR HANG

Home Treatment: RICE, as for other strains. Wear a sling to cradle your arm until your shoulder can bear its weight. As soon as you have no pain when you move your shoulder normally, stretch and strengthen your rotator cuff with door hangs—by hanging from a doorjamb or chinning bar using only your affected arm.

Prevention Stretch the rotator cuff with posture clasps and birds. Perform crossovers to strengthen the muscles which bring your shoulder toward and away from your body.

Crossovers: Lie on your back with a dumbbell in the hand of your injured arm. Straighten your arms out to the sides, then slowly bring the injured arm across your chest until the weight touches the floor next to your healthy arm. Reverse the movement to return the weight to the starting position for one rep. Do ten reps a day. Start with a 2-pound dumbbell and work up to 8 or 10 pounds.

Shoulder Bursitis

Description: Exquisite pain over the cap or the back of the shoulder where it meets the upper arm, then moderate persistent pain with the merest twinge of movement. Swelling, heat, and tenderness to the touch. Occasionally, you may hear or feel "gravel" in your shoulder cap, and you may even be able to feel little lumps with your fingers. May be caused by a blow or fall, but often caused by chronic tendinitis. The inflamed tendon develops calcium deposits and extrudes them into the bursa. If there is no swelling or heat, see **Rotator Cuff Strain.**

Home Treatment: As for any bursitis, RICE during acute pain. Carry your arm in a sling. Move your arm as soon as the acute pain is gone in order to prevent a frozen shoulder. (Your body will respond to the inflammation by forming scar tissue to wall off the inflamed area. Unless you keep the joint moving through its entire range of motion, the shoulder may stiffen up.) Bursitis is occasionally accompanied by little calcified or fibrous granules; if you feel such lumps, have them checked by a doctor, just to be on the safe side.

Prevention: Stretch your shoulders daily with posture clasps and birds. Strengthen them with arm sprints and dips. If you have no history of a blow or fall on the shoulder, assume you have shoulder tendinitis, find the cause, and cure it.

Shoulder Tendinitis

Description: Also called swimmer's, thrower's, skier's, tennis, racquetball, or . . . shoulder, depending on your sport. Acute or nagging constant pain in the front or back of the shoulder, especially during movement. Typically, it hurts to touch the inflamed spot on the tendon. There may also be some tenderness inside or behind the collarbone, where the biceps insert into the shoulder blade. As a general rule, the pain is more intense when you first wake up than after you move around and warm it up. May be accompanied by a gravelly sound or feeling (crepitus) when you move the shoulder, or by small lumps you can feel with your fingertips. These lumps indicate calcium deposits in chronically inflamed and irritated tendons. Swimmer's shoulder is a special problem because it is not the simple biceps tendinitis it once was thought to be. It now appears that one or more of three structures (the biceps tendon, the rotator cuff, or the bursa overlying these two) snags under a bridge of ligament (coracoacromial ligament) that is anchored to two bony outcroppings near the top of your shoulder blade. As these structures rub, they become irritated, inflamed, and eventually worn, like a rope frayed from rubbing on a rock.

Home Treatment: As for any tendinitis, RICE. Look for trigger points. Support your arm in a sling until the shoulder no longer hurts when the arm hangs free. Tendinitis will not go away unless you rest it. As soon as the acute pain has passed, move your shoulder gently to prevent frozen shoulder (see **Shoulder Bursitis**).

Prevention: Determine the cause. After the age of thirty-five, the forward and backward movements of your shoulders become limited unless you conscientiously stretch those muscles every day. Your movements also become restricted when you repeatedly use one set of muscles in the shoulder without using the others equally. You strengthen, shorten, and tighten one set while their antagonists remain weak and long. If you have favored one set of muscles by practicing hundreds of tennis serves, for example, or racquetball ceiling shots, stretch the muscles you have strengthened, and strengthen the muscles you have ignored. Posture clasps, door leans, and birds stretch most of the shoulder muscles. Strengthen your trunk flexors with killer sit-ups. If you have pain in the front of your shoulder, strengthen the rear shoulder muscles with push-ups. If you have pain in the back of your shoulder, strengthen the front of your shoulder girdle with push-ups, chin-ups, pull-ups, and crossovers. If you have an injury or imbalance anywhere along your body, you may compensate by placing enough stress on your shoulder to provoke a tendinitis. (Any injury anywhere in your body forces you to shift your posture and make adjustments all the way to your shoulders. Dizzy Dean, the St. Louis Cardinals' pitcher, broke his toe but continued to pitch by adjusting his style. This compensation ultimately damaged his arm and ended his baseball career.) If your legs are unequal in length, place a heel lift in the shoe of the shorter leg. Tendinitis may also come from simple overtraining. If this is the case, you have no alternative but to slow down. You can't "play through" tendinitis; it only gets worse. Continue to play, but don't do any vigorous movements that bring on pain. If necessary, modify your form to avoid any pain-provoking movements or to correct improper style. Don't fling your arm about when you stroke a ball. Instead, put your whole body behind each swing. If you have tennis shoulder, avoid overhead shots. Instead, allow the ball to bounce so that you hit ground strokes. Hit the ball at its lowest possible point, and serve with a lower toss and less exaggerated backswing. If you have racquetball shoulder, ceiling shots may be your nemesis. Shoot them underhanded from now on, instead of overhanded. If you have swimmer's shoulder, don't bring your stroking arm too far across your body. Instead, roll your body toward your arm as it strokes through the water. If the pain is in your dominant arm, alternate sides as you breathe. The arm on the breathing side always works harder. If the tendinitis is chronic, ice down your shoulder for ten minutes after each workout and again at night—whether or not the pain is severe. Unless you want to stop playing until your shoulder heals, avoid cortisone shots. Steroids reduce pain and swelling, but they weaken your tendons for forty to sixty days and make you more susceptible to tendon tears. Surgery is rarely necessary for swimmer's shoulder unless you've tried everything else over a period of a year or two.

Little League Shoulder

Description: Acute, then persistent dull pain in the shoulder joint or in the uppermost part of the upper arm in children and young adolescents. May be muscle fatigue from improper warm-up or overuse, or may involve damage to the growth plates of the upper arm bone (humerus). When you repeatedly stress the weak cartilage growth plates near the ends of bones, their blood supply is cut off, and the bone may fracture or develop irregularly.

Home Treatment: RICE for two or three days. If the pain subsides, warm up much more carefully in the future and do not overtrain. If the pain is still constant after three days, see your doctor, because any damage to the growing surfaces (epiphyses) of the bone may lead to permanent deformation or chronic tendinitis. If your doctor does diagnose an epiphysial injury, the outlook for complete recovery is still good if you rest your shoulder for a couple of months.

Collarbone Fracture

Description: Agonizing pain in the collarbone, chest, or front of shoulder, accompanied by swelling and a depression in the collarbone (clavicle), as the result of a direct fall on the point of the shoulder or a blow pushing the shoulder forward. See a doctor. If the depression in the clavicle is very deep, or if you can't breathe easily, the collarbone may be pushing into your chest. See a doctor *immediately.*

Sternoclavicular Sprain

Description: Sharp pain toward the center of, or on the bumps of, the collarbone, accompanied by tenderness anywhere along the collarbone or at the junction of collarbone and sternum (the front of the rib cage). No marked swelling or depression. This rupture of the ligaments holding the collarbone to the front of the rib cage is caused by a fall on the end of your shoulder.

Home Treatment: RICE, with as much compression as possible during the first twenty-four hours. Then, if the swelling and pain are reduced, begin to move your shoulder gingerly through its full range of motion. Continue to ice it down three times a day for three days. When the pain is only a minor inconvenience, start stretching; stand with your back to a door and grab the doorknob with your hands behind your back. Lean forward slowly until you feel a gentle pull. (Make sure the door is firmly shut.) If the pain is severe after twenty-four hours, see your doctor.

Dislocated Shoulder

Description: Also called glenohumeral dislocation. Sudden severe pain in the front or side edge of the shoulder, accompanied by swelling and the feeling that the shoulder is out of joint; arm must be held away from body after injury. The upper arm bone (humerus) has been twisted backward out of its socket at the end of the shoulder by a blow from the rear or a fall on the extended arm. The fall pushes the arm back while it is stretched out to the side, as in a football arm tackle; may also occur during skiing or as the result of a sharp gymnastic move on the uneven parallel bars.

Home Treatment: None. See your doctor. Do not try to reduce (reset) the humerus in its socket this first time unless you have no access to medical aid in the reasonable future. If you have someone push or pull on the dislocation, you may be permanently crippled.

Recurrent Shoulder Dislocations

Description: Symptoms are the same as dislocated shoulder. Once you have dislocated your shoulder, you are likely to do it again and again, and each time will be alarmingly easier than the last. Overhand throws, tennis serves, football tackles, or any motion that twists your arm back may pop it out of its socket.

Home Treatment: After your first dislocation, your doctor will probably show you how to reduce the dislocation yourself. You will need a friend. While you lie on your back and relax your arm, your friend firmly grasps your forearm with both hands, placing one hand on the inside of your elbow and the other hand lower on the forearm. She lifts your arm so that the elbow points toward the ceiling and the fingers point toward your head. While pulling up on your arm at the elbow, she gently rocks the forearm from side to side until the humerus slips back into place. If the pain increases, stop. Once you have reset the shoulder, rest it by carrying your arm in a sling until the pain is gone. If you dislocate your shoulder once in a while, eliminate the activities which pop your arm out of joint. If you dislocate your shoulder frequently, or if the pain is overwhelming, you may choose to have your shoulder surgically stabilized. However, this will interfere with your game because it will limit the shoulder's range of motion.

Trick Shoulder

Description: Also called recurrent shoulder subluxation, recurrent glenohumeral subluxation, or apprehension shoulder. Upper arm pops in and out of its socket in a partial shoulder dislocation. ("Luxation" is a synonym for dislocation.) When the arm pops out, pain is moderate and the shoulder feels frozen. You may actually be able to feel the head of the humerus with your hand when the arm is "out." The feeling is very brief, however, for the shoulder pops back in as soon as you move it. The tendons have temporarily slipped out of their grooves because the shoulder capsule has become lax. The capsule is a fibrous sac filled with lubricating fluid. The pain stops as soon as the arm is back in place and activity stops; this distinguishes it from shoulder tendinitis.

Home Treatment: None. If you can't pop the shoulder back in place, see your doctor.

Prevention: Strengthening exercises work only rarely, but they are worth a try: Strengthen the deltoids with arm sprints or dips, the rotator cuff muscles with door hangs and crossovers, and the supraspinatus with arm lifts.

Arm Lifts: Stand up with your affected arm at your side. Slowly lift your arm straight out to the side while a friend presses down with her hands on your forearm. She should apply only enough resistance to make the lift difficult—not impossible. When you reach shoulder level, return, without resistance, to your starting position for one rep. Perform ten reps every day.

If only one activity forces your arm to pop out, avoid it or change your style (see **Shoulder Tendinitis**). If this doesn't help, switch sports. It is possible that recurrent subluxations may lead to a full-blown dislocation. If the condition is serious, you

may need surgery to stabilize the shoulder, but this will probably restrict the movement in the joint.

BREASTS

Blows or Trauma

They don't lead to breast cancer.

Home Treatment: As for any other bruise, RICE.

Prevention: Wear chest protector.

Chest-Muscle Pull

Description: Dull ache behind one or both breasts. No trauma. Caused by overtraining or continuous strenuous exercise. May also be caused by strained Cooper's suspensory ligaments.

Home Treatment: As for any muscle pull, RICE for a couple of days; then warm baths during which you exercise your arm and shoulder.

Prevention: Wear a supportive bra or bind your breasts against your chest with scarves.

Strained Cooper's Suspensory Ligaments

Description: Ache in breasts close to surface of skin. No trauma. The Cooper's suspensory ligaments run from your skin to the glandular material of your breast. Because your breasts have no muscles inside them, your skin and your Cooper's suspensory ligaments are all that support them. If your breasts bounce too much, the ligaments become overstretched and hurt.

Home Treatment and Prevention: See **Chest-Muscle Pull.**

ARMS

Traumatic Bursitis

Description: Also called olecranon bursitis, water on the elbow, student's elbow, and beer drinker's bursitis. Swelling at the tip of the elbow with acute burning pain or little or no pain. Elbow joint looks as if it has a floating sac of water inside it because the padding sac (bursa) over the elbow has become inflamed after bumping the elbow on a hard surface, falling on it, or repeatedly rubbing it. May also be caused by infection or gout.

Home Treatment: RICE immediately, and on and off for twenty-four hours. If the swelling hasn't gone down by then, your doctor may have to drain the sac for you.

Forearm Fracture

Description: Severe pain or cramping in the forearm, swelling around sore spot, depression or hard bulge in or on the spot, inability to use the arm. See your doctor.

Forearm Splints

Description: Pain and cramping, burning and tenderness in the muscles of the forearm after a workout has begun. There is no pain in the elbow. Stretching may make it worse. This is probably the arm sports' equivalent of shin splints, and occurs when you support your weight on your arms while you pull, lift, or swing with them. If there is a single identifiable point of tenderness, you may have a stress fracture.

Home Treatment: RICE. Look for trigger points.

Prevention: Like shin splints, forearm splints are very stubborn. Stretch those muscles with pigeon crawls and strengthen them with wrist curls. Wear sleeves or tubes over your forearms to keep your muscles warm. Check for pronation (arm turned so that thumb is rotated toward body) and arm-length discrepancies and adjust your technique to balance them.

Funny Bone

Description: Also called crazy bone. Sharp searing pain in the elbow, or pain radiating from the elbow down the forearm, sometimes accompanied by numbness or tingling in the outside of the hand and in the little and ring fingers. A funny bone is really a bruised ulnar nerve. The nerve runs close to the skin through a groove between the two bony protuberances of the elbow, and down to the

ring and little fingers. The pain is caused by a blow to the elbow or pressure from leaning on it. Bicyclists often suffer funny bones after leaning on their handlebars with their elbows bent for long periods.

Home Treatment: Ice pack for a few minutes. If the pain or tingling persists, see your doctor.

Prevention: Wear elbow pads; straighten your elbow frequently to relieve pressure on it.

Little League Elbow

Description: Also called humerus fracture or medial epicondylar epiphysial avulsion. Pain, swelling, and tenderness when bending the elbow, turning the forearm so that the palm faces the floor when the elbow is bent, or rotating the forearm so that the palm faces behind when the arm hangs down at the side. Occurs only in children and adolescents and is not the direct result of trauma. Repeated throwing or other bending and rotating movements performed with great force crack or pop off the lower end of the upper arm bone (humerus). If the child cannot completely straighten her injured arm, she probably has an abnormality in her growth plate. This occurs only in children because their ligaments are too lax to hold the elbow firmly in place.

Home Treatment: Stop throwing. RICE for pain. See a doctor within twenty-four hours.

Racquetball Elbow

Description: Also called medial epicondylitis, bowler's elbow, spotting elbow, thrower's arm, forehand tennis elbow, or cross-country skier's elbow. Pain and tenderness, sometimes accompanied by swelling on the inside of the elbow (the side running down to the little finger). Hand is weak. Pain intensifies when you try to grip something. Even shaking hands may be excruciating. May be accompanied by numbness in the forearm, wrist, and hand if the major nerve of the forearm (the median nerve) is pressed during play. Pain is actually elicited when you move your wrist. However, you feel the pain in your elbow, not your wrist, because the wrist muscles originate at the elbow and pull on that joint. Caused by sharply snapping, pushing, or flexing your wrist, as in racquetball wrist flicks, baseball knuckle and spit balls, gymnastics assisting (spotting), or booming tennis serves. Highly trained or professional tennis players are more susceptible to this variety of tennis elbow, whereas weekend players usually suffer from the classic tennis elbow (lateral epicondylitis). This tendinitis shows up as an inflammation of the tendons attached to the muscles used for bending your wrist. These tendons attach to the epicondyles, the lumps at the lower end of your humerus; thus the English translation of this injury: inflamed epicondyles.

Home Treatment: ICE. Doctors recommend rest too (and therefore RICE), but many athletes won't stop playing. Athletes who continue to play should stretch before and after with posture clasps and birds and rub on a heat-producing ointment to warm up and loosen the joint. Wear a toeless sock or sleeve over the elbow to keep it warm, and a wrist support or pressure bandage just below the elbow. Look for trigger points.

Prevention: One or more of the following suggestions may help. Conscientiously stretch several times a day with pigeon crawls, posture clasps, and birds. Strengthen your forearm muscles with wrist curls and grip-strength exercises. Use the strong muscles which straighten your wrist (wrist extensors) instead of your weaker wrist flexors. In gymnastics spotting, for example, flip your students with the back of your hand rather than your palm. Don't flick your wrists. In racket sports, use your entire arm instead of wrist action alone. Hit from the shoulder and keep your wrist stiff. Relax your grip between strokes. Use a lighter racket or club with a smaller handle, less tension on the strings, or a lower sweet spot (center of percussion). Play with lighter balls. All these suggestions reduce the shock transmitted to your arm.

Tennis Elbow

Description: Also called lateral epicondylitis, radiohumeral bursitis, backhand tennis elbow, golfer's elbow, quarterback's elbow, badminton el-

bow, violinist's elbow, plumber's elbow, pitcher's elbow, javelin thrower's elbow, bareback rider's elbow, woodchopper's elbow, gardener's elbow, carpenter's elbow. Pain on the outside of the elbow, sometimes running down toward the thumb and forefinger. Pain may be intermittent at first, then persistent. Gripping anything, even shaking hands, is excruciating. The area is tender to the touch. You feel pain when you straighten your arm against resistance; little or no pain when you bend your arm against resistance. Moving your wrist muscles triggers the pain, but you feel the pain in your elbow because the wrist muscles attach there. Pain may be due to a tendinitis of the forearm tendons used to straighten your arm, pull up your wrist, and open your fingers. Or it may involve an inflammation of the lubricating lining of the joint or small tears in the tendon unit near its attachment to the outside, or lateral epicondyle. (See **Racquetball Elbow.**) It is also possible that tiny nerve fibers are exposed during the injury and transmit pain at the slightest provocation. Whatever the pathology, the injury is the result of one violent or several repeated minor stresses on the forearm muscles, when the arm is suddenly and jerkily straightened out while it is pronated (arm turned so that thumb is rotated toward the body). This is the classic tennis elbow and afflicts more women than men, and more middle-aged people than any other age group. Weekend tennis players are more susceptible to this type of tennis elbow, while highly trained and professional players are more susceptible to medial epicondylitis. The heavier you are, and the more you play, the more likely you are to come down with it.

Home Treatment: ICE. Although doctors recommend rest (and therefore RICE), most victims won't stop playing. *If* you continue to play, stretch your forearm muscles thoroughly before and after each workout with posture clasps and birds. Rub on a heat-producing ointment to loosen up the arm, wear a toeless sock or sleeve over the arm to keep it warm, and wear a pressure bandage just below the elbow. Look for trigger points from your elbow to your wrist down the length of each affected muscle. Press each point to relax the spasm. Only 7 percent of all tennis elbows require surgery. However, the injury is stubborn and is likely to recur.

Prevention: One or more of the following suggestions may help. Conscientiously stretch your forearm and wrist muscles several times a day with posture clasps, birds, and pigeon crawls. Strengthen your forearm muscles with wrist curls and your grip strength with grip-strength exercises, chin-ups, pull-ups, or door hangs. (According to *the physician and sportsmedicine,* Chinese badminton coaches claim you can cure tennis elbow if you hold a push-up position for as long as you can while gripping a cylinder about the size of a tennis ball can in each hand.) Eliminate the recoil stress placed on your forearm muscles when you push a ski pole, hammer, racket, or other long lever against a resistance. You may accomplish this in any of several ways. Wear a brace on your upper forearm; this also spreads out the pull of the muscle, reducing the pain. Use a two-handed backhand stroke. Tennis elbow is virtually unknown among players with a two-handed swing, and the style could be adopted by carpenters. Use a lighter racket with a smaller grip, looser strings, and lower sweet spot (center of percussion). Use lighter balls. Avoid dead or wet balls. Relax your grip between strokes. Hit from your shoulder and use your whole arm instead of your wrist. Swing or otherwise apply force with your elbow slightly bent and your thumb facing foward a little. (Rotating your thumb outward a little prevents pronation of the forearm.) Check your posture. If your neck or shoulders are stooped, you may be pressing your arm muscles or using them incorrectly to compensate for the imbalance. In this case, try head twisters, heat to relax the neck muscles, and good posture (ears over your shoulders, crown of your head held high as if pulled from above by a puppeteer's string). Although anti-inflammatory steroid shots such as cortisone mask the pain, they weaken the joint: Because you can't feel the pain, you overwork the weakened joint and permanently disable yourself.

Pitcher's Elbow

Description: Also called bicipital tenosynovitis. Pain in the hollow of the elbow, running down the outside (little-finger side) of the forearm. Tenderness, swelling, and occasional gravel or clicking noises. This inflammation of the sheath and tendon connecting the biceps muscle to the ulna, the larger of the two forearm bones, is provoked by forcing your elbow to bend upward against a resistance, as in a racquetball ceiling shot or a chin-up.

Home Treatment: ICE. Doctors recommend RICE as for tendinitis—rest your arm in a sling until the pain is gone. If you won't stop playing, stretch your biceps with door hangs and birds. Strengthen your triceps with pull-ups, unless they hurt.

WRISTS AND HANDS

Wrist Fracture

Description: Pain, with or without swelling or deformity, as the result of a fall.

Home Treatment: Varies with location of the pain. Gently grasp the wrist with your other hand. If there is a tender spot around the bone at the base of your thumb, you probably have a navicular fracture. Ice it down. After twenty-four hours, if it still hurts when gently grasped, see your doctor. Navicular fractures are serious because they heal very slowly—four to six months is common—and they sometimes require not only splinting and casting but surgical implantation of a pin. If they don't heal properly, they may lead to arthritis. Occasionally, these breaks don't show up on x-rays because the fracture line is so thin. If your doctor tells you that the wrist is sprained, and it doesn't improve in two weeks, request another set of x-rays or a bone scan. By this time, the bone will have destroyed the broken cells and absorbed them, leaving a gap visible on x-rays. If you grasp your wrist, and you feel minor pain and swelling anywhere else on the wrist, and you feel no bone sticking up or crushed down, treat the injury as a wrist sprain. If RICE, including the use of a sling to cradle your arm, doesn't significantly alleviate your pain in two days, see your doctor.

Wrist Sprain

Description: Pain, tenderness, or swelling anywhere on your wrist as the result of a fall.

Home Treatment: Unfortunately, it is difficult to know whether you have sprained or fractured your wrist unless you x-ray it. If the pain, swelling, and discomfort are minor, and there is no specific tenderness at the base of your thumb, treat as for any sprain; apply RICE, and cradle your arm in a sling. If your wrist is significantly better in twenty-four hours, continue with this treatment and move the wrist gently throughout its entire range of motion. However, if the pain persists after twenty-four hours, or if you have particular tenderness at the base of the thumb, ice the area down and see your doctor. Pain at the base of the thumb may indicate a navicular fracture; see **Wrist Fracture.** To play it safe, your doctor may want to splint your wrist to immobilize it for three weeks or a month. Ask about an air splint (see **Ankle Sprain**) to exercise those muscles while they're immobilized. This will prevent muscle atrophy.

Karate Wrist

Description: Stiffness when you try to bend your wrist up, down, or in both directions as the result of repeatedly breaking stacks of wood with the side of your hand.

Home Treatment: None, although stretching exercises may increase your mobility slightly. Do standard pigeon crawls and then inverted pigeon crawls: Put the backs of your hands on the floor, and lower your weight onto them.

Prevention: Don't break stacks of wood with the side of your hand.

Swinger's Wrist

Description: Also called racket wrist and golfer's wrist, depending on location. Pain, swelling, and tenderness may be centralized in the hand and wrist in a straight line from the little finger, across the top of the wrist, or high on the thumb side of the wrist where the two arm bones meet. No history of trauma. May be caused by tendinitis, ligament inflammation, or overloading an already unstable wrist joint as the result of repeatedly twisting your wrist against a resistance. Bending your wrist while you hit a ball with a heavy racket and then turning your wrist over during the follow-through is the most common offender.

Home Treatment: The standard treatment, as for all tendinitises, is RICE. Carry your arm in a sling for a month. Many players, however, don't want to stop playing for that long and just apply RICE (including the sling) for a day or two. After that, they wear an elastic wrist band to remind them not to twist their wrist when they swing. A firmer supportive wrist brace prevents injury but also restricts your shot-making ability.

Prevention: Strengthen your forearm with wrist curls and your hand muscles with grip-strength exercises. Stretch those same muscles with pigeon crawls and posture clasps. Use a lighter racket with a smaller grip, looser strings, and lower sweet spot (center of percussion). Use lighter balls. Keep your wrist straight, not bent, at the moment of impact during each stroke. Don't use the two-handed backhand, because it forces the wrist to roll although it protects your elbow. (People with tennis elbow who favor their tennis elbows often give themselves swinger's wrist.)

Trigger Finger

Description: Also called Quervain's disease or stenosing tenosynovitis (stenosing means constricting; tenosynovitis means an inflammation of tendons and their sheaths). Marked by pain in the wrist and hand above the thumb pad, local tenderness, and occasionally a nodule or bump you can feel with your fingers; may be accompanied by snapping or locking up when you use your thumb and wrist at the same time. No immediate trauma is involved. The tendons extending the thumb become inflamed and then constricted inside the narrow canal of fibers between the forearm and the hand, after repeated thumb-wrist movements such as those in table tennis and racket sports. Much more common in women than men.

Home Treatment: If mild, RICE. Taping the thumb and wrist into a relaxed natural position sometimes helps to relieve pain. If the pain is intense, see your doctor. Your thumb and wrist may be splinted, or, in severe cases, the fibers of the canal may be cut to release the pressure on your thumb tendons.

Prevention: Stretch the muscles with pigeon crawls and strengthen them with wrist curls and grip-strength exercises. Stroke with less thumb movement.

Carpal Tunnel Syndrome

Description: Numbness, tingling, pain, and a feeling of weakness or clumsiness in the thumb, index, and middle fingers; hand tends to fall asleep; tingling and discomfort may extend up the forearm to the elbow and are worse at night. Extremely common among middle-aged women and fairly common among pregnant women, suggesting it may be related to a glandular disturbance. Symptoms are caused by compression of the median nerve which runs from the spinal cord in your neck down the inner side of your arm and into your thumb and first two fingers. If the nerve is squashed between the bones at the back of the wrist and the watchband-like strip of tendons across the base of your palm, your hand starts tingling. The compression may arise from inflammation of the sinewy tendons above your wrist, an old improperly healed wrist fracture, repeated trauma, overuse of the wrist, or arthritis.

Home Treatment: Splint your wrist in a position which keeps the pressure off the nerve, and wear the splint whenever you are inactive—sleeping, resting, or watching television. If splinting doesn't help and the condition becomes insufferable, your doctor may cut the circular wristband-like tendon called the retinaculum.

Calluses

See **Corns and Calluses.**

Ulnar Neuropathy

Description: Pain, tingling, weakness, numbness, and stiffness along the heel of your hand (the outside edge) and into your little and ring fingers. A compression of the end of the ulnar nerve (the one that runs down the elbow and causes funny bone), this condition results from leaning on the outside part of the palms of your hands for long periods or from absorbing the vibrations of your front bicycle wheel as they are transmitted through unpadded handlebars.

Home Treatment: Rest for a few minutes or a few hours.

Prevention: Wear warmer gloves. (Cold exacerbates the problem.) Pad your handlebars with foam tubing. Insert foam pads inside your cycling gloves. Shift the position and grip of your hands on the handlebars every five minutes. Loosen your backpack straps; they may be pressing on some nerves. Get a smaller bicycle. (If your bicycle is too tall, you put too much weight on your hands when you ride.) Tilt your handlebars so that the drops are slightly below horizontal.

Black Fingernail

Description: Crushed finger or thumb with discoloration and bleeding under the nail, as the result of a blow or other crushing trauma.

Home Treatment: Immediately, press the nail and fingertip for five minutes to prevent pooling of blood. If this doesn't work, relieve the pressure and pain by drilling the nail with a red-hot paper clip (see BLACK TOENAIL). If the pain continues after the fluid has drained, or if the pain is *inside* the fingertip, you may have fractured your finger. See your doctor.

Sprained Finger

Description: Also called jammed finger, stoved finger, and proximal interphalangeal finger sprain. Pain, tenderness, bruising, and moderate swelling. This partial or complete tear of the ligaments tying the bones of your finger together may be accompanied by an inflammation of the lubricating tissues of the joint. The injury is the result of twisting or bending the finger, or jamming it against an implacable resistance.

Home Treatment: As for any sprain, RICE, frequently, the first twenty-four hours. If the pain has diminished, no bones feel out of place, and there is no tender depression in the bone (indicating a fracture), continue with RICE for another two days. Splinting the finger in a comfortable position may reduce the pain. However, the sooner you move a sprained joint through its full range of movement, the faster it heals. If the pain and tenderness persist after seventy-two hours, see your doctor.

Fractured Finger

Description: Pain, tenderness, and swelling in a finger or thumb after a blow, a smashing or crushing accident, or a fall forcing the digit to bend at an odd angle.

Home Treatment: If the finger is not bent oddly out of position, and the pain is endurable, apply RICE frequently for twenty-four hours. If the pain is unbearable, the bone sticks up or feels crushed into a depression at one point, the pain persists after twenty-four hours, or the swelling is worse; see your doctor. *Note:* My orthopedist once told me that it is not always necessary to x-ray a potentially fractured finger as long as there is no evidence that bones are displaced. The treatment for many simple finger fractures and sprains is the same, so the x-ray and that dose of radiation are superfluous. Many doctors order needless x-rays not to confirm a diagnosis but to use for evidence in case they are used for malpractice later on. Always ask your doctor whether an x-ray is necessary.

Dislocated Finger

Description: Also called interphalangeal finger dislocation. Pain, swelling, and stiffness in a finger joint; the bone wiggles loosely in the joint or is visibly out of its normal position. There are two types: The finger is dislocated at the knuckle where it joins the hand, or the finger is dislocated in a middle joint of the finger. Both are caused by a fall on the hand or by catching your finger in something which is then yanked away.

Home Treatment: If you have dislocated your finger where it joins the hand, do not try to put it back in place. This type of dislocation is very difficult to reduce and should be done by a doctor. If you have dislocated one of the middle joints in your finger, you have a choice. You may wait for your doctor to pull your finger back into position. Or you may do it yourself: Gradually pull the finger outward once; after it pops back into position, splint it in a flexed position and apply RICE; see your doctor to be on the safe side. So many coaches have reduced this kind of dislocation that the injury is often called "coach's finger." If it hurts unbearably when you pull your finger, don't do it. If the finger doesn't pop back into place after one try, don't pull it again. See your doctor. (Some doctors advise against trying to reduce any dislocated finger, especially a child's. Christine Haycock, M.D., however, says that an athlete, a coach, or a friend can safely reduce simple dislocations of middle finger joints.)

Baseball Finger

Description: Also called jammed finger, hammer finger, or mallet finger. Pain, on the top of the farthest bone of the finger, and inability to straighten the last joint in your fingertip; fingertip is stiff and bent down at an odd angle. Either a tendon has ruptured or the bone has fractured as the result of a head-on blow to the fingertip from a baseball or other piece of sports gear. May also be caused by forcibly extending the fingertip against an immovable resistance. If you can't straighten your finger at all, you may have a fracture or complete tendon rupture.

Home Treatment: If the pain is tolerable, treat as a sprained finger with RICE. If the pain persists after a couple of days, or if you cannot straighten your finger at all, see your doctor, who will probably splint your finger in a hyperextended (backward-arched) position. You will have to wear that splint night and day for six to eight weeks, for without complete immobilization this kind of fracture and rupture doesn't heal.

Boxer's Knuckle

Description: Also called boxer's fracture. Swollen and bruised knuckle; pain occasionally radiates into little finger or thumb. Knuckle exquisitely tender. May be a feeling or sound of gravel (crepitus) inside the knuckle joint, and a bone may appear to be out of place. This fracture is the result of hitting something or someone with your fist.

Home Treatment: If the pain is bearable and all bones appear to be in place, apply RICE. See your doctor in a day or two if the swelling persists. If the pain is unbearable or a bone is out of place, see your doctor right away. If this fracture doesn't heal properly, you may develop stiffness or arthritis in that joint.

Pulled Nail Bed

Description: Entire nail pulled from under cuticle. Clean nail and nail bed gently, then tenderly replace it under the cuticle. Keep it clean and in place with a bandage.

Burning Hands

After a blow, fall, or collision in which the back or neck is involved.

Caution! **Burning hands are a symptom of spinal cord injury. DO NOT MOVE THE PERSON. Get experienced medical emergency aid immediately.** Occasionally, burning hands are the *only* evidence of spinal cord injury.

Frisbee Finger

Description: Severe cuts, scrapes, discoloration, or mutilation of the fingernail; occasionally, separation of the fingernail from the finger. Caused by constantly rubbing the area, as during multiple Frisbee tosses.

Home Treatment: See **Black Toe.**

Prevention: Wear gloves, moleskin, or polyfoam adhesive padding and bandages to pad the area. Keep your fingernails short.

Gamekeeper's Thumb

Description: Also called skier's thumb. Pain along the pad of the thumb, swelling, and tenderness, often accompanied by an inability to firmly pinch something between the thumb and forefin-

ger. The ligaments of the thumb are damaged or ruptured as the result of some trauma pulling your thumb outward: A ski pole applies leverage against your thumb pad during a fall; you catch your thumb on a piece of clothing and yank the thumb forcefully upward; a racket is wrenched out of your hand, also pulling your thumb outward. It is called gamekeeper's thumb because British game wardens killed rabbits by twisting their necks between thumbs and forefingers.

Home Treatment: RICE for one or two days, as for any sprain. Then slowly move your thumb in circles for flexibility and faster healing. If the pain, tenderness, and weak pinch persist after two days, see your doctor, who may immobilize your hand in a cast or, in very serious cases, repair the ligaments surgically.

Prevention: While this is an overuse injury for gamekeepers, it is usually a traumatic injury for athletes. If, however, the symptoms are caused by repeatedly overloading and stretching the ligaments of your thumb, strengthen your grip with grip strength exercises and strengthen the thumb extensor muscles by pushing your thumb against your other hand, permitting your thumb to push the hand away with effort.

Bowler's Thumb

Description: Pain and swelling at the base of the thumb. Occasionally, thumb becomes numb. No history of trauma. An inflammation of the muscle, tendon, and sometimes the nerve, in the area as the result of repeatedly straightening and pushing the thumb out from the hand against resistance.

Home Treatment: RICE, as for tendinitis. Don't play until the swelling is down. Use heat after four days to relieve any residual pain and speed the healing process.

Prevention: Strengthen your grip muscles with grip-strength exercises to take some of the workload off your thumb. Stretch the affected muscles by gripping your thumb with your other hand and gently pulling it out, in, down—every direction—to exaggerate its normal range of motion. Strengthen your thumb extensor muscles by extending your thumb into a fully spread position while pushing against it with the palm of your other hand; return to starting position, for one rep. (The thumb should win this pushing contest, but with effort.) Do as often as possible. If your bowler's thumb actually comes from bowling, move the thumb hole closer to the finger holes so that you grip the ball with all three digits. Round the edge of the hole or wear moleskin or other padding where the ball presses against the thumb. If the thumbhole is too large or too small, adjust it. Don't put as much spin on the ball.

NECK

If someone hurts her neck, head, or back as the result of a blow, fall, or other trauma, do not move her. If you do, you may interrupt the path of nerve fibers down the spinal cord below the injury, and the victim will be paralyzed for life. Get experienced emergency medical aid immediately. If the victim is unconscious, do not use smelling salts to revive her because the violent head tossing and other movements she makes when she comes to may further damage her spinal cord.

Racquetball Neck

Description: Stiff neck, especially in the rear neck muscles; pain may travel to shoulder or down one arm. No history of trauma. Possible causes: overuse, muscle strain, irritation and inflammation of muscle or tendon units compressed between neck joints as the result of rapidly and repeatedly arching the neck to look up at the ceiling or sky. Affects tennis and badminton players too.

Home Treatment: RICE as for tendinitis. Massage the stiff muscles after each application of ICE. Stretch and relax the muscles with head twisters, posture clasps, birds, and king of Siam kowtows. Look for trigger points and relax them.

Prevention: Use heat or ice packs before and after each game. (Heat works best for most people.) Continue to stretch the affected muscles every day.

Strengthen them with the neck extensions, lateral neck flexions, neck flexions, and rotary necks in chapter 7. They are based on Nautilus exercises that high school, college, and professional football players perform to develop neck musculature strong enough to withstand the force of tackles, blocks, blows, and spearing. Perform three sets of each exercise during each workout, and do these exercises three times a week. When you finish your last set, stretch with head twisters, posture clasps, birds, and king of Siam kowtows. When you play your sport, avoid arching your back. Hit the ball at a lower point in its arc or let the ball bounce. Relax your neck muscles frequently during each game by rotating your neck through its entire range of motion.

Cyclist's Neck

Description: Low-grade pain in the shoulders and neck as the result of hunching over or cycling for long periods.

Home Treatment: See **Racquetball Neck.**

Prevention: Straighten up frequently. Strengthen the extensors of your back and neck with locusts and neck extensions.

Neck Spasm or Stiff Neck

Description: Pain anywhere in neck, not associated with trauma, lifting, hunching, or rapidly moving your head. May be caused by walking, running, or standing on legs of uneven length (see **Leg-Length Discrepancy**).

Home Treatment: Arrest the spasm as soon as it begins by stretching with head twisters, posture clasps, birds, king of Siam kowtows, or door hangs. Apply ice to dull the pain, then massage or stretch again. Look for trigger points on the front, sides, and back of the neck and on each side of the vertebral column, particularly along any hard, ropy muscles. Work down into the trapezius muscles in the shoulder and along the spine of the back, because the neck muscles are connected to vertebrae well down the spine. If you find any trigger points, release them. Once the spasm ends, rest your neck for a couple of days, applying RICE if necessary. After two days, apply heat instead.

Prevention: If you have a leg-length discrepancy, put a heel lift in the shoe of your functionally shorter leg. If you don't, correct your posture and routinely stretch your neck and back muscles with the exercises mentioned. Do them several times a day, during your daily activities as well as before and after every workout.

HEAD

If you hurt your eyes, ears, or head in a traumatic accident, see your doctor immediately. If you suddenly develop convulsions, see your doctor immediately. If you suspect a concussion or skull fracture, see your doctor immediately. If someone sustains a blow to the head and doesn't recover consciousness within a minute or two, get experienced emergency medical aid immediately.

Concussion

Description: Also called cerebral concussion. There are three levels of severity, beginning with mild or first-degree, involving momentary mental confusion, mild ringing in the ears, brief or no memory loss, mild dizziness, and no loss of consciousness. Moderate or second-degree involves brief amnesia and loss of consciousness, slight mental confusion, ringing in the ears, moderate dizziness, and moderate unsteadiness. Severe or third-degree concussion involves prolonged unconsciousness, amnesia, mental confusion, ringing in the ears, dizziness, and marked unsteadiness. All are caused by a direct blow to the head. Possible complications: cerebral hemorrhage, vulnerability to subsequent head injuries, chronic headaches, ear ringing, dizziness, disorientation, and epilepsy.

Home Treatment: None. Immediate medical aid is essential.

Headache

Description: No muscle aches; no history of trauma. Headache that occurs after exercising is probably due to heat.

Home Treatment: Splash on cool water or apply cool cloth compresses. Drink cool water.

Prevention: As for any heat injury. Wear a hat or sun visor.

Footballer's Migraine

Description: Searing, throbbing, unbearable headache, beginning on one side of the head within a minute or two of deliberately striking the head against moderate resistance, as in heading the ball in soccer, being punched in boxing, or spearing in football. May be accompanied by nausea, vomiting, chills, and dizziness. Bright lights intensify the pain. Lasts for two hours or two days. A migraine headache is the result of a seizure within the mechanism controlling the muscles inside the cranial blood vessels. First the arteries in the head and neck constrict, and then they dilate. As well as from blows to the head, migraines may develop from sunlight, overtraining, anxiety, smoking, allergies to foods or pollens, food additives, and drugs. Typically, you have no previous history of migraines, although once you get one footballer's migraine, you are likely to get more.

Home Treatment: The first time a footballer's migraine hits you, see your doctor to rule out head injury. If you get recurrent migraines, treat them yourself. As chronic migraine sufferers know, it is far easier to arrest a migraine in its early stages than to get rid of it once it's full blown. Aspirin works for a few people, but most must take powerful, addictive, prescription painkillers. However, doctors and nurses at UCLA Hospital and Clinic and at Herrick Memorial Hospital in Berkeley, California, use acupressure to relieve the symptoms of full-blown migraine and tension headaches. This form of acupressure is actually a variant of trigger-point therapy: Pressure on pairs of points° releases the headache spasms. The pressure itself is close to excruciating, but lasts for only thirty seconds per point—a small price to pay for hours or days of deliverance.

Headache Acupressure: To apply headache acupressure, sit in a comfortable chair. In the order listed, press each of the following pairs of points° with the end of your thumb for thirty seconds each. (You may have to file down your fingernails.) Press firmly, but not hard enough to cut your skin with your thumbnail. Use a solid, unremitting pressure for the whole thirty seconds, or pulse the pressure on and off every second or two, depending on what works for you. Even if you feel better after pressing one or two points, complete the series.

Point pair one: Press into the muscle bulging above the web between the thumb and forefinger of each hand, pushing toward the bone behind your index finger knuckle. Do one hand first, and then the other.

Point pair two: Stretch the fingers and thumb of one hand as far apart as you can. Elevate the thumb slightly until two tendons along the top of the thumb stand out. At the wrist end of the bottom tendon, there is a round bone. About an inch or two up your arm, in a direct line from this bone, is a small depression, and that's your point. It is very hard to find; the easiest way is to probe firmly with your finger or thumb until you hit a tender spot. When you do find the point, it will ache and may even shoot a tingling pain into your thumb or up the line of the radius, the bone rising above your thumb. Once you find the point, apply pressure first on one arm, then the other.

Point pair three: Press into the small, tender depression on the outer edge of each eye socket. This point lies just above the corner of your eye, between the eye socket and the larger soft spot on each temple. Using both hands, press both points at the same time.

Point pair four: Using three or four fingers of each hand, find the soft spot or depression at the back of your neck and the base of your skull. These spots lie lateral to the massive muscle ridges flank-

° These points were suggested by LaVada Staff, registered nurse at Herrick Memorial Hospital in Berkeley, California. They resemble some of those used in *Quick Headache Relief Without Drugs* by Howard D. Kurland, M.D. (see Selected Readings.)

ing your neck vertebrae. Push in and up toward the base of the skull. Press both points at the same time.

Prevention: After your first migraine, you will recognize an aura, a group of signals that tell you a killer headache is about to hit. You may lose your appetite, become nauseated or depressed, hear ringing in your ears, see stars or flashing lights, have tingling hands or feet, or break out in goose bumps or eye twitches. At this point, aspirin and bed rest in a quiet, darkened room may prevent an attack, as may meditation. Violent sustained exercise or a long sneezing fit (brought on, perhaps, by a pinch of snuff) may also intercept the spasm. If these don't work, however, you may have to resort to propranolol or ergotamine tartrate. Taken in small doses at the first sign of a migraine, these drugs are relatively safe and effective. However, both have side effects harmful to good sports performance. Propranolol makes you feel weak, tired, dizzy, short of breath, nauseated, or short of breath. Ergotamine raises your blood pressure by constricting your blood vessels and causes nausea, vomiting, drowsiness, and muscle cramps in some people. Some professional football and soccer players disregard the side effects and take propranolol before each practice or game to prevent migraines. However, some neurologists believe that recurring migraines are a convulsive disorder and feel that migraine sufferers shouldn't play contact sports.

Swimmer's Eye

Description: Red, stinging eyes after swimming in a chlorinated pool.

Home Treatment: Rinse with commercial nonprescription eyedrops or a mild sterile saline solution (available over-the-counter at drugstores catering to soft contact lens wearers).

Prevention: Wear swim goggles. Swim in a pool whose acidity is under 8.0.

Black Eye

Description: Also called shiner, mouse, or periorbital hematoma. Swelling, tenderness, soreness, black and blue eyelids and skin above and below the eye as the result of a direct blow to the bony eye socket.

Home Treatment: RICE, as for any bruise.

EYE GUARDS

Caution: **If you bleed through the skin of the eyelid or from the eyeball itself, or if you hemorrhage under the surface of the eye and can't see clearly, see your doctor.**

Wear eye guards whenever you play any sport featuring sticks, rackets, flying balls, pucks, or other objects. Eye injuries are rare in athletics because every reflex you possess protects your eyes. When they do occur, the results are disastrous. Wear a top-quality eye guard with clear, unbreakable plastic frames, a wide elastic band to hold them close to the back of your head, and unbreakable, nondistorting, polycarbonate lenses about three millimeters thick. Your optician can insert prescription lenses into any of these frames if you normally wear eyeglasses. (Mention the three-millimeter thickness at the center of each unbreakable lens.) Do not use open, lensless guards, which are nothing more than a thin plastic frame. They protect your eye from most assaults by a racket or stick, but not from balls or pucks.

Subconjunctival Hemorrhage

Description: Bleeding (hemorrhaging) inside the white of the eye (sclera) accompanied by swelling and bruising of the eyelid. No pain in the eyeball itself, and vision is normal. One of the tiny blood vessels in the membrane surrounding the front of the eyeball and the lining of the eyelid has ruptured as the result of a blow to the eye by an object larger than the eyeball—a ball, puck, hockey stick, elbow, or fist. If your eyeball hurts, your vision is blurred or altered, or your eyeball or eyelid is cut, see your doctor.

Home Treatment: Ice pack on and off for twenty-four hours to reduce the spread of the hemorrhage, and then warm compresses to encourage the absorption of the hemorrhage. Condition should clear up within two weeks. Since your sight is involved, if you have any doubts, see your doctor.

Corneal Abrasion

Description: Also called scratched eyeball. Unbearable pain in the eye, blurred vision, sensitivity to light, copious tearing.

Home Treatment: None. See your doctor, who will probably administer soothing eyedrops and apply a pressure eye patch. Should heal in a couple of days.

Sunburned Eyes

Description: Also called snowblindness. Dry eyes, sandy feeling, pain when you move your eyes or when you look at light, swollen eyelids, excessive tearing. This occurs after spending time in the snow, even on a cloudy day; the rays reflected by the snow have sunburned the surface of your eye.

Home Treatment: Apply cold compresses to your eyelids. Rest in a darkened room or in the shade. See your doctor.

Prevention: Wear goggles, wraparound sunglasses, or side blinders to shield your eyes from direct and angled rays of the sun.

Swimmer's Ear

Description: Also called otitis externa. Itching, acute pain, swelling, inflammation just inside the ear; burning sensation; sometimes accompanied by ringing in the ears or impaired hearing. You probably have swimmer's ear if it hurts when you press your finger lightly in your ear, gently tug on your earlobe, or move your jaw from side to side. A discharge from the ear indicates a severe infection. Symptoms often show up hours or even a day or two after water entered the ear. (This distinguishes swimmer's ear from diver's ear, whose symptoms are felt immediately during the descent phase of a dive.) Swimmer's ear is caused by a bacterial infection egged on by a secondary fungus infection when the normal skin oils, ear wax, and layers of skin protecting the ear are washed away, or when the ear is weakened by allergies or exposed to contaminated water. If you swim in warm water, such as the water in a heated pool, you have a five times greater risk of developing ear infections than the general population because bacteria and fungi love to grow in warm, moist environments. If you have unusually curvy, narrow, or obstructed ear canals, you have trouble expelling water from your ear and so are susceptible to infections. Water settling in the ear lowers the acidity of the ear canal and encourages the growth of bacteria. If you remove the wax from your ear by washing it away or making a minute scratch with your fingernail, you remove the ear's protective barrier to microorganisms. Once you suffer a bout of swimmer's ear, you are likely to get it again and again because each infection scars and partially destroys some of the wax glands assigned to protect your ear. Serious infections migrate into your middle ear and can permanently damage your hearing and sense of balance.

Home Treatment: If you have a minor infection—simple itching, moderate pain, tenderness and ringing in the ears—gently wash your ear four times a day with white distilled vinegar. Do not use cider or other types of vinegar. Use it full strength if it's not too painful; otherwise dilute it with boiled and cooled-to-lukewarm water, anywhere from equal parts water vinegar and water to one part vinegar to five parts water—whatever you can stand. If this doesn't help in two or three days, or if your symptoms get worse, see your doctor. If you have any discharge, be it green, gray, or brown, or if you have swelling, fever, severe pain, or tenderness, see your doctor; you may need a cotton wick inserted into your external ear canal, an exceedingly painful but minor procedure. For a day or two, the wick transfers antibiotics and other medications past the inflammatory barrier to the infection. Once the swelling is gone, most of the pain leaves too.

Prevention: Unless you take some or all of the following precautions, you will probably suffer recurring bouts of swimmer's ear. Get all water out of your ear after you swim or shower. Shake your head, jump up and down, lean over and hit the side of your head with the heel of your hand, or dry your ear canal with the warm air from a hair dryer. Don't dive, for that forces the water into your ear. Keep the external ear canal dry and acidic by placing glycerine drops in your ear before and after each swim. After your swim, put a small wad of cotton *over* (not in) the hole into your ear for an hour. As an alternative, acidify and dehydrate your ear before and after each swim with two drops from an eyedropper of the following mixture: ¼ teaspoon distilled white household vinegar, an acid; 3 drops rubbing (isopropyl) alcohol, a dehydrating agent; 2 tablespoons cooled boiled water. This works well for some people, but others find it leaves their ears wet and more susceptible to infection. See what works for you. Do not wear earplugs or Vaseline-coated cotton because they don't form a complete seal; your ear still gets wet. What's more, unless they are custom-fitted, the earplugs may exert pressure of their own and force the water farther into your ear. If none of this works, your doctor can prescribe an antibiotic for you to use before and after every swim.

Diver's Ear

Description: Also called ear squeeze. Pain, ringing in the ears, and impaired hearing, occasionally accompanied by dizziness, ruptured blood vessels in the middle ear, and a ruptured eardrum. The pain strikes immediately during the descent of the scuba dive. This distinguishes it from swimmer's ear, which hurts minutes or hours after the swim is over. This is a water-pressure injury, resulting when the pocket of air becomes blocked inside the eustachian tube connecting the middle ear and the pharynx. If the compressed air the diver breathes cannot enter the middle ear, the pocket of air trapped inside the middle ear remains at a much lower pressure than that of the surrounding water, causing immediate symptoms.

Home Treatment: Don't dive until the pain is gone. Over-the-counter decongestants such as Sudafed may help. A small hole in the eardrum heals in a few days. If pain is severe, or you are dizzy, see your doctor. A large rupture in your eardrum may require a surgical graft.

Prevention: Stop your descent if you feel even mild ear discomfort. Clear your eustachian tubes to equalize pressure by exhaling through your nose while it is pinched almost shut. A light popping or squeak tells you that you're cleared. Other methods: Turn your head from side to side and swallow; yawn with your mouth shut; jut your jaw back and forth; flood your mask, then blow the water out by exhaling through your nose. Start clearing within the first six feet of descent. Don't dive when you have a cold, hay fever, or other allergies. Many divers take decongestant tablets before every dive as a preventive; Sudafed is so popular, in fact, it stands next to the cash register in many dive shops. However, even mild decongestants make some people drowsy and should be used cautiously.

Surfer's Ear

Description: Intermittent loss of hearing; itching; pain; ringing in the ears; feeling that your ear is plugged up or full of wax; recurrent bouts of swimmer's ear. Swimming in cold water for months or years causes bony growths inside the ear canal. Often has no symptoms.

Home Treatment: If you have no pain or other symptoms, and your doctor discovers the bony growth in the course of a routine checkup, don't worry. There's no reason to have them removed because they are entirely benign. However, if you have pain, recurrent swimmer's ear, or loss of hearing, your doctor can remove the growths without damaging your hearing in the slightest.

Ruptured Eardrum

Description: Sudden pain, ringing in the ear; loss of hearing; possible bleeding. The eardrum, the thin membrane which transmits sound to the inner ear, is torn by a blow to the ear or by increased pressure, as in diving from a high tower or scuba diving.

Home Treatment: None. See your doctor. During the month or so it takes for your eardrum to heal, do not dive, get the ear wet, blow your nose violently, or fly in an airplane. Competition

divers who consider their next meet more important than their hearing sometimes wear custom-molded earplugs or Silly Putty in their ears.

Prevention: See *Diver's Ear.* If you are not susceptible to swimmer's ear, over-the-counter swimmer's earplugs may prevent a buildup of pressure. However, some divers complain that the earplugs destroy their sense of balance.

Runner's Ear

Description: Temporary hearing loss or deafness accompanied by a feeling that your ears are plugged up, occurring during the late stages of a strenuous workout, or afterward. When you have a cold or allergy, or gasp for air during exercise, mucus builds up in your pharynx and blocks your eustachian tube, causing a dry-land version of diver's ear.

Home Treatment: Clear your eustachian tubes and equalize the pressure in your middle ear using the techniques suggested in *Diver's Ear.* The condition should clear up and your hearing return after a few minutes of rest. If not, a decongestant might do the trick, as long as it doesn't make you drowsy or trigger an allergic reaction. If the pain or deafness persists, see your doctor. You may have ruptured a membrane in your middle ear.

Prevention: Clear your ears periodically while you exercise. Take an over-the-counter decongestant, as long as it doesn't interfere with your performance.

Wrestler's Ear

Description: Bruise or inflammation and tolerable pain anywhere on the external ear or earlobe as the result of a blow, fall, scrape, or other trauma.

Home Treatment: Ice packs and compression. If the swelling is not down after twenty-four hours, see your doctor. If the swelling or bruise is significant or the pain is severe, do not try to treat the ear yourself. Your doctor will have to drain the swollen area and then apply pressure dressings in order to prevent the permanent deformity called cauliflower ear.

Prevention: If you wrestle and play other sports in which ear injuries are likely, wear ear pads.

Sinus Squeeze

Description: Sharp pain or pinch above the eyes or behind the nose while diving underwater; occasionally, your nose bleeds into your face mask. Symptoms are caused by low internal pressure and rupture of tiny blood vessels in the sinuses as the result of unequal pressure between the sinuses and the water during a scuba dive.

Home Treatment and Prevention: See **Diver's Ear.** Do not dive when you have a cold or any nasal congestion. Swollen tissue and mucus can block your sinuses completely. When you try to clear, you force fluids into your inner ear, causing dizziness, ringing in the ears, and hearing loss.

Nosebleed

Description: Also called epistaxis. Bleeding from the nostrils as the result of a blow, fall, or other trauma to the nose.

Home Treatment: If you can breathe normally, and the nose does not appear to be crooked or to wiggle any more than it normally does, sit up and relentlessly squeeze the front of your nose with a small ice pack for fifteen minutes. If this doesn't stop the bleeding, squeeze all the way to the doctor. If your nose wiggles, is crooked, or out of alignment, it is probably broken; see **Broken Nose.**

Prevention: If you have recurrent nosebleeds, especially in the winter or in desert climates, your nasal membranes may be dry and cracked. A vaporizer or humidifier may help. Or try lightly misting the air around you with water.

Broken Nose

Description: Pain, bleeding, and swelling. Nose wiggles, is crooked, or is out of alignment. It is difficult to breathe through your nose. Later on, you may develop a black eye. Caused by a blow, fall, or other trauma to the nose. Sit up, apply an ice pack and a small amount of pressure, and see a doctor immediately. For optimal healing, broken noses should be reset within the first few hours after injury. After that, the nose begins to swell and is next to impossible to straighten. Most doctors will not reset a swollen nose. They wait three or four days until the swelling has gone down.

Runny Nose

Description: Mucus streaming from your nostrils or remaining stuffed uncomfortably up in your nose when you exercise strenuously. Mucus may trickle down your throat and cause you to choke or gag. In moderate amounts, mucus is a normal response to strenuous exercise and is caused by increased blood flow or inhaling extra airborne particles. If you wheeze and are uncomfortably stuffed up, you may be allergic to air-borne particles, pollutants, pollens, or foods. This reaction is also triggered when you breathe dry or cold air.

Home Treatment: Carry a handkerchief.

Prevention: Wear a ski mask to filter the air and keep your breath warm and moist. In your pre-exercise meals, eliminate wheat, milk, eggs, or any other food you might be allergic to. Some doctors recommend taking decongestant tablets, but they may make you drowsy. Decongestant sprays solve the problem temporarily, but after they wear off they leave you more stuffed up than before.

Cuts and Scrapes Inside the Mouth

Home Treatment: Very little for minor injuries. Your mouth has a rich array of blood vessels and so heals very quickly. If you think dirt was introduced into the cut, dab on peroxide as an antiseptic. According to the U.S. Food and Drug Administration, peroxide is the only substance that safely and effectively can be used to clean injuries of the mouth and gums. Neither it nor any over-the-counter nonprescription product actually promotes healing. Do not use peroxide for more than seven days straight, and see your doctor if you have any irritation, inflammation, infection, or fever.

Toothache

Acupressure temporarily relieves the pain of any toothache quickly and effectively. Pressing and massaging a key point (similar to a trigger point) short-circuits the pain more thoroughly than aspirin without any side effects. The operative point is the first pressure point for migraine headaches; see **Footballer's Migraine.** Find the point on the hand corresponding to the side of your sore tooth. Press it

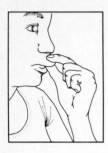

ACUPRESSURE FOR TOOTHACHE

very firmly for thirty seconds. Then massage an ice cube into the same spot for another ten to thirty seconds. Time is dictated by how much cold you can stand. Relief lasts for fifteen to thirty minutes. Repeat the acupressure as often as necessary until you see your dentist.

Tooth Pain

Description: Also called aerodontalgia. During airplane flying or scuba or skin diving. No trauma. Caused by a change in the pressure of the environment around you. May be due to blocked sinuses.

Home Treatment: Clear your sinuses as for diver's ear.

Prevention: Clear frequently before you feel pressure. See discussion of decongestant tablets under **Diver's Ear.**

Tooth Knocked Out

Description: The result of a blow or other trauma.

Home Treatment: Clean it off with your own saliva (but don't scrape off any tissue) and put it back into place immediately. If you are too hurt or upset to do it yourself, have someone else reinsert it immediately. If you can't get the tooth back into its socket, tuck it between your lower lip and teeth to keep it warm and bathed in saliva. See a dentist immediately. If you and your tooth are treated within thirty minutes, it may be possible to reimplant the tooth in its socket, where it will take root again as if nothing ever happened. After thirty

minutes, there is little chance that the tooth can be reimplanted successfully.

Tooth Pushed Out of Line

Description: The result of a blow or other trauma.

Home Treatment: Carefully and gingerly push it back into its correct position. If the tooth is pushed up into the gum, do nothing. In either case, see your dentist immediately.

Tooth Cracked or Broken Off

Description: The result of a blow or other trauma.

Home Treatment: None. See your dentist immediately, particularly if you can see a pinkish spot.

Tooth Bumped

Description: Pain but no outward signs of injury. If tooth continues to hurt, or if it becomes sensitive when you apply pressure to it, or changes color, see your dentist.

SKIN

Abrasion

Description: Also called scrape, strawberry, cinder burn, floor burn, grass burn, mat burn, skid burn, or slide burn. Friction or scraping of the skin provokes localized pain, stiffness, tenderness, oozing, swelling, and loss of top layers of skin. Possible complication: infection.

Home Treatment: Cleanse wound thoroughly and keep it clean as it heals. A cleansing method described in the journal *the physician and sportsmedicine* by D. R. McVeigh, cycling coach for St. Mary's Academy in Winnipeg, Manitoba, is said to cut healing time by 50 percent. Wash and rinse the abrasion with ordinary soap, then apply a disinfectant such as Neosporin. Prick a 400 I.U. vitamin E capsule, spread the oil over the whole area, and cover it with a patch of household plastic wrap. Smooth the surface of the plastic to press out all air bubbles, and then fasten it in place with adhesive tape. The next day, remove the plastic patch and gently and carefully blot up the gray paste that has formed over the sore. Gauze, facial tissue, or a paper towel work best. This paste is a combination of oil, damaged tissue, and dirt. Reapply vitamin E oil and plastic wrap once or twice more, or until the oil no longer becomes gray. From then on, keep the wound clean and dry, and it should heal in six or seven days.

Many people swear by aloe vera. The juice or gel from the inside of a broken aloe vera leaf does appear to speed the healing of a cut or burn, but the juice must be fresh. Commercial preparations containing stabilizers and other additives appear to be toxic to human cells and delay the healing process. Aloe vera grows happily in the house, and one medium-sized plant purchased from a health food store or plant shop should provide all the healing an average household needs.

I like to cover abrasions and burns with Spenco Second Skin, a cut-to-size sheet of plastic that holds water within it. I store it in the refrigerator, so that it feels cool and soothing when I apply it, and its hydrophilic, or water-retaining, properties keep the wound pliable while letting air in so the sore breathes and heals quickly. Second Skin is available in many drugstores and sporting goods stores.

Blister

Description: A sac of skin usually filled with fluid. Occurs as a result of friction between a piece of clothing or equipment and your skin. The friction separates the top layers of skin from those underneath and permits fluid to accumulate. Possible complication: infection.

Home Treatment: If the blister is small, doesn't hurt, and hasn't popped, gently clean it, then leave it alone. If you must continue to irritate it, protect it with a bandage, a piece of moleskin, or Spenco Second Skin, a water-filled plastic. Remove the covering and expose the blister to the air whenever possible. If the blister is large, painful, and hasn't popped, clean it thoroughly with soap and water and an antiseptic such as alcohol or Bactine. Prick it a few times along its edges with a needle sterilized in a flame. Do not remove the flap of skin—it acts as a painless, sterile dressing. Dry the blister and cover it with a sterile bandage. If the blister has torn or popped, carefully cut away the shredded skin, wash the area, allow it to air-dry, then apply a sterile dressing. If the area becomes reddened or more painful, or if red streaks appear around the blister, see a doctor immediately.

Prevention: Wear properly fitted, well-broken in shoes, gloves, and other clothing. Keep your skin dry by powdering it or wearing dry socks or other dry fabric linings. Tape vulnerable spots. Coat your skin with petroleum jelly before long sweaty workouts. Don't wear wet shoes, gloves, or other equipment. Wet shoes often form blisters with a thick, white skin on top and little or no fluid.

Bruise

Description: Also called zinger or contusion. Tissue damage involving pain, swelling, discoloration, stiffness and tenderness. Blood oozes out of small broken blood vessels and pools in the tissues of the skin. May start out as a raised red circle with a white center and only later turn into a multicolored bruise that lasts two or three weeks. Usually caused by a direct on-target hit. Complications are rare, but bruises do occasionally calcify or turn into small nonmalignant (noncancerous) bony masses.

Home Treatment: RICE.

Laceration

Description: Also called cut, gash, cleat wound. A painful, tender, bleeding open wound in the skin. Caused by some sort of tearing force or trauma. Possible complications: infection.

Home Treatment: Clean wound with soap and water and an antiseptic. Cover it with gauze or a bandage to keep it clean. Change dressing frequently, and expose wound to the air whenever there is no chance of contagion.

Bicycle Burn

Description: Scrape or abrasion of the skin after falling off a bicycle or other moving object.

Home Treatment: As for any abrasion.

Saddle Sores

Description: Also called saddle burns. Irritation or open sores on the buttocks overlying bones as a result of riding a bicycle or horse for long periods.

Home Treatment: As for any abrasion.

Prevention: Sew chamois or other padding into the seat of your pants. Place seams away from all areas of friction. If your pants become sweaty during a long ride, change them. Apply baby powder, cornstarch, or other absorbent powder to the area to absorb moisture. Or smear petroleum jelly on vulnerable areas before each ride, but wash it off afterward to expose your skin to the air. Adjust your bicycle seat. If it is too high or too low, you slide or bounce from side to side and increase the rubbing on your backside.

Chapped Lips and Skin

Description: Dry air during wintry or windy weather shrinks the tiny blood vessels supplying your skin with moisture.

Home Treatment and Prevention: Your skin lacks water, not oil. Therefore, trap water next to your skin so that the skin cells can soak it up. Moisten your skin with water and blot off the drippy excess. While the skin is still wet, seal the water next to your lips with beeswax, lip gloss, or dechapper containing simethicone. Seal the water to the rest of your skin by spreading on a cream with the same ingredients or using a thin layer of petroleum jelly. Moisturize your office or home with a humidifier or cold-mist vaporizer. If you develop deep cracks in your lips or skin, lay a thin strip of Spenco Second Skin over the sore and cover with a bandage.

Cold Sores

Description: Also called fever blisters. Group of tiny blisters on a red base around the mouth, which eventually pop and form a soft crust which soon hardens; itching or burning. You may catch fever blisters by touching someone else's cold sore, but there are other as yet unknown avenues of contagion. The sores are caused by a *Herpes* virus which lies dormant in your system until sunlight, fever, cold weather, dry air, nervous stress, or any number of other factors stimulates an eruption. Once you come down with cold sores, you are likely to get them again and again, for the virus never leaves your body. It lies in wait in your nerve ganglia (relay stations in your nerves) until something triggers it into activity. As of this writing, there is no cure for *any Herpes* infection.

Home Treatment: A person with recurring cold sores feels a warning itch, tingle, or burning sensation on the spot around the mouth before the actual lesion erupts. When you feel this warning signal (prodrome), apply an ice cube to the spot for ten minutes or more and repeat several times during the day. This arrests the cold sore before it develops. If you have a fully developed fever blister, avoid over-the-counter cold-sore medications, for they may spread the lesions or make them worse by keeping them moist. Antibiotics don't work because *Herpes* is a virus, not a bacterium. Drying the lesion with a hair dryer minimizes the pain and speeds healing. Many people report miraculous success with a product called L-Lysene, whose active ingredient is the essential amino acid lysine.

Prevention: Use a PABA sunscreen (see **Sunburn**) or zinc oxide ointment around your mouth whenever you are about to exercise in the sun. Keep your lips dry. Do not spread the virus when you have lesions by kissing others or by touching a lesion and then touching something else.

Herpes Rash

Description: Stinging, burning, or otherwise painful tiny masses of blisters on a reddened base of skin anywhere on the body; blisters later pop and form a soft, then a hard crust; itching; sometimes accompanied by chills, headaches, fever, and body aches; sores may occur in the eyes, in and around the vagina and cervix, and on any spot of skin. These are caused by a *Herpes* infection, as cold sores are, and are spread by a variety of factors. One of the most common in athletics is skin-to-skin contact in basketball, wrestling, and other bare-skin contact sports. Once you contract *Herpes*, it lies dormant in your ganglia (the masses of nerve cells throughout your body), waiting to be provoked into another episode by sunlight, fever, cold weather, dry air, nervous stress, or other stimuli. As of this writing, *Herpes* is incurable and will recur throughout your life.

Home Treatment and Prevention: See **Cold Sores.** Shingles, which is a kind of *Herpes*, is treated with DMSO in Europe. *Herpes* in the vagina and cervix is particularly dangerous because birth defects or even infant death may occur in babies who pass through an infected birth canal. Until there is a cure for *Herpes*, the only way to control the spread of the virus is to avoid skin-to-skin contact. If you have an active outbreak, do not let anyone else touch your lesions. Either cover them with bandages or don't play until your skin has completely healed. (In competition wrestling, wrestlers with *Herpes* are prohibited from practicing or competing, because the virus may be spread by contaminated mats as well as skin-to-skin contact.)

Nighttime Hot Flashes

Description: Also called nocturnal erythromelalgia. Reddened feet or legs or, less frequently, hands, accompanied by a burning sensation during sleep after a day of strenuous exercise. Your blood vessels dilate as if you are overheated, in much the same fashion as they do during menopausal hot flashes. May be a disorder in its own right or it may be a symptom of diabetes, gout, or high blood pressure.

Home Treatment: Take vitamin E, pantothenic acid, or pyridoxine (vitamin B6). Sleep with your feet uncovered. Treat as for menopausal hot flashes (chapter 8). If the symptoms don't abate, see your doctor.

Bites and Stings

Description: Symptoms vary with the insect or arachnid (spider or scorpion) and with your sensitivity to the chemical injected into your system: sudden sharp pain, swelling, redness, itching; occasional blistering, pins-and-needles prickling sensation or numbness of site and adjacent area. If you are allergic to the venom of bees, wasps, yellow jackets, hornets, or ants (all members of the order Hymenoptera), you may suffer hives, wheezing, swollen lips and face, and shock. Without immediate medical care, you may die. (This, not heart attack, may be one cause of sudden death among trained athletes during exercise.) Black widow spider bites look like two pinpricks surrounded by red swelling. The toxin affects the nerves, bestowing intense pain and muscle spasm in the abdomen. A small percentage of black widow spider bites are fatal. Brown recluse spider bites produce intense pain and blistering, accompanied by fever, rash, tingling, numbness, overall weakness, and breakdown of red blood cells. Scorpion stings first produce acute pain and pins-and-needles prickling in the immediate area, then progress to numbness and weakness in the affected limb, inflammation of the lymph nodes, itching in the mouth and upper throat, speech impairment, twitching, vomiting, and convulsions. Death can occur within three hours in small children or already ill adults.

Home Treatment: If you are not allergic to Hymenoptera stings, remove the stinger without squeezing its attached venom sac by scraping it out with a dull knife drawn across the skin. Wash the area with soap and water, then apply ice packs for ten minutes several times a day. Calamine lotion may soothe the itching; aspirin, acetaminophen, or oral antihistamines may reduce the pain and swelling. If you suffer the more serious generalized allergic reaction, see your doctor immediately. If you already know you are allergic, carry a prescription insect-sting emergency kit such as Ana-Kit, containing a syringe of epinephrine, a tourniquet, and some antihistamine tablets whenever you venture out into Hymenoptera country. Use the epinephrine immediately to forestall shock and see your doctor within thirty minutes (when the epinephrine wears off). Centipede bites hurt but don't progress to generalized damage. After cleaning with soap and water, apply cool compresses. If you've been bitten by a black widow spider, see your doctor for an injection of antivenom. Your doctor can prevent the full-body effects of brown recluse spider toxin by giving you steroids and antihistamines within twenty-four hours of the bite. For scorpion stings, pack the site in ice to slow the absorption of the toxin; apply a tourniquet above the area for five-minute intervals, allowing at least a minute between each interval for blood to enter the limb. (If you are traveling in scorpion country, carry an aerosol can of ethyl chloride to use as an ice-pack substitute.) See your doctor immediately for scorpion antivenom.

Prevention: Wear shoes (not sandals) and, if possible, high socks, long pants, and long-sleeved shirts, especially in scorpion country. Bright or vividly patterned clothes or flashy jewelry attract bees. Instead, wear white, light green, tan, khaki, or other light colors. Avoid perfumes and scented toiletries. If you are attacked by Hymenoptera, don't flail or swat at them. Retreat slowly or lie face down and cover your head with your hands and arms.

Poison Ivy, Poison Sumac, or Poison Oak Rash

Description: Red weeping blisters, burning, itching, swelling; in severe cases, accompanied by headache and fever. Only half of all human beings are allergic or sensitive to urushiol, the irritating oil in the leaves, stems, roots, flowers, and berries of these plants. No season is risk-free—the oil lurks even in the leafless, unidentifiable stems of dormant plants.

Home Treatment: Very little helps. Calamine provides temporary relief, as does a cool cornstarch bath: Mix one cup of cornstarch with four cups of water, then dump this gel into a tub of cool water and soak for several minutes. Colloidal oatmeal, sold under the brand name Aveeno, also gives welcome though temporary relief. Follow the directions on the label. Air drying prevents infection. Rub crushed fresh plantain leaves on the rash to dull the itch and speed healing—provided you can find fresh plantain leaves in a nearby field or lawn. Do not cover lesions while they are weeping. Air drying prevents infection. Although scratching the blisters will not spread the rash, it may infect the lesions.

Prevention: If you are sensitive to these plants, wear long pants and long-sleeved shirts whenever you go hiking and don't let hanging branches brush

your face. Poison oak, in particular, grows into large, trailing vines, capable of reaching exposed skin anywhere on your body. If you think you have touched a suspicious plant, wash your skin within an hour with cool water and ordinary soap (if you have it). However, if you are several hours away from mild soap and a bathtub, wade or dive into a river or lake, even if you have to do it with your clothes on. Do not use hot water or harsh soaps because they wash away your skin's protective oils and make it easier for the urushiol to penetrate. If you have no water available, gasoline, alcohol, or acetone will rinse away urushiol, although it also washes away your skin's natural oils. Prescription and over-the-counter desensitizing preparations don't work, and many have unpleasant or dangerous side effects.

Sunburn

Tender, stinging, occasionally swollen skin; color varies from light pink to bright, almost lobster red. Caused by exposure to the ultraviolet rays of the sun. These rays penetrate clouds and can burn light-skinned people even on overcast days. If you exercise or sunbathe in snow or near water, you are twice as likely to get sunburned, for you are exposed to the direct rays of the sun and the reflected rays bouncing off the snow or water. Even if you have dark skin and are normally resistant to sunburn, you may become very sensitive to ultraviolet rays if you are taking birth-control pills, antibiotics (tetracycline, sulfa drugs, and griseofulvin); thiazide diuretics for high blood pressure (Aldoril, Anhydron, Diuril, Hydrodiuril, and hydrochlorothiazide); oral hypoglycemics; tranquilizers (Thorazine, Stelazine, Compazine, and chlorpromazine); or using deodorant soaps.

Home Treatment: Soak for twenty minutes in a cool bath with or without cornstarch (see **Poison Ivy**), then smooth on a thin coating of a cream or ointment containing allantoin or vitamins A and D. A paste of one tablespoon each of baking soda and cornstarch mixed in a small amount of water may also relieve the pain. Try four aspirin or acetaminophen tablets every four hours, during a meal or with milk to minimize stomach upset, but don't take them if you are sensitive to aspirin. Or try Ecotrin or another coated (enteric) aspirin.

Prevention: Don't sunbathe. Use a strong sunscreen whenever you work or play outdoors. Even suntanning prematurely ages your skin, and sunburn does it grievous injury, making it leathery, hard, wrinkled, and loose. (Ever notice that your buttocks and belly are less wrinkled than your face? That's because your buttocks aren't exposed to the sun as often.) The ultraviolet rays of the sun dry out the elastic fiber in your skin and thicken the skin cells. They also cause both curable and incurable forms of skin cancer. Skin cancer is second only to lung cancer in its rise in this country. The fairer your skin, the more susceptible you are to skin cancer and the more you need a sunscreen, but no matter how dark or tan your skin, you need a sunscreen if you spend hours in the sun.

The most effective sunscreens contain PABA (para-aminobenzoic acid), benzophenone, or both. The FDA now requires every tanning lotion and cream to list its Sun Protection Factor. The SPF indicates how much longer it will take you to tan with the screen than without it. Choose your SPF by combining the usual time it takes you to burn with the estimated time you expect to be in the sun. If it usually takes you thirty minutes to burn, and you expect to stay at the beach for four hours, wear a sunscreen with an SPF of eight; instead of burning in thirty minutes, you'll start to burn in eight times thirty minutes, or four hours. If you tan well and rarely burn, you may prefer an SPF of four or six. Wearing a sunscreen, you tan, but more slowly. Apply the sunscreen before you go out into the sun, and reapply it if you sweat or swim. If you are fair and are traveling to the tropics or embarking on a long ski trip, apply the sunscreen to your skin every night for a week before you leave, and every night during the trip, as well as frequently during each day. If you take tetracycline or other drugs to prevent traveler's diarrhea, you will be even more sensitive to the sun and will need a stronger sunscreen. Wear sunscreen during the winter whenever you are in the snow. Snow is a very efficient reflector of sunlight. *Note:* People allergic to sulfa drugs may also be sensitive to PABA. There are a few effective sunscreens made without PABA. Check the labels.

Sun Poisoning

Description: Also called sun allergy. Rash, itching, and (in moderate to severe cases) blisters, immediately or a few days after short or long exposure to the sun. May be triggered by an ordinary allergy, by the same drugs that make you susceptible to sunburn, or by first-aid creams, deodorant soaps, detergents, cosmetics, or toiletries containing Bithionol or Tribromsalan. PABA sunscreens may start a rash in people allergic to sulfa drugs. Just touching carrots, celery, and parsnips—all members of the same family—may also set off a sun reaction.

Home Treatment: Treat as for poison ivy. For mild cases, cold compresses and calamine lotion dry the skin and soothe the itch. If the blisters or rash are severe, or if your condition doesn't improve in three days, see your doctor.

Prevention: Pinpoint the allergen. Wear a sunscreen. Stay out of the sun.

HEAT

Heat Cramps

Description: Excruciatingly painful cramps in the muscles most used (calf muscles in runners, for example), accompanied by profuse sweating during exercise on very hot or humid days; cramps do not relax when you stretch or massage the muscle. Heat cramps are the first signs of heat injury and result from the excessive loss of body salts via sweating. They strike men more often than women because men sweat more than women, but women taking diuretics for high blood pressure, premenstrual water retention, or swelling are susceptible.

Home Treatment and Prevention: See **Heatstroke.**

Heat Exhaustion

Description: Also called heat prostration or heat syncope (syncope means fainting). Symptoms are heat cramps, inexplicable anxiety, headache, nausea, fatigue, a vague but pervasive feeling of discomfort, heart palpitations, breathlessness, dimness or blurring of vision, dizziness, chills and goose bumps, feeling faint, numbness in hands and feet; oral body temperature may be elevated to 100 to 105 degress Fahrenheit in water-depletion heat exhaustion but normal in salt-depletion heat exhaustion; profuse sweating, rapid pulse, low blood pressure, gray, clammy, cold, wet skin; stupor or shock. (If the effective temperature is well below 70 degrees, these symptoms probably indicate hypoglycemia.) In mild cases of heat exhaustion, you may feel as though you have had a cold for several days. This is the second stage of heat injury. These symptoms result from exercising in hot or humid weather and are usually so uncomfortable that you can't keep going. Heat exhaustion is common but rarely fatal.

Home Treatment and Prevention: See **Heatstroke.**

Heatstroke

Description: Also called sunstroke. Dizziness, vomiting, diarrhea, dilated pupils, eyes very sensitive to light, head throbbing; skin usually hot and dry, although may be covered with sweat and chilled; fainting; mental confusion or anger; oral body temperature 105 degrees Fahrenheit or above; low blood pressure; rapid, weak, diminishing pulse; snoring while breathing. In the most severe heatstrokes, the victim collapses and is unresponsive to any external stimulation. This is the final, most serious stage of heat injury and, if left untreated, is fatal.

When you exercise, you produce heat. Since your body runs best at its normal temperature of 98.6 degress Fahrenheit, it uses several mechanisms to get rid of excess heat: It transfers it to a cooler atmosphere or cools your skin by producing sweat. In fact, sweat evaporating off your skin is the most efficient form of body cooling there is for humans and most other mammals. However, if the weather is humid, the air is already saturated with water vapor and can't absorb enough of your sweat to cool your skin. Your heart pumps faster and faster, vainly carrying more blood to the ski for cooling. You sweat profusely to no avail and, in the process,

lose so much water that your blood becomes concentrated. The heart works harder to pump that thickened blood, placing still greater strain on your cardiac muscle. Furthermore, the thickened blood can't carry enough oxygen to nourish your internal tissues. To aggravate this vicious cycle, the heavy sweating depletes your body of so much water it can't get rid of the wastes your muscles churn out during exercise. All these factors together start producing the symptoms of heat injury. When your internal temperature rises, you become an oven and the heat cooks the protein in every tissue and organ in your body. Like a hardboiled egg or a piece of grilled steak, a cooked brain or heart cannot be uncooked. For this reason, full-fledged heatstroke is fatal about 80 percent of the time, and people who do survive usually suffer permanent damage.

It is possible to suffer serious heat injury while exercising when the outdoor temperature is mild and balmy. To the air temperature, add 10 to 20 degrees if the humidity is high to very high. Add another 10 or 20 degrees if the day is bright and cloudless, and another 5 or 10 degrees if there is no wind to evaporate the sweat off your skin, or if the wind is a tail wind. Following winds do not cool you nearly as effectively as head winds. Thus, for example, a calm, bright, humid 70-degree day has an effective temperature of 95, much too hot for any all-out effort. If you are not used to heat, or if you are dehydrated from drugs, illness, or other causes, or if you've recently lost a lot of weight, you may be susceptible to heat injury. Obesity also increases your chances of heat exhaustion or heatstroke because the thick layer of fat under your skin acts as an insulating layer to hold your heat deep inside you. A woman is more susceptible to heat injury than a man because she sweats less. She compensates by more readily dilating the blood vessels close to the skin, so that the heat in the blood is transferred to the skin. As she moves through the air, the air and wind cool her skin and the blood beneath it. This cooler blood then returns to the body core to cool her internal organs. However, this convection cooling mechanism isn't very effective if the temperature of the outside air is too high to cool anything, or if there is little or no wind. Phenothiazines (Compazine, Mellaril, Stelazine, Thorazine, Tindal, Repoise) and other anti-cholinergic drugs used to control vomiting and nausea, reduce motion sickness, increase heart rate, relax the muscles of the bronchial tubes, bladder and bowel, or to act as tranquilizers inhibit sweating and the body's ability to regulate its temperature, and so, make you more susceptible to heat injury.

Home Treatment for Heat Cramps: Rest in the shade. Drink four ounces or more of lightly salted cool or cold water every fifteen minutes. Cool or cold water is absorbed more quickly than warm water, and cools you in the process. Massage the cramps away. You should recover in about an hour, although you may feel weak for a few days.

Home Treatment for Heat Exhaustion: Lie down in the shade and elevate your feet eight to twelve inches higher than the rest of your body. Loosen your clothes. Soak under wet clothes. Have someone fan you. Drink four or more ounces of cool or cold water every fifteen minutes. Lightly salt it if you think you are suffering from salt-depletion heat exhaustion.

If you observe someone else faint or suffer any other symptoms of true heatstroke, get her out of the sun, remove her clothes, and rapidly lower her body temperature by immersing her in a tub of ice cubes or cool water. If you don't have a tub available, apply cool wet cloths continually. If you don't have even that available, fan her with a piece of paper, a shirt, or whatever is at hand. If you wait for medical aid before trying to lower her body temperature, she may suffer brain damage or die before the medics arrive. Whenever a heat injury is accompanied by fainting, changes in behavior, or any other symptoms of true heatstroke, see a doctor even if you seem to recover quickly.

Prevention: Women who have just begun to exercise after many sedentary years must adjust themselves to the heat. According to Fred Kasch of San Diego State, many sedentary women lose their ability to sweat but can train themselves over several months to sweat again by gradually increasing

their amount of aerobic exercise in heat each day. If you don't sweat *at all* when you exercise, take sauna or steam baths once or twice a week to start your sweat glands going. Don't use deodorants or antiperspirants when you exercise. Throughout the day drink extra water during hot weather, and increase your water intake still more when you exercise. Even if you are physically fit, you can acclimate yourself to the heat by using steam baths and saunas for a month before the hot weather is scheduled to begin. Once the heat is upon you, work out for only short periods at first, and build up to your usual workout only after ten days or two weeks. Once acclimated, your heart rate will decrease during exercise in heat, and your sweat production and blood flow will increase. The cooling mechanisms will start operating sooner; you will cool your body more efficiently. At first, your sweat glands will exude large quantities of salt in your perspiration, but once you are used to exercising in heat, they will reabsorb much of the salt, so that you are less likely to suffer from salt-depletion heat stress.

When you exercise, wear as little clothing as possible. The more skin you have exposed, the more surface area is cooled by any available breeze and by evaporation. What clothes you wear should be white to reflect the rays of the sun. Wet your clothes and your skin with cool water. Do not wear a hat if you want your scalp to release heat, but wear a white mesh hat with a visor if you want to shield your face and reflect the rays of the sun from your head.

Slow down. For every five degrees above 70 degrees Fahrenheit, add about 5 or 10 percent to your time. If the weather is humid, calm, or cloudless, slow down even more.

Drink water continuously throughout the day; drink as much water as you can hold and then a little more before beginning your workout. Some athletes drink two or three glasses of water two hours before a long workout or big race. An hour to an hour and a half later, they have urinated away the excess. Then, just before they start exercising, they fill up again, although not to overflowing. Because the kidneys shut down during strenuous exercise, you rarely have to urinate during short exercise bouts. If you wait until you feel thirsty, you're already down about two quarts of water. Thirst is an unreliable signal during exercise; some people on their way to heatstroke never feel thirsty at all. Drink about a cup of cold water every fifteen minutes during an exercise session. Some athletes carry lightweight waistband water packs with them. Others drink from a thermos they have standing open and ready. Marathoners practice techniques for grabbing cups of water and drinking on the run. (Sticking two fingers into the cup as they grasp the outside seems to be the favorite.) Many people simply slow down or stop while they drink, knowing that they will make up the time later when the racers who spilled half their water or skipped a water stop collapse from heat cramps. If you are bicycling in hot weather, you may not feel the loss of fluid because your wind speed evaporates your sweat. Remind yourself to drink periodically. Although children don't sweat at an adult rate until the age of twelve or thirteen, their high ratio of skin surface to internal organs gives them a large surface area for cooling. As long as they drink enough water to keep their blood diluted, they are not likely to suffer from heat injury. A child exercising in heat should gulp water until she can't drink anymore.

Drink plain cold water. It is absorbed most quickly into your system. Many people drink sugar water, soft drinks, or so-called sports drinks for fluids and energy, but the sugar in these beverages actually dehydrates you instead of replenishing your water supply. (See chapter 3.) Furthermore, if you drink sugar solutions immediately before you exercise, it triggers an insulin reaction, temporarily lowering your blood-sugar level. This lowered blood sugar forces the muscles to absorb glucose too quickly, hastening their exhaustion. If you drink the sugar during your workout, the sugar will be too concentrated for your body to absorb unless you have an excess of fluids in your system—an unlikely event on a hot day. Thus you will become exhausted about 20 percent faster than if you had drunk plain cold water.

Electrolyte replacement drinks are not as effective as water. They claim to replace the electrolytes or body salts you sweat away during exercise. However, each drink has its own odd balance of sodium, potassium, calcium, magnesium, phosphorus, sulfur, chlorine, and other minerals. Since you have your own unique needs, no single drink can supply them in proper balance. In addition, many of these drinks contain too much sodium and too little potassium and zinc. The sugar slows the absorption of the water into your blood and slows the time it takes for the liquid to get out of your stomach and into your system. For this reason, it takes thirty minutes or more for these drinks to have any effect.

Don't take salt tablets to prevent heat injury. You probably consume far more sodium in your normal diet than you need. Salt tablets require great quantities of water to dissolve. If you don't drink enough water to dilute them, they won't dissolve for four hours, will draw water out of your brain, and overtax your kidneys.

Alcohol reduces your heat tolerance. One beer lowers your tolerance for the next twenty-four to forty-eight hours. Three beers continue to affect you for the next four to ten days.

After your workout, drink cold water until you feel cool, refreshed, and thirstless, and replace any lost minerals by drinking a glass of orange juice and eating a normal diet.

If you have ever suffered a heat injury, you are likely to suffer one again. No one is certain yet whether recurring heat exhaustion is due to a faulty internal thermostat or damage caused by the first heat injury, but the effect is the same. Avoid exercising in heat, and take precautions against heat exhaustion even on moderate days.

Hitting the Wall

Description: Sudden muscle aches, loss of coordination, and fatigue; arms and legs so heavy you can't move them. The glycogen stores in your muscles are exhausted by exercising beyond your capacity or in hot weather. When you work at 75 percent or more of your maximum heart rate, and your muscles aren't trained to this pace, you deplete your muscle sugar stores in an hour or an hour and a quarter. Because your muscles burn glycogen faster in heat, you hit the wall sooner. Once you hit the wall, you may be able to continue exercising, but you'll go slower, and every movement will be agonizing.

Home Treatment: None. Stop exercising, rest, and eat and drink normally. You'll recover without incident. However, your muscles may ache for a couple of weeks.

Prevention: Build up your training schedule gradually to teach your muscle fibers to store more glycogen and burn an optimal balance of fat and sugar. Depletion runs or carbohydrate loading may increase your stores of glycogen, but then again they might not. (See chapter 3.)

Hypoglycemia

Description: Also called the bonk or (in England) the knock. Symptoms are dizziness, shakiness, anxiety, anger or mental confusion, disorientation, loss of coordination, and cold sweat. Your liver's supply of sugar fuel has been depleted as the result of extended endurance exercise. Your blood sugar drops and your brain can't function properly. (These symptoms are similar to cold and heat injury. If the weather is mild and you don't have uncontrolled shivering and your skin doesn't feel cold, rule out cold injury. If the weather is mild and dry and you don't have muscle cramps, nausea, heart palpitations, or breathlessness, rule out heat injury.) Experienced athletes rarely bonk.

Home Treatment: Eat a simple carbohydrate immediately. This raises your blood sugar and brings you out of the bonk right away.

Prevention: Eat simple carbohydrates every fifteen minutes during long endurance workouts or races.

COLD

Frost Nip

Description: Cold, white, firm patches on the face, fingers, or toes during or after exposure to cold weather. This is the first stage of frostbite.

Home Treatment: Rewarm yourself immediately. Move into a 70- to 80-degree room. Apply clothes soaked in warm (100- to 108-degree) water.

Bathe in warm water. Do not use hot water. Usually has no lasting effect.

Prevention: See **Frostbite.**

Frostbite

Description: Earliest symptoms are cold, white, firm patches on nose, cheeks, ears, fingers, toes; no pain. Second stage: Affected area begins to tingle or sting. Third stage: Affected area turns gray and numb; there is no pain or sensation because the cold has damaged the nerves and constricted the small blood vessels in the tissues. However, once rewarming begins, the pain in the affected area becomes excruciating. In frostbite, your tissues are actually frozen. Ice crystals form in the cells of your skin just as they do in a frozen steak. Frostbite is a result of a low effective temperature, the combination of the actual temperature and the amount of wind blowing. This is called the Wind-Chill Factor. Wind cools your skin by evaporating moisture from its surface. Thus, you feel cooler at 25 degrees with a ten-mile-per-hour wind than with no wind at all. As you can see from Table XIV, if the air temperature is 45 degrees Fahrenheit and the wind is blowing at thirty miles per hour, it feels as if it is 21 degrees Fahrenheit outside. If the air temperature is 15 degrees Fahrenheit and the wind is blowing at fifteen miles per hour, the effective temperature for your body is −11 degrees Fahrenheit. Whereas 15 degrees Fahrenheit might seem a reasonable winter temperature, −11 degrees Fahrenheit is not. The lower the temperature, the quicker you freeze. At 20 degrees Fahrenheit, on a calm day, it takes an hour of continued exposure to freeze exposed skin. At −25 degrees Fahrenheit, on a still day, it takes one minute. You can achieve −25 degrees Fahrenheit by skiing in 5-degree weather into a fifteen-mile-per-hour wind. What's more, you can create your own wind by moving quickly. Skiing in 5-degree weather at ten miles per hour into a five-mile-per-hour breeze creates an effective skin temperature of −25 degrees Fahrenheit, as does bicycling on a calm 10-degree day at twenty miles per hour.

Home Treatment: Don't rewarm your frozen skin unless you can keep it warm. If you must stay

TABLE XIV: WIND-CHILL FACTOR: EFFECTIVE TEMPERATURE ON EXPOSED FLESH*

Air Temperature

Wind Speed	45	40	35	30	25	20	15	10	5	0	−5	−10	−15	−20	−25	−30	−35	−40
5	43	37	32	27	22	16	11	6	0	−5	−10	−15	−21	−26	−31	−36	−42	−47
10	34	28	22	16	10	3	−3	−9	−15	−22	−27	−34	−40	−46	−52	−58	−64	−71
15	29	23	16	9	2	−5	−11	−18	−25	−31	−38	−45	−51	−58	−65	−72	−78	−85
20	26	19	12	4	−3	−10	−17	−24	−31	−39	−46	−53	−60	−67	−74	−81	−88	−95
25	23	16	8	1	−7	−15	−22	−29	−36	−44	−51	−59	−66	−74	−81	−88	−96	
30	21	13	6	−2	−10	−18	−25	−33	−41	−49	−56	−64	−71	−79	−86	−93		
35	20	12	4	−4	−12	−20	−27	−35	−43	−52	−58	−67	−74	−82	−89	−97		
40†	19	11	3	−5	−13	−21	−29	−37	−45	−53	−60	−69	−76	−84	−92			

(The label WIND CHILL appears vertically along the left side of the data rows.)

☐ Exposed flesh may freeze in one minute   ☐ Exposed flesh may freeze in thirty seconds

† Wind speeds above 40 mph have little additional chilling effect.
* Adapted from a table prepared by the National Oceanic and Atmospheric Administration.

out in the cold, keep it frozen. If you rewarm and then refreeze it, your skin will be more severely damaged than if it had stayed frozen until you reached a warm haven. Don't rub or massage the area with your hands or with snow because you will push the sharp corners of the ice crystals through the membrane walls of your cells and permanently damage them.

For the earliest stages of frostbite, rewarm as for frost nip. If you are far from warm water, rewarm your whole body by bundling up with someone in a sleeping bag or blankets. Once the part is thawed, it may hurt. If you have an advanced stage of frostbite, see your doctor; probably your whole body should be rewarmed in warm water rather than just the affected area. Whole-body warming dilates all the body's blood vessels and stimulates the circulation. You will also be given painkillers and antibiotics if necessary. The last ten minutes of rewarming are intensely painful. If you can't reach a doctor, rewarm your whole body in a warm (100- to 108-degree) bath until the skin returns to its normal color. Do not use hot water or fire because your skin is numb and you won't feel it if you burn yourself. If you can't bathe in a tub of warm water, rewarm only the frostbitten area in lukewarm or warm water, or in your mouth, or under your armpits. See a doctor or expert in treating cold injury as soon as you return to civilization.

Note: Not all doctors are up-to-date on the techniques for treating frostbite and hypothermia. After the frostbitten area is rewarmed, it should be kept warm and clean and should be treated with whirlpool baths to stimulate circulation and with antibiotics to arrest infection. Don't let a doctor amputate a frostbitten finger or toe until you have given your digit several months to heal itself. Surgeons used to believe that a severely frostbitten finger or toe had to be amputated immediately in order to save the whole hand or foot. Now, however, experts know that it is impossible to determine the extent of damage to a finger or toe for months, no matter how ugly and smelly the dead and dying tissue may appear. In four to six months, most of the dead tissue sloughs off and new tissue replaces it, frequently making amputation unnecessary. The doctor's job is to keep your decaying digit free of infection while it is healing.

Prevention: Cover every inch of your body. Wear hats, ski masks, mittens (not gloves), woolen socks. Don't let anything interfere with your circulation. Wear loosely fitting clothes in layers (see **Hypothermia**), and loose bindings, laces, and straps on skis, shoes, snowshoes, and backpacks. Don't smoke. Nicotine impedes the circulation to your fingers and toes and cuts down on your blood's ability to carry oxygen. Wiggle. Clench and unclench your fingers and toes to stimulate your circulation. Swing your arms in full circles. Don't get hungry or overtired. Don't get wet—even if the moisture comes from your own sweat. Work on a buddy system: Watch your buddy's face for the first white patches of frostbite, and have her watch yours.

Hypothermia

Description. Also called cold injury. Early stages: slurred speech, uncontrollable shivering; clumsiness in fingers and hands progressing to lethargy, with or without shivering. May be accompanied by high blood pressure. You may not feel cold but your skin feels cold to the touch. Middle stage: previous symptoms plus pale blue or pinkish-blue skin; skin may be puffy; poor coordination; no shivering. Advanced stage: previous symptoms plus inability to walk without stumbling; slow pulse; low blood pressure; shallow, slow breathing; taut or rigid muscles; pupils small or slow to constrict when exposed to light. Acute stage: unconsciousness; victim appears to be dead, although a faint pulse and faint breathing *may* be detectable.

Cold not only freezes and destroys the internal and external tissues of your body, it causes the heart to beat weakly and irregularly until it fails. Below-zero effective temperatures cause cold injury (see **Frostbite**) but so does high altitude. When you exercise at high altitudes, you breathe more rapidly and lose body moisture with every exhalation. Dehydration combined with the reduced amount of oxygen in the air makes the air temperature feel much lower to your body and increases your chances of hypothermia. If your clothes get wet from sweat or clinging snow, or if you are tired or overexerted, you are even more susceptible. However, very cold weather is not the only cause of hypothermia. Swimming and skin or scuba diving in cold water also cause cold injury. It is possible, with the right combination of factors, to suffer cold injury in air temperatures as high as 50 degrees. If the atmosphere feels cold to you, it *is* cold, no matter what anyone around you says. Women are more susceptible to cold injury than men; they readily dilate the blood vessels close to the skin and dissipate warmth from their blood into the atmosphere.

Home Treatment: Always rewarm gradually.

Mild Cases: If you have access to a bathtub, rewarm yourself by taking a body-temperature or lukewarm bath. Then put on dry clothes, snuggle in blankets, and sip warm (*not* hot) soup or cocoa. If you are out in the wilds, change into warm dry clothes and wrap yourself in blankets or a sleeping bag. Drink warm nonalcoholic liquids. Alcoholic beverages won't hurt you if you're mildly hypothermic, but they won't help either because they dehydrate you and decrease your body heat.

Moderate cases: Remove your clothes and bundle up in blankets or a sleeping bag with another naked but non-hypothermic body. Sip warm (*not* hot) soup or cocoa. If you are uncoordinated and cannot hold a cup yourself, someone else should very carefully pour the liquid down your throat. You don't want to choke while recovering from hypothermia. Use warm rather than hot liquids, because rewarming should be gradual, and because you are too numb to feel when you are getting burned. Don't use alcoholic beverages to rewarm moderately or severely hypothermic people. Alcohol increases body heat loss by dehydrating tissues and increasing the flow of warm interior blood to the surface of the skin. See a doctor as soon as possible.

Severe cases: Do not rewarm a victim of advanced or acute hypothermia unless expert medical help is too far away. Rewarming in these cases is much more complicated because the blood near the skin is too acidic for the heart muscle. If this acidic blood reaches the heart through incorrect warming procedures, or because the victim has moved her muscles, the heart will beat irregularly (fibrillate). More than 50 percent of hypothermia victims in this situation die. Keep the victim perfectly still—don't handle her roughly; don't let her move any part of her body. If possible, don't do anything to her. Just rush her to the doctor. If you must remove wet, freezing clothes, do so without any muscular help from the victim. If you are trapped in the wilderness and it's a matter of life and death, rewarm the victim gradually with a lukewarm immersion bath or by bundling her naked body with a succession of naked non-hypothermic bodies and then rush her immediately to the hospital, but remember: It is *extremely* dangerous for nonmedical personnel to rewarm a severely hypothermic person.

Prevention: Wear adequately warm clothing in layers so that the air spaces between each layer insulate you the way the air space in a thermos bottle insulates the liquid inside. The layer next to your skin should act as a wick to draw sweat away from your skin. Although cotton is absorptive, it doesn't transfer moisture away from your body. Wool, polypropylene, or fishnet underwear works better. (Fishnet underwear does have cotton in it, but little of it touches your skin.) In very cold weather, wool is comfortable because its scratchy fibers rub your skin and warm it. However, if you don't sweat much, you can wear cotton or cotton angora underwear next to your skin. The next layer should be cotton or thermal long underwear, or a cotton turtleneck T-shirt, or the equivalent. Over that, wear wool clothes. Wool is a good insulator, even when wet, and dries from the inside out. If you need a waterproof outer layer, use something made of Gore-Tex or another porous fabric. Nonporous windbreakers or rain suits become miniature steam baths when you exercise. All clothes should fit loosely. Tight-fitting clothes, boots, or equipment cut off your circulation and lead to cold injury. (After all, the freely circulating fresh supply of warm blood from your heart keeps your body warm.) Cover every bit of skin with scarves and ski masks, mittens (not gloves), thermal socks, and insulated hats. Hats are extremely important; at least 30 percent of your body heat is lost through your scalp because the blood vessels in your head don't constrict when they become cold. (The vessels in the rest of your body do.)

Drink at least two quarts of water a day. Cold draws moisture out of your system, as does heavy breathing, and the subsequent dehydration reduces the amount of blood feeding oxygen to your tissues. Get plenty of rest. Stay dry. Don't smoke. (See **Frostbite.**) As you get older, you become susceptible to cold. Drugs to treat anxiety, depression, and nausea also alter your ability to warm yourself. Build up resistance to the cold over a period of four to six weeks by exercising a few minutes longer each day. If you feel yourself getting cold, move around. Stamp your feet and wiggle your toes. Warm your hands by clenching and unclenching them and by swinging your arms in circles. If your hands become too cold, your body stops shivering. The rapidly contracting and relaxing muscles during shivering are essential for producing body heat in cold weather.

ALTITUDE

Altitude Sickness

Description: Also called mountain sickness. Early stages: shortness of breath, mild pounding, headache, blurred vision, weakness, sleeplessness, irritability, nausea, vomiting. These symptoms occur hours after you ascend to any altitude above 6,500 feet. However, most people don't suffer altitude sickness until they reach altitudes of 10,000 to 14,000 feet. The higher you go, the more the air pressure decreases. At 10,000 feet, for example, the pressure is reduced by 30 percent. The less air pressure, the thinner the air is, and the wider apart the oxygen molecules are. With less oxygen available to nourish your tissues, your heart pumps more blood to supply the same amount of oxygen, and so beats faster. Your lungs breathe faster and deeper in order to inhale the necessary amount of oxygen, but still your tissues get less and less oxygen, do less and less work, and you lose moisture and become dehydrated from panting. Your muscles shift into an anaerobic phase (see chapter 2) to work without adequate oxygen, and you produce lactic acid wastes which tire your muscles further. If you are adjusted to the altitude, the alkalinity produced by deep breathing balances the lactic acid, and the acidity of your blood remains in the normal level. If either the alkaline byproducts or the lactic acid wastes predominate, however, you get sick. You also get sick if you don't get enough oxygen to power your basic bodily processes.

Home Treatment: Go back down to a lower altitude; drink water to replace any fluids you lose. If your only symptom is a mild headache, aspirin may relieve it.

Prevention: Ascend gradually, taking two or three days to reach the summit. Stop at intermediate levels to sleep. Maintain a heart rate of under 140 if you are under thirty-five years old, and under 120 if you are older. If you have an acid taste in your mouth as you climb, you may be susceptible to type R (acid imbalance) mountain sickness. Chew enough Tums, Rolaids, or other soda mint tablets to neutralize that taste. You may need anywhere from four to twenty-four tablets. Along with the stomach mints, drink water almost constantly to maintain an abundant urine output. Eat two and a half ounces of any sugar per hour.

Acute Altitude Sickness

Description: Wheezing, coughing, blood in sputum, difficulty in breathing, pneumonialike symptoms. *Most severe stage:* Previous symptoms plus severe headache, mental and emotional upset, hallucinations, palsied movements or staggering, visual disturbances. The respiratory symptoms are caused by fluid accumulating in the lungs. The headaches and mental symptoms are caused by a buildup of fluid within the brain. Symptoms can occur as low as 8,200 feet but usually occur within one to three days after rapid ascent above 14,000 feet.

Home Treatment: Descend immediately to a lower elevation and get emergency medical aid. The medics will probably place you in a pressurized chamber and administer oxygen.

Prevention: Ascend gradually; sleep overnight at intermediate levels. Some mountain climbers climb high and sleep low, descending to a lower base camp each night. They are up and down so quickly they don't have time to develop mountain sickness. Your doctor can prescribe acetazolamide (Diamox) to prevent the loss of acidity that leads to symptoms. Its effects are temporary, but they last long enough for your body to adjust on its own. However, this sulfa drug may induce numbness or tingling in the lips and fingers, temporary nearsightedness, and other side effects.

Appendix A: Sources of Information

I: THE BASICS

Sports Questions

Looking for a local basketball, soccer, or football league? Can't find a gymnastics coach experienced in teaching adults? Need information on athletic scholarships, college recruiting, sports organizations which welcome the handicapped, or how to become an Olympic athlete? The Women's Sports Foundation has established a toll-free Sportsline to answer questions for and about women in sports. Funding was arranged by Jess Bell of Bonne Bell, Inc., the telephone bills to be paid by a $1.00 surcharge added to the entrance fee for each racer on the Bonne Bell Women's Amateur Track Circuit. In the continental United States, call 800-227-3988; in California, call 800-652-1455. Open from noon to 5 P.M. (Pacific Time) weekdays. Toll free except in Hawaii and Alaska.

If you feel you, or your mother, or your daughter is the victim of discrimination in athletics, contact SPRINT, Women's Equity Action League Educational Defense Fund (WEAL Fund), Suite 822, 805 15th Street NW, Washington, D.C. 20005, 800-424-5162 (toll free). It is a national clearinghouse of information on equal opportunity in sports, and the toll-free SPRINTline handles requests for information in athletic programs and complaints about discrimination.

And don't forget to check with the nearest YMCA, YWCA, or Jewish Community Center.

Most of them have wide-ranging sports and exercise programs. The YWCAs are often smaller than the YMCAs, but those that have the facilities, such as the YWCA of the City of New York (610 Lexington Avenue, New York, New York 10022) are more likely to offer gymnastics, fencing, badminton, and other activities designed for adult women.

If you think you have a serious vitamin or mineral deficiency, or if you are looking for a doctor with a solid background in nutrition, contact the International Academy of Preventive Medicine, 10409 Town and Country Way, Suite 200, Houston, Texas 77024 (713-468-7851) for member physicians in your area.

Special Programs

Senior Olympics/Senior Sports International Association, 5670 Wilshire Boulevard, Suite 360, Los Angeles, California 90036. Sports include archery, badminton, basketball, body building, boogie boarding, bowling, canoeing/kayaking, cross-country running, cycling, decathlon, diving, fencing, gymnastics, handball, ice hockey, marathon running, Asian martial arts, ocean aquatics, Olympic lifting, power lifting, racquetball, recreational ice skating, rifle shooting, roller skating, rugby, sailing (multi-hull and sunfish), scuba and skin diving, soccer, slo-pitch softball, swimming, tennis, track and field, volleyball, water polo, wrestling, skiing, and speed skating.

National Senior Sports Association, Inc., 1900 M Street NW, Suite 350, Washington, D.C. 20036. Acts as a clearinghouse, discount purchase plan, and tournaments sponsor for people over the age of fifty. (Monthly subscription to *Senior Sports News* included in membership fee.)

Special Olympics, Inc., 1701 K Street NW, Washington, D.C. 20006. Sponsors an international program of physical fitness, sports training, and athletic competition for mentally retarded children and adults.

United States Association for Blind Athletes, 55 West California Avenue, Beach Haven Park, New Jersey 08008. Promotes sports and organizes regional and national competitions for blind and visually impaired people.

American Blind Bowling Association, 150 Bellaire Avenue, Louisville, Kentucky 40206. Official sanctioning body for blind bowlers and blind bowling leagues in the United States.

National Wheelchair Athletic Association, 40-24 62nd Street, Woodside, New York 11377. Organizes and sanctions wheelchair sports in the United States, with the exception of wheelchair basketball.

National Wheelchair Basketball Association, 110 Seaton Building, University of Kentucky, Lexington, Kentucky 40506.

North American Riding for the Handicapped Association, Inc., P.L. Box 100, Ashburn, Virginia 22011. Advisory and sanctioning body for riding programs, instruction, and research into horseback riding for the handicapped.

National Handicapped Sports and Recreation Association, 4105 East Florida Avenue, Denver, Colorado 80222. Promotes and encourages participation in sports and other recreational activities for the handicapped.

II: SPORTS AND EXERCISE

Alpine Skiing

United States Grass Skiing Association, Bryce Mountain, Basye, Virginia 22810.

United States Ski Association, P.O. Box 100, Park City, Utah 84060. National governing body for competition; local affiliates sponsor trips and instruction.

Woman's Way Ski Seminars, P.O. Box 1182, Tahoe City, California 95730. Presents five-day ski courses in major ski areas throughout the country.

Badminton

United States Badminton Association, P.O. Box 237, Swartz Creek, Michigan 48473.

Basketball

Amateur Basketball Association of the United States, 1750 East Boulder Street, Colorado Springs, Colorado 80909. Although this organization is the governing body for amateur basketball in this country, it actually is active only at the upper levels of competition. It may be difficult for the average woman who is not affiliated with a school to find anything more than pick-up games to play. Try your local Y, community center, or even the chamber of commerce. (Many local businesses sponsor teams for local leagues.) Some high school and college basketball coaches know where the local adult basketball action is.

Bicycling

Bikecentennial, P.O. Box 8308, Missoula, Montana 59807. Nonprofit membership-sponsored service organization for cycle tourists. Creates and provides maps for bicycle trails all over the United States. Its *Cyclist's Yellow Pages* (free with membership) lists resources, clubs, publications, inns, and much more. There is no more thorough organization in the United States.

International Bicycle Touring Society, 2115 Paseo Dorado, La Jolla, California 92037. Plans and organizes bicycle tours throughout the United States and Europe.

League of American Wheelmen, P.O. Box 988, Baltimore, Maryland 21203. Oldest and most active lobbyist for the protection and support of bicycles as transportation. Sponsors rallies, organizes tours, and provides insurance and legal advice for members on cycling-related issues. Subscription to *American Wheelmen* (with good how-tos and history) included in membership. Despite its name, women participate actively.

United States Cycling Federation, 1750 East Boulder Street, Colorado Springs, Colorado 80909. Governing body of the sport of bicycle racing. Every competitor must have a USCF racing license before registering for a sanctioned race. Membership includes a subscription to *Cycling U.S.A.*, which lists the results of all racing events.

Board Sailing

International Windsurfer Class Association, 1955 West 190th Street, Torrance, California 90509. Governs national and international competition in board sailing in the United States.

Canoeing and Kayaking

American Canoe Association, P.O. Box 248, Lorton, Virginia 22079. Organization for canoeists and kayakers at every level of skill. Sanctions races, provides educational and training services, works toward conservation or waterways. Member of the United States Olympic Committee and the International Canoe Federation.

Circuit Training and Exercising

Aerobic Dancing, Inc., 18907 Nordhoff Street, P.O. Box 6600, Northridge, California 91328. Exceedingly well-designed nationwide program of dancing, running in place, and calisthenics, based on sound aerobic and medical principles. One of the few programs that incorporate warm-ups, cooldown, monitoring your pulse, and individualized pace. Instructors must be certified. Routines change every twelve weeks. Classes are reasonably priced.

Nautilus Sports/Medical Industries, P.O. Box 1783, De Land, Florida 32720, will send you the address of your nearest Nautilus center.

Cross-Country Skiing

Ski Touring Council, West Hill Road, Troy, Vermont 05868. Promotes noncompetitive, recreational cross-country skiing.

United States Ski Association, P.O. Box 110,

Park City, Utah 84060. A member of the Amateur Athletic Union and the governing body for competitive amateur Nordic and Alpine skiing in this country.

Fencing

Amateur Fencers League of America, 601 Curtis Street, Albany, California 94706. Organizes and conducts fencing tournaments, sponsors training camps, publishes *American Fencing* magazine.

Field Hockey

United States Field Hockey Association, 4415 Buffalo Road, North Chili, New York 14514. Promotes interest in field hockey, organizes exhibition games, sponsors training camps, and acts as governing body for the Olympic sport.

Figure Skating

United States Figure Skating Association, 20 First Street, Colorado Springs, Colorado 80906. National governing body for figure skating.

Football

National Women's Football League, 2714 Bryden Road, Columbus, Ohio 43209.

Gymnastics and Acrobatics

United States Association of Independent Gymnastics Clubs, 235 Pinehurst Road, Wilmington, Delaware 19803.

United States Gymnastics Federation, P.O. Box 12713, Tucson, Arizona 85732. National governing body for competitive gymnastics.

United States Gymnastics Safety Association, 424 C Street NE, Washington, D.C. 20002.

United States Sports Acrobatics Federation, P.O. Box 7, Santa Monica, California 90406.

Handball

United States Handball Association, 4101 Dempster Street, Skokie, Illinois 60076.

Ice Hockey

Amateur Hockey Association of the United States, 2997 Broadmoor Valley Road, Colorado Springs, Colorado 80906. National governing body for competition from beginning youth levels through U.S. Olympic and national teams and into senior and oldtimers' hockey.

Ice Skating

Amateur Skating Union of the United States, 4423 West Deming Place, Chicago, Illinois 60639.

United States International Speed Skating Association, Deggs Isle, Oconomowoc, Wisconsin 53066. National governing body for competitive speed skating.

Lacrosse

Lacrosse Foundation, Inc., Lacrosse Hall of Fame Museum, Newton H. White, Jr., Athletic Center, Homewood, Baltimore, Maryland 21218. Promotes and develops the game in this country.

United States Women's Lacrosse Association, P.O. Box 1289, State College, Pennsylvania 16801. At the women's request, the women's governing association is independent of the men's.

Mountain Climbing

Alpine Club of Canada, P.O. Box 1026, Banff, Alberta, Canada's national mountaineering club: organizes climbing, skiing, and social activities; publishes the *Canadian Alpine Journal*, distributed to members; maintains huts throughout the mountains of western Canada.

American Alpine Club, 113 East 90th Street, New York, New York 10028. A nonprofit educational and scientific organization whose library, research programs, and publications serve experienced mountaineers in the United States and several other countries.

American Women's Himalayan Expeditions, 900 Darien Way, San Francisco, California 94127. Organized the Annapurna and Bhrigupanth expeditions. Partially funded women's expeditions to Peru, Greenland, and Nepal. Compiling a directory of women climbers.

Appalachian Mountain Club, 5 Joy Street, Boston, Massachusetts 02108. The oldest mountaineering and conservation group in the United States. Publishes the semiannual journal *Appalachia* and the monthly *Appalachia Bulletin;* maintains huts and camps in the Northeast; sponsors hikes, bicycle trips, ski tours, canoe and kayak trips, backpacking, climbing and mountaineering instruction, and excursions.

Outward Bound, Inc., 384 Field Point Road, Greenwich, Connecticut 06830. The six Outward Bound Schools in the United States teach wilderness survival techniques over a variety of terrains. A third of the participants in these demanding courses are women, and many of them are in their thirties, forties, and fifties. The schools stress that there is no upper age limit.

Race Walking

Athletic Congress of the United States of America, 155 West Washington Street, Suite 200, P.O. Box 120, Indianapolis, Indiana 46204. This is the governing organization for amateur track and field competition.

United States Association of Women's Race Walking, 276 South El Molino Avenue, Pasadena, California 91101.

Racquetball

United States Racquetball Association, 4101 Dempster Street, Skokie, Illinois 60076. Governs amateur racquetball, publishes official rules, and sponsors local, regional, and national tournaments.

Roller Skating

United States Amateur Confederation of Roller Skating, 7700 A Street, P.O. Box 83067, Lincoln, Nebraska 68501. Promotes the sport of artistic skating and governs national competitive roller skating.

Rowing

National Women's Rowing Association, 2015 24th Avenue East, Seattle, Washington 98112. Governing body for the sport of women's rowing; conducts regional and national championships. Six regions. Member of the National Association of Amateur Oarsmen, the national governing body for U.S. rowing, and liaison with international and Olympic federations.

Rugby

Because the United States of America Rugby Football Union does not compile a list of women's rugby clubs, Paula Cabot at the Women's Sports Foundation has taken over the task. For a list of rugby sites in your area, write Women's Sports Foundation, 195 Moulton Street, San Francisco, California 94123.

Running

American Medical Joggers Association, P.O. Box 4704, North Hollywood, California 91607. Aimed at running doctors. Membership includes subscription to the quarterly *AMJA Newsletter*, featuring medical articles on the physiological and psychological effects of running.

American Running and Fitness Association, 2420 K Street NW, Washington, D.C. 20037. Clearinghouse for information on injury prevention, nutrition, training, and programs for men and women at all levels of fitness. Publishes sports medicine clinic directory. Not oriented toward racing.

Canadian Orienteering Federation, 333 River Road, Vanier, Ontario, Canada.

Masters Sports Association (member of the Athletic Congress of the U.S.A.), 3400 West 86th Street, Indianapolis, Indiana 46268. For track and field athletes thirty years old and older. The Athletic Congress of the U.S.A. sponsors and accredits races. You must be a member before entering many of the races in this country.

North American Network of Women Runners, P.O. Box 924, Shaker Heights, Ohio 44120. A nonprofit action group dedicated to providing resources (money, coaches, child care) to help women participate in sports.

Road Runners Club of America, 3203 Agnes

Boulevard, Alton, Illinois 62002. Promotes noncompetitive jogging events, as well as competitive long-distance races, and operates running clinics throughout the country.

United States Orienteering Federation, P.O. Box 1081, Athens, Ohio 45701.

Skin and Scuba Diving

National Association of Underwater Instructors, 785 Colton Avenue, Colton, California 92324. Trains and certifies divers.

Professional Association of Diving Instructors, 2064 North Bush Street, Santa Ana, California 92706. Trains and certifies scuba instructors and divers.

YMCA, 445 Grace Avenue, Panama City, Florida 32401.

Soccer

Soccer Association for Youth, P.O. Box 921, Cincinnati, Ohio 45201. Organizes nationwide soccer leagues for children; similar to Little League in baseball.

United States Soccer Federation, 350 Fifth Avenue, Suite 4010, New York, New York 10001. National governing body for soccer at all levels of the game. Organizes the most important and comprehensive leagues for children and women.

Women in Soccer, 242 East 75th Street, New York, New York 10021.

Women's International Soccer, 409 East Franklin Avenue, El Segundo, California 90245.

Softball

Amateur Softball Association of America, 2801 NE 50th Street, Box 385, Route 4, Oklahoma City, Oklahoma 73111. Governing body for softball teams and leagues.

Squash

National Squash Tennis Association, 50 Vanderbilt Avenue, New York, New York 10017.

United States Women's Squash Racquets Association, member of the United States Squash Racquets Association, 211 Ford Street, Bala-Cynwyd, Pennsylvania 19094. Promotes the sport, oversees rules, and governs national competitions.

Surfing

National Scholastic Surfing Association, P.O. Box 1245, Huntington Beach, California 92647. Promotes surfing competitions for high school and collegiate surfers. Conferences in California, Texas, Florida, Hawaii, North and South Carolina, New Jersey, Illinois, and Rhode Island.

United States Surfing Federation, 11 Adams Point Road, Barrington, Rhode Island 02806. Governing body for amateur surfing in this country.

There are no national surfing associations for the recreational surfer.

Swimming

International Swimming Hall of Fame, 1 Hall of Fame Drive, Fort Lauderdale, Florida 33316. Library, bookstore, and resource center.

Masters Swimming Program, F. H. Haartz, Chairman, 155 Pantry Road, Sudbury, Massachusetts 01776.

National Institute for Creative Aquatics, Elaine Douma, President, 12 Washington Lane, West Milford, New Jersey 07480.

Team Handball

United States Team Handball Federation, 1750 East Boulder Street, Colorado Springs, Colorado 80909. Governing body for the sport in the United States. Has a strong educational campaign to promote team handball, provides teams with instructional movies, and sets up regional or local clinics to teach the game.

Tennis

American Platform Tennis Association, P.O. Box 901, Upper Montclair, New Jersey 07043.

United States Tennis Association, 51 East 42nd Street, New York, New York 10017. Sanctioning body for tennis in the United States: conducts amateur and professional tournaments, ranks players, maintains rules, promotes tennis at all levels of play.

Volleyball

United States Volleyball Association, 1750 East Boulder Street, Colorado Springs, Colorado 80909. Governing body for amateur competitive volleyball at all levels of expertise.

Walking

American Hiking Society, 1255 Portland Place, Boulder, Colorado 80302. Active in preserving wilderness areas and promoting hiking and backpacking.

International Backpackers Association, Inc., P.O. Box 85, Lincoln Center, Maine 04458. Works on conservation and outdoor recreation.

Inward Bound Adventures, Inc., 1613 West Greenleaf Street, Chicago, Illinois 60626. Wilderness trips throughout the country for women novices over the age of thirty.

National Outdoor Leadership School, P.O. Box AA, Lander, Wyoming 82520.

National Speleological Society, Inc., Cave Avenue, Huntsville, Alabama 35810. Studies, explores, and lobbies for conservation of caves.

Outward Bound, Inc., 384 Field Point Road, Greenwich, Connecticut 06830. Teaches courses in outdoor survival techniques, wilderness skills, mountaineering, campcraft, and first aid. Six schools in the United States.

The Sierra Club, 530 Bush Street, San Francisco, California 94108. Lobbies for conservation of wilderness areas. Sponsors outdoor activities, including day hikes, backpacking trips, and rock climbing.

Wilderness Society, 1901 Pennsylvania Avenue NW, Washington, D.C. 20006. Conservation group lobbying for preservation of public lands.

Water Polo

Amateur Athletic Union, Water Polo, U.S. National Sports Building, 1750 East Boulder Street, Colorado Springs, Colorado 80909.

Waterskiing

American Water Ski Association, P.O. Box 191, Winter Haven, Florida 33880. Promotes waterskiing for recreation and competition, governs tournaments, publishes information on techniques and equipment.

Weight Lifting, Power Lifting, and Body Building

National Physique Committee, 27280 Southfield Road, Suite 3, Lathrup Village, Michigan 48076.

United States Weight Lifting Federation, 3400 West 86th Street, Indianapolis, Indiana 46268.

Women's Bodybuilding Association, International Federation of Bodybuilding, 2875 Bates Road, Montreal, Canada.

Wrestling

New England Women's Amateur Wrestling Association, P.O. Box 1435, Torrington, Connecticut 06790. Although located on the East Coast, NEWAWA has been active in establishing wrestling groups throughout the United States and in Great Britain. It is also a referral service connecting women with other wrestlers throughout the world. No dues for membership or instruction.

United States Wrestling Federation, 504 West Hall of Fame Avenue, Stillwater, Oklahoma 74074. Governs amateur wrestling, sets rules, and organizes tournaments.

III: THE INNER WOMAN

Pregnancy and Childbirth

American Society for Psychoprophylaxis in Obstetrics, 36 West 96th Street, New York, New York 10025. For Lamaze method classes in your area.

Cesarean Birth Council, P.O. Box 6081, San Jose, California 95150.

C/Sec Inc., 66 Christopher Road, Waltham, Massachusetts 02154.

International Childbirth Education Association, P.O. Box 20852, Milwaukee, Wisconsin 53220. For information on many of the different organizations dedicated to their own philosophies of prepared childbirth and family-centered maternity care.

IV: SPORTS MEDICINE

To find a sports-medicine specialist near you, write:

American College of Sports Medicine, 1440 Monroe Street, Madison, Wisconsin 53706. For general problems.

American Academy of Podiatric Sports Medicine, P.O. Box 31331, San Francisco, California 94131. For problems relating directly or indirectly to the foot.

American Orthopaedic Society for Sports Medicine, 70 West Hubbard Street, Suite 202, Chicago, Illinois 60610. For bone or joint problems.

National Association of Underwater Instructors, P.O. Box 630, Colton, California 92324. For doctors with diving expertise.

American Physical Therapy Association; 1156 15th Street NW, Washington, D.C. 20005.

American Osteopathic Academy of Sports Medicine, 1551 Northwest 54th Street, Seattle, Washington 98107.

For information on biomechanics, write:

American Society of Biomechanics, Savio L.-Y Woo, Ph.D., Secretary-Treasurer, Division of Orthopedic Surgery, University of California at San Diego, M-004, La Jolla, California 92093.

International Society of Biomechanics, Richard C. Nelson, Ph.D., President, Biomechanics Laboratory, Pennsylvania State University, University Park, Pennsylvania 16802.

Biomechanical analysis is so complicated and expensive that only elite and professional athletes can afford the full array of tests. A full analysis should not only describe an idealized style but also adjust that style to the individual athlete's weight, stature, limb length, hereditary joint looseness, age, medical history, and many other complex factors. The cut-rate diagnoses available for about $75 are too generalized and cursory to help many people.

Appendix B: Mail-Order Sources for Equipment and Other Supplies

I: THE BASICS

Skin-fold calipers

Fat-O-Meter, Health and Education Services, Division of Novel Products, 80 Fairbanks Street, Addison, Illinois 60101.

The Slim Guide Skinfold Caliper, Creative Health Products, 9135 R General Court, Plymouth, Michigan 48170.

Vitamins

Commercial multivitamin preparations approximating Dr. Roger J. Williams's guidelines:

Vitamin and Mineral Formula, Bronson Pharmaceuticals, 4526 Rinetti Lane, La Canada, California 91011.

Strong Cobb and Arner, ICN Pharmaceuticals, 222 North Vincent Avenue, Covina, California 91722.

Milk Intolerance

Lact-Aid to break down milk sugars is made for SugarLo Company, P.O. Box 1017, Atlantic City, New Jersey 08404.

Altitude training stimulator

PO_2 Aerobic Exerciser is manufactured by Inspirair, Inc., 2630 Townsgate Road, Suite I, Westlake Village, California 91361. Available by mail from Pacific Athletic Trading Company, P.O. Box 5038, Thousand Oaks, California 91360, or Sweat Inc., P.O. Box 567, 3219 Close Court, Cincinnati, Ohio 45201.

II: SPORTS AND EXERCISE

Sports Bras

The Lady Duke Sports Bra, Royal Textile Mills, Yanceyville, North Carolina 27379.

Jogbra, SLS Inc., P.O. Box 661, 24 Clarke Street, Burlington, Vermont 05402.

Playtops, International Playtex, Inc., 700 Fairfield Avenue, Stamford, Connecticut 06902.

Running Bra, Formfit Rogers, 530 Fifth Avenue, New York, New York 10017.

The Sport Bra, Lily of France, 90 Park Avenue, New York, New York, 10016.

The Serious Running Bra, Flexees, 16 East 40th Street, New York, New York 10016. (They also make the Step-In Bra.)

Run Around, Splendor Form Brassiere, Inc., 632 Broadway, New York, New York 10012.

Clothing Manufacturers

Damart Thermawear, 1811 Woodbury Avenue, Portsmouth, New Hampshire 03805. Specializes in exceedingly warm, light, comfortable under- and outerwear for all sizes, even petites and extra-talls. Sold only at the showroom or by mail.

Moving Comfort, 890-G South Picket Street, Alexandria, Virginia 22304. Manufactures women's running clothes in designs also useful for roller skating and for playing soccer, tennis, and racquetball. Sold through sporting good stores.

QP-Pants by Sarah, 3300 Atlantic Boulevard, Jacksonville, Florida 32207. Hiking slacks and shorts tailored for a woman's proportions but with crotch seams fastened together with Velcro instead of stitches. When nature calls, you don't have to strip off your pants; you just open the Velcro crotch. Sold by Outdoor Gal or by mail order.

Sierra Designs, 247 Fourth Street, Oakland, California 94607. Outdoor clothing made of wool, down, Thinsulate, and other light, warm fibers, fitted for women as well as men. Sold direct by mail order or from other retail suppliers.

Silva Company, 1 Marine Midland Building, P.O. Box 966, Binghamton, New York 13902. Sells armored socks to ward off thorns and other attacking vegetation. Also sells other orienteering equipment.

Women on the Run, 2087 Union Street, San Francisco, California 94123. Athletic clothes constructed specifically for women. Available from sporting goods and department stores.

Mail-Order Houses

Eddie Bauer, Fifth and Union, P.O. Box 3700, Seattle, Washington 98124. Hiking, backpacking, and casual clothes. Stocks small sizes and will custom-make catalogue items in nonstandard sizes.

L. L. Bean, Freeport, Maine 04033. Casual, outdoor, and backpacking, inner- and outerwear. Open twenty-four hours a day, 365 days a year. Refunds for damaged or unsatisfactory goods as prompt as delivery of merchandise.

Early Winters Ltd., 110 Prefontaine Place South, Seattle, Washington 98104. Outdoor and camping clothing and equipment, including a plethora of fascinating gadgets. Offers a search service for hard-to-find items not in their catalogue. Good source for polypropylene underwear.

Eastern Mountain Sports, Vose Farm Road, Peterborough, New Hampshire 03458. Outdoor, camping, cross-country skiing, and mountaineering clothing and equipment.

Outdoor Gal, 116 East Chestnut Street, Burlington, Wisconsin 53105. Clothing designed specifically for women. Sells QP-Pants.

Recreational Equipment Co-op, Inc., P.O. Box C-88125, Seattle, Washington 98188. Costs $5 to join this co-op, but members receive cash dividends at the end of each year. Serious camping, hiking, backpacking, mountaineering, and cross-country skiing clothes and equipment. Sells own products and well-known quality brands. Good source of polypropylene underwear. No small or large sizes.

Sierra Designs (see Clothing Manufacturers).

Women's Sports Center, 555 Washington Street, Wellesley, Massachusetts 02181. Clothes, uniforms, and equipment for the woman athlete in almost any sport, including curling, lacrosse, track and field, ice hockey, field hockey, and soccer. Particularly strong in racket sports. Features women's athletic shoes and clothing in large sizes. No catalogue. You request the size and type of item and they send it to you.

Shoes

If possible, buy your shoes and boots in person rather than by mail. Fitting footwear by drawing foot outlines and estimating shoe size is a tricky business.

Eddie Bauer (see Mail-Order Houses). Hiking boots.

L. L. Bean (see Mail-Order Houses). Hiking, walking, and running shoes and boots.

Danner Shoe Manufacturing Company, P.O. Box 22204, Portland, Oregon 97222. Hiking boots and walking shoes designed especially for women.

Fabiano Shoe Company, 850 Summer Street, South Boston, Massachusetts 02127. Hiking, cross-country skiing, and mountaineering boots; some women's sizes, some unisex sizes.

Outdoor Gal (see Mail-Order Houses). Hiking boots and running shoes.

Recreational Equipment, Inc. (see Mail-Order Houses). Large selection of rock-climbing, backpacking, mountaineering, and hiking boots in women's sizes, as well as women's walking, leisure, running, and court shoes.

Relayce, P.O. Box 2643, Scottsdale, Arizona 85252. Manufactures rubberized shoelaces which give wherever an athletic shoe feels tight.

Tall Gals Shoecraft, 603 Fifth Avenue, New York, New York 10017. Shoes and socks for large feet.

Vasque Shoe Company, 419 Bush Street, Red Wing, Minnesota 55066. Manufactures no-nonsense walking shoes as well as hiking, rock-climbing, and mountaineering boots which meet the toughest specifications; some models designed especially for women. No mail order; write for retail store nearest you.

Women's Sports Center (see Mail-Order Houses). Shoes for most sports.

Safety Equipment

Spex Sports Opticians, 575 Boylston Street, Boston, Massachusetts 02116. Mail-order prescription swimming, waterskiing, surfing, and skiing goggles as well as prescription wraparound eye protectors for racket and contact sports and prescription lenses fitted inside scuba and skin-diving face masks.

Alpine Skiing

Inside Edge Ski and Bike Shop, 624 Glen Street, Glen Falls, New York 12801. (Mail-order company at same address is called Reliable Racing Supply.) Competitive ski gear.

Recreational Equipment Inc. (see Mail-Order Houses).

Bicycling

Bell Helmets, 15301 Shoemaker Avenue, Norwalk, California 90650. Manufacturers of the safest helmets on the market as of this writing.

Bikecology, Inc., 12509 Beatrice Street, P.O. Box 66–909, Los Angeles, California 90066. Sell a very large stock of their own and name-brand equipment, accessories, including the Mirrycle, and clothes.

Bike Warehouse, 215 Main Street, New Middletown, Ohio 44442.

Cycles Peugeot (U.S.A.) Inc., 555 Gotham Parkway, Carlstadt, New Jersey 07072 *or* 18805 Laurel Park Road, Compton, California 90220. Wholesalers for imported bicycle parts, including Mafac and Weinmann short-reach brake levers for

small hands. Write them for distributor nearest you.

Lickton's Cycle City, 310 Lake Street, Oak Park, Illinois 60302.

Canoeing and Kayaking

Baldwin Boat Company, Hoxie Hill Road, Orrington, Maine 04474. Kayaks, canoes, and sailing kayaks, assembled and in kit form.

Perception, Inc., P.O. Box 686, Liberty, South Carolina 29657. White-water canoes, kayaks, and accessories.

Circuit Training and Exercising

The following list of manufacturers of indoor exercisers accept mail orders. They will also provide you with a list of distributors in your area. If possible, buy your equipment from a nearby store. With few exceptions, dumbbells and exercise equipment are heavy and expensive to ship.

Advanced Fitness Equipment of Northern California, 703 Grandview Drive, South San Francisco, California 94080. Reliable mail-order department featuring top-quality brands of stationary bicycles, rowing machines, home gyms, free weights, and other equipment.

Amerec Corporation, 1776 136th Place Northeast, Bellevue, Washington 98005. Distributors of Tunturi and Amerec 610 stationary bicycles and rowing machines.

AMF-Whitely, 29 Essex Street, Maywood, New Jersey 07607. Manufacturers of chest pulls, hand grips, jump ropes, and more.

Diversified Products Corporation, 309 Williamson Avenue, Opelika, Alabama 36801. Manufacturers of dumbbells, barbells, wrist and ankle weights, and other weight-lifting equipment.

Dynavit, Keiper U.S.A., 5600 West Dickman Road, Battle Creek, Michigan 49015. Distributes Dynavit, a very expensive ultra-modern stationary bicycle that paces your pedaling according to your age, weight, and sex.

Exer-Genie, Inc., 1628 South Clementine Street, Anaheim, California 92802.

Lifeline Gym (see Lifeline Rope under Rope Jumping).

Mini-Gym, Inc., 1026 South Powell Street, East Independence, Missouri.

Nautilus Sports/Medical Industries, P.O. Box 1783, DeLand, Florida 32720.

Schwinn stationary bicycles, Excelsior Fitness Equipment Company, 613 Academy Drive, Northbrook, Illinois 60062.

Total Gym, Total Medical Systems, 7161 Engineer Road, San Diego, California 92111. Sturdy, expensive incline board and pulley system for sliding resistance training with a *small* amount of aerobic conditioning.

Universal Gym, Centurion Sales Company, P.O. Box P, Mountain View, California 94042.

Cross-Country Skiing

Akers Ski, Andover, Maine 04216.

Early Winters (see Mail-Order Houses).

Eastern Mountain Sports (see Mail-Order Houses).

Inside Edge Ski and Bike Shop (see Alpine Skiing). Large selection of training and racing supplies, including roller skis.

Nordic Sports, 218 West Bay Street, East Tawas, Michigan 48730. Discount prices on large selection of racing and touring equipment and accessories.

Recreational Equipment, Inc. (see Mail-Order Houses). In addition to offering a wide selection of equipment, they provide workshops on choosing proper skis, poles, bindings, and boots.

Lacrosse

These two manufacturers make non-contact lacrosse games:

STX-ball, STX-Inc., 1500 Bush Street, Baltimore, Maryland 21230.

McWhippet, Brine Company, 47 Sumner Street, Milford, Massachusetts 01757.

Mountain and Rock Climbing

See under Mail-Order Houses, Eastern Mountaineering, Recreational Equipment, and Sierra Designs.

Rope Jumping

Goodleg Jumper Company, P.O. Box 363, Graton, California 95444. Sells adjustable small and large nylon jump ropes in a selection of vibrant colors.

Lifeline Rope, Lifeline Production and Marketing, Inc., 30 North Charter Street, Madison, Wisconsin 53715. Sells adjustable ropes weighted with beads for a better arc (and more painful bruises when they hit your shins) and ropes with digital counters in the handle.

Rugby

As of this writing, no rugby boots or clothing are made specifically for women. Patrick boots, like most other French-made shoes, have a narrow last suitable to many women. Mitre boots, like most British shoes, have a wider last.

Matt Godek Rugby Supply, P.O. Box 565, Merrifield, Virginia 22116. Boots, jerseys, and equipment in unisex sizes and styles.

Grizzly Sports Supply, P.O. Box 3858, San Rafael, California 94912. Complete selection of uniforms, equipment, accessories, and shoes in unisex sizes and styles.

Rugby Imports, 1019 Waterman Avenue, East Providence, Rhode Island 02914. Supplies, books, and films.

Running

Because of the popularity of the sport, running shoes, clothing, and accessories are available in almost any part of the country and in almost every mail-order sporting goods catalogue.

Silva Company, 1 Marine Midland Building, P.O. Box 966, Binghamton, New York 13902. Supplies compasses, bramble-proof high socks, and other orienteering equipment.

Soccer

Like rugby players, women soccer players must be satisfied with men's shoes. If you wear a shoe smaller than a size six, you may have to settle for the lacrosse shoe sold by the Women's Sport Center.

Both of the following stores sell extensively by mail to women's teams all over the country:

Fishers of Florissant, 75 South Florissant Road, Florissant, Missouri 63031.

Mr. Soccer, 14027 Floyd Road, Dallas, Texas 75240.

Swimming and Diving

Each of the following mail-order houses supplies a wide variety of competitive and recreational swimming and diving suits, goggles, nose clips, caps, and training equipment:

The Finals, 149 Mercer Street, New York, New York 10012.

National Aquatic Service, 1425 Erie Boulevard East, Syracuse, New York 13210. Also sells scuba gear.

The Swim Shop, 1400 Eighth Avenue South, Nashville, Tennessee 37203.

Uglies Unlimited, 1617 East Highland, Phoenix, Arizona 85016.

Team Handball

These companies supply nets, balls, uniforms, coaching manuals, and training films:

Jayfro Corporation, P.O. Box 400, Waterford, Connecticut 06385.

U.S. Team Handball Supply Company, 400 Hillside Avenue, Hillside, New Jersey 07205.

Walking

See under Mail-Order Houses, Eddie Bauer, L. L. Bean, Early Winters, Eastern Mountain Sports, Recreational Equipment, and Sierra Designs.

III: SPORTS MEDICINE

Ambeze, Whitestone Products, 40 Turner Place, Piscataway, New Jersey 08854.

Ana-Kit, Hollister-Stier Laboratories, 3525 North Regal Street, Spokane, Washington 99207. First aid for insect stings.

Spenco Medical Corporation, P.O. Box 8113, Waco, Texas 76710. Manufactures flexible and firm arch supports, shock-absorbing insoles, cold/hot packs, and Second Skin, a film filled with watery gel that protects blistered or burned skin.

Unpetroleum Jelly, Pure Body Creations, Londonderry Plaza, Londonderry, Vermont 05148. Protects skin longer than Vaseline and other petroleum jellies.

Notes

INTRODUCTION

Page

1–2   Figures are based on statistics from: The *President's Council on Physical Fitness and Sports Newsletter*, December 1980, p. 7; *The Perrier Study: Fitness in America,* a survey conducted by Louis Harris & Associates, Inc. Published in January 1979.

CHAPTER 1—CHOOSING YOUR
PERSONAL FITNESS PROGRAM

7–8   Endorphins and exercise are discussed in "Physical Conditioning Facilitates Exercise-Induced Secretion of Beta-Endorphins and Beta Lipotropins in Women," *The New England Journal of Medicine,* September 3, 1981: 560–563 and "What Makes Us Run?" pp. 578–579 of the same issue.

9   Dr. Allan J. Ryan reviews the history and explanations of athletes' enlarged hearts in "Heart Size and Sports" in *the physician and sportsmedicine,* vol. 8, August 1980: 29–38. For another discussion, see "Echocardiography and the Athlete's Heart" by Francois Peronnet, Ph.D., Ronald J. Ferguson, Ph.D., Helene Perrault, M.Sc., Giuseppe Ricci, M.Sc., and Daniel Lajoie, M.Sc. in *the physician and sportsmedicine,* vol. 9, May 1981: 103–112.

Page

18–22   Most of these strength and flexibility tests are explained in *Total Woman's Fitness Guide* by Gail Shierman, Ph.D., and Christine Haycock, M.D. Mountain View, California: World Publications, 1979, pp. 9–12.

26   The evaluation of stress tests ran in *The New England Journal of Medicine,* October 4, 1979: 792–793.

CHAPTER 2: FOURTEEN
PRINCIPLES OF CONDITIONING

30   The classic oxygen debt theory, developed by 1922 Nobel prize winners Hill and Meyerhof, states that lactic acid is a dead-end waste product during exercise. However, George Brooks and Glenn Gaesser, writing in the *Journal of Applied Psysiology* (vol. 49, December 1980: 1057–1069), claim that their research shows that under some conditions, muscles burn lactic acid (in the presence of oxygen) as a source of quick fuel for muscles. The figure for Grete Waitz's max VO_2 comes from "The Pulse Rate Game" by Amby Burfoot, *Runner's World,* July 1981: 86.

36–37   University of Texas at Dallas scientist William J. Gonyea, Ph.D., showed that weight lifting stimulates the muscle fi-

Page
36–37
(cont.) bers in cats to multiply, as reported an article in *the physician and sportsmedicine*, vol. 8, January, 1980: 22–23. Although Dr. Gonyea is careful not to apply his findings to human beings, the chances are the mechanisms are the same. In "Muscle Fiber Composition and Performance Capacities of Women" by C. J. Campbell, A. Bonene, R. L. Kirby and A. M. Belcastro, *Medicine and Science in Sports*, vol. 11 (1979): 260–265, the fiber composition of twenty-four women is analyzed and shown to be only one small factor in how well athletes perform.

44 B. Ricci, M. Marchetti, and F. Figura of the Institute of Human Physiology at the University of Rome, Italy, explain which muscles are used during each part of the sit-up in "Biomechanics of Sit-Up Exercises" in *Medicine and Science in Sports and Exercise*, vol. 13 (1981): 54–59. Alan Halpern and Eugen Gleck performed the electromyographic studies showing how active the abdominal muscles are in each type of sit-up, as published in "Sit-Up Exercises: An Electromyographic Study" in *Clinical Orthopedics and Related Research*, no. 145: 172–178.

CHAPTER 3: SOUND NUTRITION

51 *Dietary Goals for the United States, 1977*, the report released by the Senate Select Committee on Nutrition and Human Needs, is sold for $.95 by the Superintendent of Documents, Government Printing Office, Washington, D.C. Ask for stock number O52-070-3913-2. *Nutrition and Your Health*, a free twenty-page booklet from the Office of Governmental and Public Affairs, U.S. Department of Agriculture, Washington, D.C. 20250, is a 1980 update issued jointly by the Departments of Agriculture and Health, Education and Welfare.

Dr. Michael Colgan's work is introduced by William Gottlieb in "Supple-

Page
menting Your Performance," *Women's Sports*, September, 1981: 50–51.

57 After years of medical scepticism about the efficacy of vitamin C, recent research has supported much of the early work done by Dr. Williams and Linus Pauling. William Gottlieb reports on the work on vitamin C and exercise in "The Ascorbic Acid Test," *Women's Sports*, October, 1981: 48. The beneficial effects of taking extra vitamin C—including lowered cholesterol levels and resistance to infection (and perhaps even some cancers), are reported in "Multiple Vitamin C Effects Described" in *Medical Tribune*, May 27, 1981: 4. *Medical Tribune*, July 22, 1981: 1, also reported that Japanese scientists have found that terminal cancer patients receiving large doses of vitamin C survive from 1½ to 15 times as long as patients receiving little or no vitamin C.

69 For a very technical exposition on the effects of alcohol, see "Smoking Habits, Alcohol Consumption and Maximal Oxygen Uptake" by Henry J. Montoye, Richard Gayle, and Millicent Higgins in *Medicine and Science in Sports and Exercise*, vol. 12 (1980): 316–321.

70–71 Sugar is discussed in "Diet, Fitness and Athletic Performance" by Angelo Bentivegna, D.Ed., R.D.; E. James Kelley, Ed.D; and Alexander Kalenak, M.D., in *the physician and sportsmedicine*, vol. 7, October 1979: 99–105; and in "Sports Nutrition: The Role of Carbohydrates" by David Costill, *Nutrition News*, vol. 41, February 1978.

75–76 Blood doping is reviewed in "Blood Doping: An Update" by Melvin H. Williams, Ph.D., in *the physician and sportsmedicine*, vol. 9, July 1981: 59–64.

76–77 Altitude simulators are explained in "Instant Altitude" by Eric Olsen, *The Runner*, August 1981: 22–23.

83 The calorie costs of many sports and household chores are listed in *Nutrition, Weight Control and Exercise* by Frank

Page

83   I. Katch and William D. McArdle, Bos-
(*cont.*) ton: Houghton Mifflin Company (1977):
        348–357; and in "Human Energy Ex-
        penditure" by R. Passmore and J. V. G.
        A. Durnin, *Physiology Review*, vol. 37
        (1955): 8091–840; and in *Human Nutri-
        tion: Its Physiological, Medical and So-
        cial Aspects* by Jean Mayer. Springfield,
        Ill.: Charles D. Thomas, Publisher
        (1972): 13–37.

86   The analysis of the activity of obese girls
        appears in "Energy Balance of Obese
        Patients During Weight Reduction: In-
        fluence of Diet Restrictions and Exer-
        cise" by E. R. Buskirk, R. H. Thompson,
        L. Lutwak and G. D. Whedon in *Annals
        of the New York Academy of Sciences*,
        vol. 11 (1963): 918–940.

CHAPTER 5: FIVE BASIC SPORTS

96–98   The features of a supportive athletic bra
        were outlined by Christine E. Haycock,
        M.D., Gail Shierman, Ph.D. and Joan
        Gillette, C.A.T., in their paper "The Fe-
        male Anatomy—Does Her Anatomy
        Pose Problems?" which was presented at
        the American Medical Association Meet-
        ing, June 1977. The subject is also fully
        covered by Gale Gehlsen, Ph.D. and
        Marge Albohm, M.S., A.T.C., in "Evalu-
        ation of Sports Bras," *the physician and
        sportsmedicine*, vol. 8 October 1980: 89–
        97.

98ff   All statistics on sports participation on p.
        98 and throughout the chapter are ex-
        trapolated from *The Perrier Study: Fit-
        ness in America*, already cited, and from
        USA Statistics in Brief, 1979. The bicy-
        cling figures are based on "Future
        Bikes" by Barney Cohen. *The New York
        Times Magazine*, August 10, 1980: 20,
        and "Bicycling Injuries," *the physician
        and sportsmedicine*, vol. 8 May 1980:
        88–96.

120   John Schubert reports on the work on re-
        flectorized suits in "Should You Be
        Wearing Early Warning?" in *Bicycling*,
        June 1981: 52–56.

Page

124   Wind resistance figures come from page
        24 of Barney Cohen's "Future Bikes" ar-
        ticle already cited.

141   "The Ultimate Study of Running Injur-
        ies" by John Pagliano, D.P.M., and
        Douglas Jackson, M.D., appeared in
        Runner's World, November 1980: 42–
        50.

CHAPTER 6: THE HOME CIRCUIT
TRAINING PROGRAM

151   Researchers have done very little work
        on women in circuit training. The two
        studies including women are "Physio-
        logical Alternations Consequent to Cir-
        cuit Weight Training" by Jack H. Wil-
        more, R. B. Parr, R. N. Girandola et al,
        in *Medicine and Science in Sports*, vol.
        10 (1978): 79–84; and *The Syracuse Cir-
        cuit Weight Training Study Report* by
        D. S. Garfield, P. Ward, R. Cobb et al.
        Houston: Dynamics Health Equipment,
        1979. For an overview, also see "Circuit
        Weight Training: A Critical Review of
        Its Physiological Benefits" by Larry R.
        Gettman, Ph.D., and Michael L. Pollock,
        Ph.D., in *the physician and sportsmedi-
        cine*, vol. 9, January 1981: 44–60.

154–155 *Rating the Exercises* by Charles T.
        Kuntzleman and the editors of *Consum-
        er Guide* devotes an entire chapter to
        useful and useless exercise gadgets. New
        York: William Morrow and Company,
        Inc. (1978): 256–271.

189   *Proprioceptive Neuromuscular Facilita-
        tion* by Margaret Knott is the definitive
        work on PNF. New York: Hoeber, 1956.
        Marjorie A. Moor and Robert S. Hutton
        validated the method in "Electromyo-
        graphic Investigation of Muscle Stretch-
        ing Techniques" in *Medicine and Sci-
        ence in Sports and Exercise*, vol. 12,
        (1980): 322–329.

CHAPTER 7: SPORTS A–W

220   The California Interscholastic Federation
        developed the guidelines on how to fit a

Page

220 football helmet, as reported in *Sports-*
(*cont.*) *medicine Digest*, August 1981, p. 3.

CHAPTER 8: MENSTRUATION
AND MENOPAUSE

277 Among the studies on athletic performance during menstruation, the following
are especially interesting: Christine L.
Wells, Ph.D. "Sexual Differences in
Heat Stress Response," *the physician
and sportsmedicine*, vol. 5, September
1977: 79–90; L. A. Stephenson, M. A.
Kolka, and J. E. Wilkerson, "Anaerobic
Threshhold, Work Capacity and Per-
ceived Exertion During the Menstrual
Cycle," a paper presented at the annual
meeting of the American College of
Sports Medicine, 1980; Mona Shangold,
M.D., "Sports and Menstrual Function,"
the physician and sportsmedicine, vol. 8
August 1980: 66–69; "Physical Activity
During Menstruation and Pregnancy,"
edited by H. Harrison Clarke, Ed.D.,
Physical Fitness Research Digest, Series
i, July 1978.

280 Michael Osterholm, Ph.D., of the Minnesota Health Department reported that
exercise was one of the few significant
factors in the Tri-State Toxic Shock Syndrome Study, as quoted in *the physician
and sportsmedicine*, vol. 9, June 1981:
21–22.

291 J. M. Aitken et al reviewed the chances for
osteoporosis after surgically induced
menopause in "Osteoporosis After Oo-
phorectomy for Nonmalignant Disease
in Premenopausal Women," *British
Medical Journal*, vol. 2, May 1973: 325–
328.

292 *The Health Letter*, vol. 18, no. 1, discusses the possible relationship of antacids and osteoporosis. Hellen M. Linkswiler reported on the relationship
between protein consumption and calcification in *Transactions of the New
York Academy of Sciences*, series 2, vol.
36, no. 4: 333–340.

Page

CHAPTER 9: BIRTH CONTROL
AND PREGNANCY

296 For the effects of birth control pills on
heart disease, see: Dennis Slone, Samuel
Shapiro, David W. Kaufman, Lynn
Rosenberg, Olli S. Miettinen and Paul D.
Stolley, "Risk of Myocardial Infarction
in Relation to Current and Discontinued
Use of Oral Contraceptives," *The New
England Journal of Medicine*, vol. 305,
August 20, 1981: 420–424; Bruce V. Sta-
del, "Oral Contraceptives and Cardio-
vascular Disease," *The New England
Journal of Medicine*, part I, vol. 305,
September 10, 1981: 612–618; part II,
vol. 305, September 17, 1981: 672–677.

397 For the effects of physical activity on
pregnancy, see Carl T. Javert, M.D.,
Spontaneous and Habitual ABortion.
New York: McGraw Hill, 1975, 240–243.
See also the same author's "Role of the
Patient's Activities in the Occurrence of
Spontaneous Abortion," *Fertility and
Sterility*, vol. 11 (1960): 550–558.

CHAPTER 10: SPORTSMEDICINE

329–330 *The Medical Letter* reviews DMSO in its
October 31, 1980, issue: 95.

332 Electrical stimulation to mask pain is reported in "Brain Electrodes Fulfilling
Pain Relief Promise," *Medical Tribune*,
May 27, 1981: 30–31; and in *Science
News*, vol. 119: 374. Electrical stimulation to promote bone healing is reviewed
in *The Medical Letter*, April 3, 1981:
35–36.

333 George Ulett discusses the efficacy of
acupuncture in "Acupuncture Treatments in Pain Relief," *Journal of the
American Medical Association*, vol. 245
(1981): 768–769.

391 The aloe vera work of Wendell D. Winters, M.D., associate professor of microbi-
ology at the University of Texas Health
Sciences Center in San Antonio, is cited
in *The Health Letter*, vol. 18, no. 5.

Selected Reading

I: THE BASICS

Exercise and Weight Control

Lappé, Frances Moore. *Diet for a Small Planet* (revised edition). New York: Ballantine Books, 1975.

Nutrition Search, Inc. *Nutrition Almanac* (revised edition). New York: McGraw-Hill Book Company, 1979.

Pennington, Jean, and Helen Nichols Church, eds. *Bowes and Church's Food Values of Portions Commonly Used* (thirteenth edition). New York: Harper & Row (Colophon Books), 1980.

Williams, Dr. Roger J. *The Wonderful World Within You*. New York: Bantam Books, 1977.

Smith, Nathan. *Food for Sport*. Palo Alto, Calif.: Bull Publishing Company, 1976.

II: SPORTS AND EXERCISE

Outside, P.O. Box 2690, Boulder, Colorado 80321. Eight issues per year. A beautiful full-color magazine filled with striking photos and literate articles about animal behavior, sports, conservation, and equipment innovations.

Women's Sports, P.O. Box 121, Mount Morris, Illinois 61054. Twelve issues per year. Publishes articles on athletes, sports techniques, health, and sports medicine for all sports.

Alpine Skiing

Ski, P.O. Box 2795, Boulder, Colorado 80302. Seven issues per year. Filled with columns and features on technique and travel.

Skiing, P.O. Box 2777, Boulder, Colorado 80302. Seven issues per year. Concentrates on technique and buying guides to equipment.

Slanger, Elissa, and Dinah Witchel. *Ski Woman's Way*. New York: Summit Books, 1979. Explains their own program, tailored exclusively to a woman's psychological and physical makeup.

Basketball

Women's Basketball, P.O. Box 11302, Chicago, Illinois 60611. Ten issues per year. Publishes scores, statistics, and articles about high school, college, and professional women's basketball.

Bicycling

Bicycle Motocross Action, Wizard Publications. P.O. Box 4277, Torrance, California 90510. Twelve issues per year. Aimed at teenage males.

Bicycling, Emmaus, Pennsylvania 18049. Nine issues per year. Racing, touring, and good how-to repairs.

BMX Plus! 2458 West Lomita Boulevard, Lomita, California 90717. Twelve issues per year. Aimed at teenage males.

City Cyclist, Transportation Alternatives, 133 West 72nd Street, New York, New York 10023. Irregular newsletter, but subscription includes free want ads.

Cuthbertson, Tom. *Anybody's Bike Book: An Original Manual of Bicycle Repairs* (revised edition). Berkeley, Cal.: Ten Speed Press, 1979.

Cycletouring, Cyclists' Touring Club, Cotterell House, 69 Meadrow, Godalming, Surrey, England GU6 3HS. Six issues per year. Good information on international touring.

DeLong, Fred. *DeLong's Guide to Bicycles and Bicycling: The Art and Science*. Radnor, Pa. Chilton Book Company, 1978.

Kingbay, Keith. *Inside Bicycling*. Chicago: Contemporary Books, 1976.

McCullagh, James C., ed. *Pedal Power in Work, Leisure, and Transportation*. Emmaus, Pa.: Rodale Press, 1977. How to produce electricity from a stationary bicycle to power televisions and other home appliances.

Sloan, Eugene A. *The All New Complete Book of Bicycling*. New York: Simon and Schuster, 1980.

Velo-News: A Journal of Bicycle Racing, P.O. Box 1257, Brattleboro, Vermont 05301. Eighteen issues per year. Results, training, personalities.

Board Sailing

Sailboarder, P.O. Box 1028, Dana Point, California 92629. Six issues per year.

Windsurfer, 1955 West 190th Street, Torrance, California 90509. Six issues per year, available with membership in the International Windsurfer Class Association. Contains instructional articles and results of national and international competitions.

Canoeing and Kayaking

Canoe, P.O. Box 10748, Des Moines, Iowa 50340. Six issues per year. Devoted entirely to canoeing and kayaking in all forms; includes consumer buying information, travel features, and articles on technique.

Cross-Country Skiing

Hixson, Edward G., M.D. *The Physician and Sportsmedicine Guide to Cross-Country Skiing*. New York: McGraw-Hill Book Company, 1980.

Cross Country Skier, P.O. Box 1203, West Brattleboro, Vermont 05301. Seven issues per year.

Circuit Training and Exercising

Anderson, Bob. *Stretching*. Bolinas, Cal.: Shelter Publications (distributed by Random House), 1980. The best, most complete, and most attractive book on sports stretching on the market today.

Hittleman, Richard. *Richard Hittleman's Yoga 28 Day Exercise Plan*. New York: Bantam Books, 1968. Step-by-step instructions for an introductory, relatively undemanding Yoga routine to loosen muscles and strengthen them very slightly.

Isaacs, Benno, and Jay Kobler. *The Nickolaus Technique*. New York: Viking Press, 1978. Thirty calisthenic and yogic exercises choreographed into an original and unusual program which both strengthens and stretches most parts of your body. Posture and physical appearance stressed over athletics. Tapes based on routines performed at Nickolaus classes in and around New York City are also available.

Dance

American Square Dance, P.O. Box 488, Huron, Ohio 44839. Twelve issues per year. Includes dancing, choreography, and calling tips as well as calendars and personality profiles.

Contact Quarterly, P.O. Box 603, Northampton, Massachusetts 01060. Four issues per year. Stresses body therapies, injury rehabilitation, holistic health, applied kinesiology, and other methods of body awareness for dancers.

Dance in Canada, 100 Richmond Street East, Suite 325, Toronto, Ontario, Canada M5C 2 9. Four issues per year. Although concerned with the developing dance scene in Canada, its articles on training and its review section have international applications.

Dancemagazine, 1180 Avenue of the Americas, New York, New York 10036. Twelve issues per year. The world's largest dance publication: includes nationwide performance calendars and reviews and a dance school directory as well as articles on technique and injury rehabilitation.

Dance Scope, American Dance Guild, 1133 Broadway, Room 1427, New York, New York 10010. Four issues per year. Subjects range from dance criticism and historical scholarship to book reviews and personality profiles of ballet, modern, and musical theater dancers.

Jacob, Ellen. *Dancing: A Guide for the Dancer You Can Be*. Reading, Mass.: Addison-Wesley Publishing Company, 1981. An encyclopedia for every dancer—beginner or advanced, male or female—covering such topics as how to find a good teacher, how to choose your own dance style, and how to avoid injuries. Discusses ballet, modern, tap, and jazz dance.

Vincent, L. M., M.D. *Competing with the Sylph: Dancers and the Pursuit of the Ideal Body Form*. Kansas City: Andrews and McMeel, 1979. An intelligent and sympathetic discussion of ballet dancers' dangerous obsession with thinness.

———. *The Dancers' Book of Health*. Kansas City: Sheed Andrews and McMeel, 1978. A treatise in plain English on dancers' special health and injury problems.

Figure Skating

Skating, 20 First Street, Colorado Springs, Colorado 80906. Eight issues per year. The official publication of the United States Figure Skating Association, but also available by subscription to nonmembers. Features results of competitions as well as articles on technique.

Ogilvie, Robert S. *Basic Ice Skating Skills*. New York: J. B. Lippincott Company, 1968.

Gymnastics and Acrobatics

Sports Illustrated Women's Gymnastics 1: The Floor Exercise Event and *Sports Illustrated Women's Gymnastics 2: The Vaulting, Balance Beam, and Uneven Parallel Bars Events*. New York: Lippincott & Crowell, Publishers, 1980. Clear, stop-action drawings and instructions of all major maneuvers.

Handball

Handball. Six issues per year. Distributed to all members of the United States Handball Association. Articles on technique, equipment, tournaments, and personalities.

Ice Hockey

Hockey and Arena, published by the Amateur Hockey Association, 2997 Broadmoor Valley Road, Colorado Springs, Colorado 80906. Seven issues per year. Available by subscription or membership in the AHA.

Stamm, Laura. *Power Skating the Hockey Way*. New York: E. P. Dutton, 1977.

Ice Skating

For $12.50, Dianne Holum sells a dry-land and ice manual she has compiled herself. Write Dianne Holum, 1035 Malory Street, Lafayette, Colorado 80026.

Karate, Kung Fu, and Tae Kwon Do

Fighting Woman News, P.O. Box 1459, Grand Central Station, New York, New York 10163. Four issues per year. Feminist magazine covering all martial arts.

Nagamine, Shoshin. *The Essence of Okinawan Karate-Do*. Translated by Susan Borger. Rutland, Vt.: Charles E. Tuttle Company, 1976.

Schroeder, Charles Roy, and Bill Wallace. *Karate: Basic Concepts and Skills*. Reading, Mass.: Addison-Wesley Publishing Company, 1980.

Mountain Climbing

Climbing, Box E, Aspen, Colorado 81611. Six issues per year.

Mountain, P.O. Box 184, Sheffield, England S11 9DL. Six issues per year.

Racquetball

National Racquetball, available with membership in the United States Racquetball Association, 4101 Dempster Street, Skokie, Illinois 60076. Twelve issues per year. Instructional articles, equipment reports, schedules, and results of tournaments.

Spear, Victor I., M.D., *Sports Illustrated Racquetball*. New York: J. B. Lippincott Company, 1979.

Roller Skating

RollerSkating Magazine, P.O. Box 1028, Dana Point, California 92629. Six issues per year. Concentrates on recreational skating, roller hockey, and speed skating but is now beginning to include instructional articles on artistic skating.

Skate, published monthly by the United States Amateur Confederation of Roller Skating, 7700 A Street, P.O. Box 83067, Lincoln, Nebraska 68501. Results of tournaments and serious how-to articles.

Rope Jumping

Prentup, Frank B. *Skipping the Rope.* Boulder, Colorado. Pruett Publishing Company (3235 Prairie Avenue), 1963. Techniques for fancy steps.

Smith, Paul. *Rope Skipping Rhythms, Routines, Rhymes.* Freeport, N.Y.: Educational Activities, Inc. 1969.

Rugby

Rugby, 527 Madison Avenue, New York, New York, 10022. Eight issues per year. Newspaper covering world rugby scene, sports medicine, and coaching.

Running

Fixx, James F. *The Complete Book of Running.* New York: Random House, 1977. Slightly outdated, but still the most entertaining and inspirational of the how-to books.

———— *Jim Fixx's Second Book of Running.* New York: Random House, 1980. A personal review of current theories about running and health.

Ullyot, Joan L. *Women's Running.* Mountain View, Cal.: World Publications, 1976. The first book to discuss style and training from a woman's perspective.

———— *Running Free.* New York: G. P. Putnam's Sons, 1980. An update of *Women's Running* with much more feminist political rhetoric.

The National MASTERS Newsletter, P.O. Box 2372, Van Nuys, California 91404. Twelve issues per year. The only national periodical devoted exclusively to track and field and long-distance running for people over thirty.

The Runner, P.O. Box 2730, Boulder, Colorado 80322. Twelve issues per year. In-depth news magazine for distance runners with explicit how-to articles as well as news of races and racers.

Runner's World, P.O. Box 366, Mountain View, California 94042. Twelve issues per year. Slick magazine of how-to articles discussing current fads and theories for the beginning and intermediate distance runner. Many of the articles are excerpted from books published by World Publications, their own publisher, and others are recycled, in slightly altered guises, year after year.

Running, P.O. Box 350, Salem, Oregon 97308. Four issues per year. Glossy, with exquisite photographs and explanations of running theories. No condescension, little faddism. Has always called itself "the thinking runner's magazine" and is now owned by Nike, the shoe manufacturer.

Running Times, 12808 Occoquan Road, Woodbridge, Virginia 22192. Twelve issues per year. No-nonsense news about runners and running, plus thorough national race calendar and results from large and small races.

Track and Field News, P.O. Box 296, Los Altos, California 94022. Twelve issues per year. The bible of track and field since 1948, listing national and international records and interviews of top performers.

Skin and Scuba Diving

British Sub-Aqua Club Diving Manual. New York: Charles Scribner's Sons, 1977.

Jeppeson Sport Diver Manual. Denver: Jeppeson, Sanderson, Inc., 1975.

Ketels, Hank, and Jack McDowell. *Safe Skin and Scuba Diving: Adventure in the Underwater World.* Boston: Educational Associates, Little Brown, 1975.

Reseck, John, Jr. *Scuba Safe and Simple.* Englewood Cliffs, N.J.: Prentice Hall, 1975.

Sleeper, Jeanne Baer, and Susan Bangasser. *Women Under Water.* Crestline, Cal.: DeepStar Publishing, 1979.

Soccer

Soccer America, P.O. Box 23704, Oakland, California 94623. Weekly magazine filled with how-tos and results of tournaments in youth and adult leagues. In cooperation with the Women's Sports Foundation, publishes a Women's Soccer Directory.

Squash

Squash News, a monthly newspaper reporting the dates and results of national and regional tournaments, is distributed to all members of the United States Squash Racquets Association, 211 Ford Street, Bala-Cynwyd, Pennsylvania 19094.

Surfing

Surfer, P.O. Box 1028, Dana Point, California 92629, Twelve issues per year.

Surfing, P.O. Box 28816, San Diego, California 92128. Twelve issues per year. Both magazines have few how-to articles but do report on equipment innovations and the pro and amateur tournaments.

Swimming

Counsilman, James E. *The Science of Swimming.* Englewood Cliffs, N.J.: Prentice-Hall, 1968.

Cuthbertson, Tom, and Lee Cole. *I Can Swim, You Can Swim.* Berkeley, Cal.: Ten Speed Press, 1979.

Journal of Masters Swimming: Lane Four, c/o Paul Hutinger, Men's Physical Education Department, Western Hall, Western Illinois University, Macomb, Illinois 61455. Four issues per year.

Katz, Jane, with Nancy P. Bruning. *Swimming for Total Fitness.* New York: Dolphin Books, 1981. A how-to book filled with techniques and training programs for anyone at any stage.

Swim-Master, 2308 Northeast 19th Avenue, Fort Lauderdale, Florida 33305. Nine issues per year.

Swim Swim, P.O. Box 5901, Santa Monica, California 90045. Four issues per year.

Swimming Technique, P.O. Box 45497, Los Angeles, California 90045. Four issues per year.

Swimming World, P.O. Box 45497, Los Angeles, California 90045. Twelve issues per year.

Synchro-Info, c/o Dawn Bean, 11902 Red Hill Avenue, Santa Ana, California 92705. Six issues per year.

Team Handball

Blazic, Branko, and Zorko Soric. *Team Handball.* 90–170 Hargrave Street, Holiday Tower, Winnipeg, Manitoba, Canada R3C 3H4. Rules, sketches, strategy, skills, and drills.

Neil, Graham I. *Modern Team Handball—Beginner to Expert.* Montreal: McGill University Press, 1976. (Available from the United States Team Handball Federation Supply Company, 400 Hillside Avenue, Hillside, New Jersey 07205.) Rules, skills, strategy, and training.

Tennis

Tennis, P.O. Box 10185, Des Moines, Iowa 50349. Twelve issues per year. Focuses on technique and tournament results, with a few personality profiles thrown in.

Walking

Fletcher, Colin, *The New Complete Walker.* New York: Alfred A. Knopf, 1974.

Walking for Exercise and Pleasure. President's Council on Physical Fitness and Sports, 400 Sixth Street SW, Washington, D.C. 20201. (Free.)

Backpacker. P.O. Box 2784, Boulder, Colorado 80302. Six issues per year.

Walking News, P.O. Box 352, Canal Street Station, New York, New York 10013.

Waterskiing

Spray's Water Ski Magazine, 2469 Aloma Avenue, Suite 218, Winter Park, Florida 32792. Twelve issues per year.

The Water Skier, published by the American

Water Ski Association, P.O. Box 191, Winter Haven, Florida 33880. Seven issues per year.

World Water Skiing, 1211 Palmetto Avenue, Winter Park, Florida 32789. Eight issues per year.

Weight Lifting, Power Lifting, and Body Building

Reynolds, Bill, *Complete Weight Training Book*. Mountain View, Cal.: World Publications, 1976. Teaches the basic resistance exercises and variations, with emphasis on proper technique, and then outlines weight-lifting programs for more than thirty-eight different sports. For the serious athlete who wants to do serious weight training.

Iron Man, P.O. Box 10, Alliance, Nebraska 69301. Twelve issues per year. Profiles of body builders and power and weight lifters; columns and features on training techniques; results of competitions.

Lady Athlete, P.O. Box 237, Pearl River, New York 10965. Twelve issues per year. Very small magazine featuring profiles and photographs of body-building stars.

Natural Bodybuilding, Yorton-Dayton Enterprises, P.O. Box 57, Fremont, California 94537. Six issues per year.

Powerlifting USA, Suite 2B, 863 Lemon Drive, Camarillo, California. Twelve issues per year.

Women's Strength and Physique Publication, P.O. Box 443, Ho-Ho-Kus, New Jersey 07423. Twelve issues per year. Offset printed homemade magazine featuring snapshots of tournament winners.

Wrestling

Spackman, Robert R., Jr. *Conditioning for Wrestling*. Murphysboro, Ill. (62966): Schwebel Printing, 1973. A thirty-nine-page no-nonsense pamphlet aimed at male high school and college wrestlers but crammed full of useful conditioning exercises for every wrestler. Other booklets in the series discuss baseball, football, golf, ice hockey, parachute jumping, swimming, and more.

The Parent's Guide to Children's Wrestling, United States Wrestling Federation, 405 West Hall of Fame Avenue, Stillwater, Oklahoma 74074.

III: THE INNER WOMAN

Menstruation and Menopause

Reitz, Rosetta. *Menopause: A Positive Approach*. Radnor, Pennsylvania: Chilton Book Company, 1977.

Seaman, Barbara, and Gideon Seaman, M.D. *Women and the Crisis in Sex Hormones* (updated revised edition). Garden City, N.Y.: Doubleday, 1980.

Birth Control and Pregnancy

Donovan, Bonnie. *The Cesarean Birth Experience* (updated edition). Boston: Beacon Press, 1977. A pioneering and reassuring book. Tells you everything to expect along the way.

Noble, Elizabeth. *Essential Exercises for the Childbearing Year: A Guide to Health and Comfort Before and After Your Baby Is Born*. Boston: Houghton Mifflin, 1976.

Garfink, Christine, and Hank Pizer. *The New Birth Control Program*. New York: Bantam Books, 1979.

Shapiro, Howard I., M.D. *The Birth Control Book*. New York: Avon Books, 1978.

IV: SPORTS MEDICINE

Bennett, Hal Zina. *Cold Comfort: Colds and Flu, Everybody's Guide to Self-Treatment*. New York: Clarkson N. Potter, 1979. The myths, the old wives' tales, the folk cures that really work, and the latest in modern medical and nutritional discoveries about colds, flus, and their viruses, combined with the hocus-pocus of biorhythms and self-growth movements.

Biermann, June, and Barbara Toohey. *The Diabetic's Sports and Exercise Book*. Philadelphia: J. B. Lippincott Company, 1976.

Frazier, Claude A., M.D., and F. K. Brown. *Insects and Allergy and What to Do About Them*. Norman, Okla.: University of Oklahoma Press, 1981.

Biermann, June, and Barbara Toohey. *The Diabetic's Total Health*. Los Angeles: J. B. Tarcher, Inc., 1980.

Holt, Robert Lawrence. *Hemorrhoids*. Laguna Beach, Cal. (95652): California Health Publications (Box 963), 1977. Medical description of hemorrhoids, and thorough discussion of useful and useless home and medical treatments.

Kurland, Howard D., M.D. *Back Pains: Quick-Relief Drugs*. New York: Simon and Schuster, 1981. Recommends acupressure therapy for stubborn back problems.

————. *Quick Headache Relief Without Drugs*. New York: William Morrow and Company, 1977. A must for anyone who gets headaches frequently, this book discusses causes as well as cures and lists acupressure points for many types of headaches.

the physician and sportsmedicine. McGraw-Hill, Inc., 4530 West 77th Street, Minneapolis, Minnesota 55435. Twelve issues per year. Although aimed at doctors, coaches, and other sports medicine professionals, this readable journal is required study for anyone serious about their health and training.

Prudden, Bonnie. *Pain Erasure the Bonnie Prudden Way*. New York: M. Evans and Company, 1980. An attractive, abundantly illustrated book about the cause and control of trigger points.

Schneider, Myles J., D.P.M., and Mark D. Sussman, D.P.H. *How to Doctor Your Feet Without the Doctor*. New York: Charles Scribner's Sons, 1980. Includes instructions on how to make your own orthotics.

Vickery, Donald M., M.D., and James F. Fries, M.D. *Take Care of Yourself* (revised and updated). Reading, Mass.: Addison-Wesley Publishing Company, 1981. Simple flow charts direct the reader through the decisions necessary for choosing when to see the doctor and when to care for yourself.

Exercise Index

General Index